D1429554

Coeliac Disease

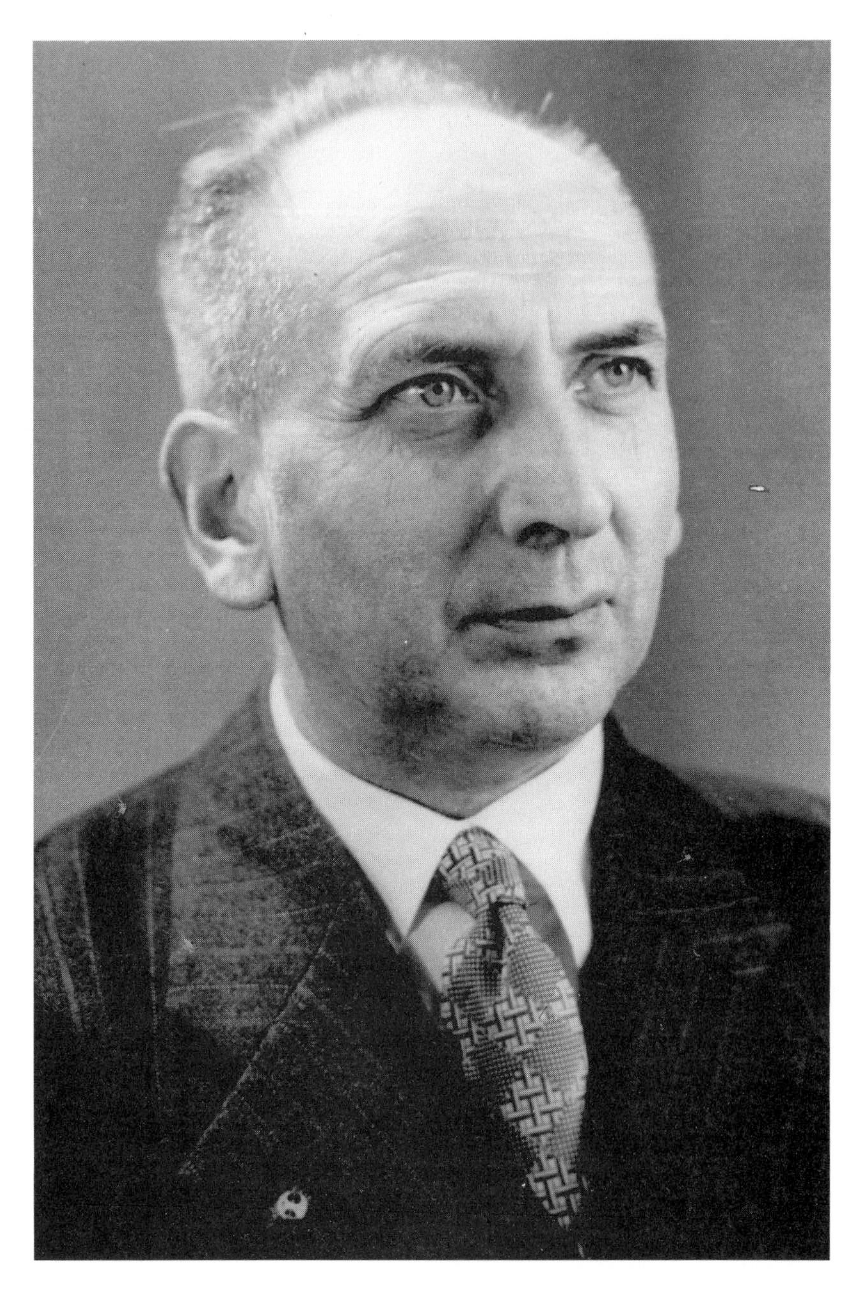

Willem Karel Dicke MD (1905–1962). '. . .he died after a well-spent life dedicated to sick children and trying to improve their health and their social situation in general. . .' [From a letter written by Mrs Agaath Dicke-Schouten, Dr Dicke's widow, to the editor of this book and published with her consent.]

Coeliac Disease

EDITED BY
MICHAEL N. MARSH
Reader in Medicine, University of Manchester

OXFORD
BLACKWELL SCIENTIFIC PUBLICATIONS
LONDON EDINBURGH BOSTON
MELBOURNE PARIS BERLIN VIENNA

Editorial Offices:
Osney Mead, Oxford OX2 0EL
25 John Street, London WC1N 2BL
23 Ainslie Place, Edinburgh EH3 6AJ
238 Main Street, Cambridge
Massachusetts 02142, USA
54 University Street, Carlton
Victoria 3053, Australia

Other editorial offices:
Librairie Arnette SA
2, rue Casimir-Delavigne
75006 Paris
France

Blackwell Wissenschafts-Verlag
Meinekestrasse 4
D-1000 Berlin 15
Germany

Blackwell MZV
Feldgasse 13
A-1238 Wien
Austria

First published 1992

Set by Setrite Typesetters Ltd, Hong Kong
Printed in Great Britain at
The Alden Press, Oxford and bound by
Hartnolls Ltd, Bodmin, Cornwall

DISTRIBUTORS

Marston Book Services Ltd
PO Box 87
Oxford OX2 0DT
(*Orders*: Tel: 0865 791155
Fax: 0865 791927
Telex: 837515)

USA
Blackwell Scientific Publications, Inc.
238 Main Street
Cambridge, Massachusetts 02142
(*Orders*: Tel: 800 759-6102
617 876-7000)

Canada
Times Mirror Professional Publishing Ltd
5240 Finch Avenue East
Scarborough, Ontario M1S 5A2
(*Orders*: Tel: 800 268-4178
416 298-1588)

Australia
Blackwell Scientific Publications (Australia) Pty Ltd
54 University Street
Carlton, Victoria 3053
(*Orders*: Tel: 03 347-0300)

A catalogue record for this title is available from the British Library

ISBN 0-632-03097-6

Contents

Contributors

CHARLOTTE M. ANDERSON MD, MSc, FRACP, FRCP, FACP
Professor Emeritus of Paediatrics, University of Birmingham, Edgbaston, Birmingham E15 2TT, UK

PER BRANDTZAEG PhD, MD
Professor and Chairman of Pathology, LIIPAT, Institute of Pathology, The National Hospital, Rikshospitalet, Pilestredet 32, N-0027, Oslo 1, Norway

LIONEL FRY BSc, MD, FRCP
Consultant Dermatologist, St Mary's Hospital, Praed Street, London W2 1NY, UK

TROND S. HALSTENSEN MD
Scientist, LIIPAT, Institute of Pathology, The National Hospital, Rikshospitalet, Pilestredet 32, N-0027, Oslo 1, Norway

GEOFFREY K.T. HOLMES MD, FRCP
Consultant Physician and Gastroenterologist, Derbyshire Royal Infirmary, London Road, Derby DE1 2QY, UK

PETER D. HOWDLE BSc, MD, FRCP
Senior Lecturer in Medicine, University of Leeds and Consultant Physician, St James' University Hospital, Beckett Street, Leeds LS9 7TF, UK

METTE HVATUM MD
Scientist, LIIPAT, Institute of Pathology, The National Hospital, Rikshospitalet, Pilestredet 32, N-0027, Oslo 1, Norway

MARTIN F. KAGNOFF MD
Professor of Medicine and Director, Laboratory of Mucosal Immunology, University of California at San Diego, San Diego, 9500 Gilman Drive, La Jolla, California 92093–0623, USA

DONALD D. KASARDA PhD
Research Chemist, Western Regional Research Center, Agricultural Research Service, US Department of Agriculture, 800 Buchanan Street, Albany, California 94710, USA

KJELL KETT MD
Intern, Medical Department A, The National Hospital, Rikshospitalet, Pilestredet 32, N-0027, Oslo 1, Norway

RICHARD F.A. LOGAN BSc, MB, MSc, FRCPE, FRCP
Senior Lecturer in Clinical Epidemiology, Department of Public Health and Epidemiology, University Hospital, Queen's Medical Centre, Clifton Boulevard, Nottingham NG7 2UH, UK

MONTY S. LOSOWSKY MD, FRCP
Professor of Medicine, University of Leeds, St James' University Hospital, Beckett Street, Leeds LS9 7TF, UK

THOMAS T. MACDONALD PhD, MRCPath
Wellcome Senior Lecturer and Reader in Intestinal Immunology, Department of Paediatric Gastroenterology, St Bartholomew's Hospital, London EC1A 7BE, UK

MICHAEL N. MARSH DM, FRCP
Reader in Medicine, University of Manchester and Consultant Physician, University Department of Medicine, Hope Hospital, Eccles Old Road, Manchester M6 8HD, UK

TORLEIV O. ROGNUM MD
Associate Professor, Institute of Forensic Medicine, The National Hospital, Rikshospitalet, Pilestredet 32, N-0027, Oslo 1, Norway

JACQUES SCHMITZ MD
Professor of Paediatric Gastroenterology, Hôpital des Enfants Malades, 149 Rue de Sèvres, 75743 Paris, Cedex 15, France

HELGE SCOTT MD
Senior Scientist, LIIPAT, Institute of Pathology, The National Hospital, Rikshospitalet, Pilestredet 32, N-0027, Oslo 1, Norway

PETER R. SHEWRY BSc, PhD, DSc
Professor, Department of Agricultural Sciences, University of Bristol and Head, AFRC Institute of Arable Crops Research, Long Ashton Research Station, Bristol BS18 9AF, UK

ARTHUR S. TATHAM BSc, PhD
Research Fellow, Department of Agriculture Sciences, University of Bristol and Principal Scientific Officer, AFRC Institute of Arable Crops Research, Long Ashton Research Station, Bristol BS18 9AF, UK

HENRY THOMPSON MD, FRCPath
Reader in Histopathology, University of Birmingham and Honorary Consultant Pathologist, Department of Histopathology, The General Hospital, Steelhouse Lane, Birmingham B3 6NH, UK

Preface

It may seem legitimate to ask, in the face of several international conferences and their published symposia, why another book on coeliac disease is justifiable or even necessary. The answer, simply, is that none of the symposia published successively over the last 20 years was designed to provide a broad, comprehensive overview of the subject, readily accessible to either the general reader or specialist. Indeed, events on many fronts relevant to this fascinating condition have continued to move so fast that a new publication seemed almost mandatory in order to provide a clearer view of those advances, and to make a reasonably authoritative statement about their significance to its aetiology and pathogenesis, diagnosis and treatment. It has been a particularly enjoyable task to assemble and edit such a book in conjunction with Blackwell Scientific Publications.

My own interest in coeliac disease stems from the late 1960s during a period in C.C. Booth's gastrointestinal unit at the Royal Postgraduate Medical School at Hammersmith Hospital, London. It was at that time, perhaps, that the field of intestinal morphology had reached a peak, and it was my abiding fascination with the microscopic organization of biological tissue that attracted me to the striking alterations in coeliac jejunum (which had so recently been described) and to their pathological basis. My debt, however, is not only to Booth but also to C.V. Harrison who then held the Chair in Pathology and Morbid Anatomy at the Postgraduate Medical School. It was one of Harrison's typical designer-engineered, end-of-staff-round remarks, meticulously timed to unfoot the majority of assembled cognescenti, which questioned the theoretical basis to standard 'quantitative' measurements of intestinal mucosae (and cell counting procedures) and hence the validity of comparisons between normal and diseased (flat coeliac) specimens. Here a major technical problem had been unearthed to which I had no satisfactory answer.

Indeed, I continued to be perturbed by this difficulty until evolving a satisfactory practical solution (many years later in Manchester) with the aid of computerized image analysis. This technique, which permits the three-dimensional reconstruction of tissue structure, proved invaluable in facilitating the quantitation of mucosal changes seen across the gluten-sensitivity spectrum, in our experimental dose–response work with Frazer's fraction III, and, currently, in evaluating the tissue response to oral challenges with various pure, synthetic oligomeric peptides of α-gliadin.

However, advances concerning gluten sensitivity are not simply confined to the morphological or immunopathological domain, despite their central importance to a proper understanding of the condition. There have also been substantial gains regarding the antibody response to gliadin and its value in diagnosis; in the molecular aspects of coeliac-associated major histocompatibility complex (MHC) class 2 specificities, of the codon switches which determine the outer (β1) polymorphisms of these molecules and which therefore influence the way in which gliadin oligopeptides are presented to (or 'seen' by) the T cell receptor; and in our knowledge of the amino acid sequences of all major prolamins which are providing useful insights into presumptive epitopic domains with disease-activating potential. These, in turn, have led to the realization that there is no single, elusive 'toxic' gliadin peptide responsible for mucosal pathology, but rather a small number of cross-reactive epitope motifs (present throughout the vast range of prolamins) all of which will evoke some kind of host response from genetically susceptible individuals. We are also becoming aware of the changes which continue to influence the epidemiology and natural history of coeliac disease; that a great deal of gluten sensitivity exists in a 'latent' and hence undetected form; and that this latent coeliac population, numerically, is surprisingly large; these issues are fully addressed in the relevant chapters of the book.

There are other detailed chapters on clinical aspects of coeliac disease in children and adults, and on dermatitis herpetiformis, and of their malignant complications. Together, this volume provides an important, up-to-date forum that will be of immense value to practising clinicians, paediatricians, gastroenterologists and histopathologists, as well as to those engaged in other scientific disciplines who may, directly or indirectly, wish to obtain a succinct state-of-the-art account of gluten sensitivity (for example, immunologists, food scientists, chemists, molecular biologists or experimental pathologists). It would appear to be the first occasion when all the many and diverse themes relevant to gluten sensitivity have been brought together into a single, comprehensive volume.

Nevertheless, this is by no means the end of the story. We still need to learn which other genes, other than MHC D subloci, predispose to coeliac disease; to determine the nature of the disease-related epitopes of gliadin and allied prolamins; to understand the kind of T cell receptors relevant to the condition and whether T cells expressing γ/δ receptors (especially within the intraepithelial lymphocyte (IEL) pool) play any role in immunopathogenesis or, as is becoming more likely, not; to isolate and clone gluten-sensitive T cells from affected mucosae, and to define their patterns of released cytokines that presumably help to mould the characteristic changes in mucosal architecture. The way now seems clear for tackling some of these remaining major problems. On the clinical front, there is an ever increasing need for a more effective means of verifying the presence of gluten sensitivity, especially in the face of growing numbers of individuals who are either asymptomatic ('latent') or who present with a variety of unusual or atypical symptoms, while further approaches to a better understanding of the mechanism(s) of end-stage, unresponsive disease need to be undertaken.

Finally, I should like to offer my sincere appreciation to Mrs Agaath Dicke-Schouten and her son, Professor Karel Dicke (of the University of Nebraska at Omaha Medical Center, NE) for allowing me to dedicate this work to the memory of the man who first revealed that gluten protein plays a central role in the aetiology of gluten sensitivity — Dr Willem Karel Dicke (1905–1962).

Michael N. Marsh

Chapter 1 / The evolution of a successful treatment for coeliac disease

CHARLOTTE M. ANDERSON

In 1887 a lecture entitled 'On the coeliac affection' was given at the hospital for Sick Children, Great Ormond Street, London, by Dr Samuel Gee, then senior physician at St Bartholomew's Hospital, and subsequently published in the St Bartholomew's Hospital Reports in 1888 [1]. This article is considered to contain the first detailed and accurate description of the condition we now refer to as coeliac disease, one of a group of conditions in which malabsorption of ingested foods is a salient feature — this was referred to by Gee. The basis of the absorptive defect has since been widely sought. Most attention in the early years after Gee's report was devoted to the mechanism of fat malabsorption; steatorrhoea having first been documented by Herter in 1908 [2]. Further understanding came slowly, however, mainly because of the limited availability of investigative techniques applicable to the gastrointestinal tract.

For the first half of the twentieth century, treatment of coeliac disease was largely empirical and consisted of dietary manipulations aimed at improving nutrition and lessening malabsorption of fat, as judged by improvement towards normality of stool frequency, colour and fat content. In Britain, removal of fat from the diet was strongly favoured, particularly by Sir Leonard Parsons [3], Professor of Paediatrics and Child Health at the University of Birmingham (Fig. 1.1). However, clinical improvement was very slow and mortality still considerable. In the USA, a restricted intake of complex carbohydrates, introduced by John Howland [4], Professor of Paediatrics at the Johns Hopkins Hospital, Baltimore, became popular because clinical improvement was more consistent and mortality considerably less. However, it was not until the late 1940s that the deleterious effect of a specific dietary ingredient, notably wheat flour, was recognized clinically by a Dutch paediatrician, Professor Wim Dicke [5] of the University of the Hague. Removal of all dietary products containing wheat, and subsequently rye, flour from an otherwise normal diet was shown by Dicke and his colleagues [6] to result in complete resumption of normal health, as well as normal fat absorption, in coeliac children.

The story of Dicke's initial discovery, and its confirmation with laboratory evidence in cooperation with his colleagues Weijers and

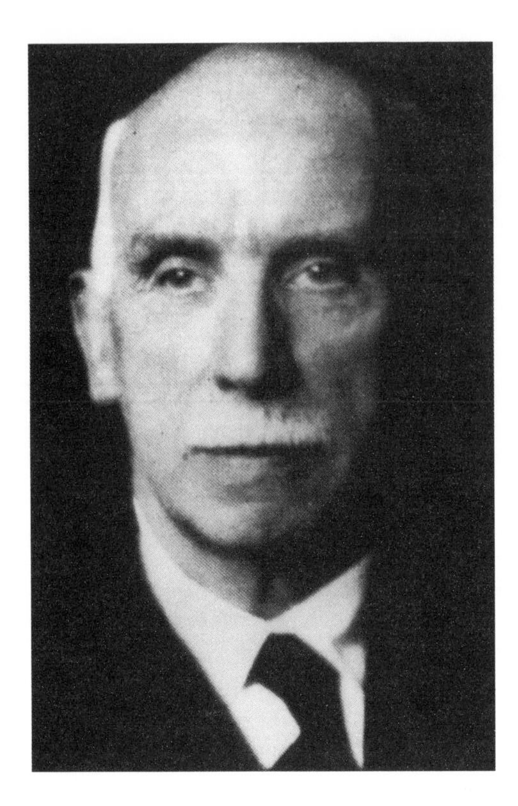

Fig. 1.1 Sir Leonard Parsons, Professor of Paediatrics in the University of Birmingham, 1927–1945.

van de Kamer (Fig. 1.2) from Utrecht, is a fascinating one. It is my memories of this exciting period that the editor of this book asked me to record, since I had close contact with these Dutch workers during my membership of a Birmingham group which quickly confirmed their findings in the early 1950s [7]. Unfortunately, the key members of that group are no longer alive, but I was privileged to meet Professor Dicke in Holland in 1951 and to have Dolf Weijers and Jan van de Kamer as friends for many years afterwards.

How did I become involved in these exciting events? The story begins in August 1950, when I first came to England seeking postgraduate experience in paediatrics, after 2 years spent as registrar in the newly created clinical research unit of the Royal Children's Hospital, Melbourne, where my interest in malabsorptive problems had first been kindled. By that time 'the wheat story' had yet to reach 'down under' and my sole experience of the treatment of coeliac children was to see them languish in hospital for months, miserable and depressed, consuming an unappetizing low-fat diet and gaining weight very slowly. The calorie content of the diet could be increased by the consumption of numerous bananas, as recommended by Haas [8] of the USA, who considered they had a specific beneficial effect. This was probably due

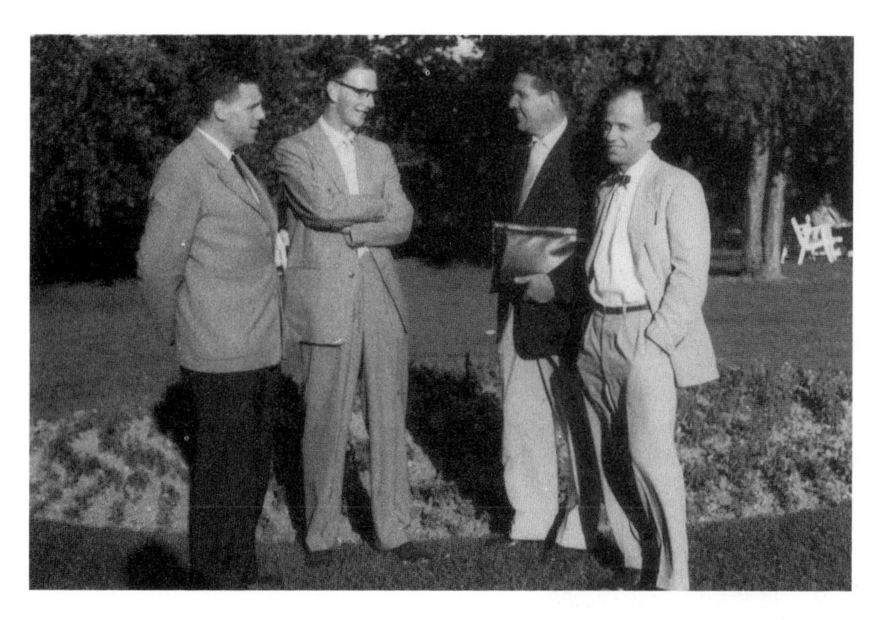

Fig. 1.2 Photograph of (left to right): Jan van de Kamer, Jack French, Dolf Weijers and a very youthful-looking Cyrus E. Rubin, taken at a Gastroenterology Congress, Washington DC in the early sixties.

to their inadvertent replacement of much of the complex carbohydrate in the diet and hence wheat products.

My first post in England was a 6-month research Fellowship at the Hospital for Sick Children, Great Ormond Street, under Sir Wilfred Sheldon, where I was made to count chylomicrons in serum as a method of estimating fat absorption. Although this was not an exciting project, it turned out to be a very fortunate one because Sheldon sent me to the Department of Pharmacology at Birmingham University to learn how to count those minute dancing particles. This department was headed by Professor Alistair Frazer, who was well known for his ideas and work on the mechanism of fat absorption. I learned to count chylomicrons under the tuition of Dr Jack French (Fig. 1.2), the Senior Research Fellow. Of more interest to me and also, as it turned out, of more importance to my future was his telling of the story of the success in treating coeliac disease with a wheat-flour-free diet which he had viewed during a visit to the Hague and Utrecht, some months previously.

He then introduced me to the first, and at that stage the only coeliac child, Judith (Fig. 1.3) who had been treated on such a diet at the Birmingham Children's Hospital. Here was a happy, well-covered little girl eating her lunch with enjoyment which, as Dr John Gerrard (Fig. 1.4), first assistant with the paediatric professorial department, pointed out with great glee, consisted of 'fish and chips' (Sir Leonard

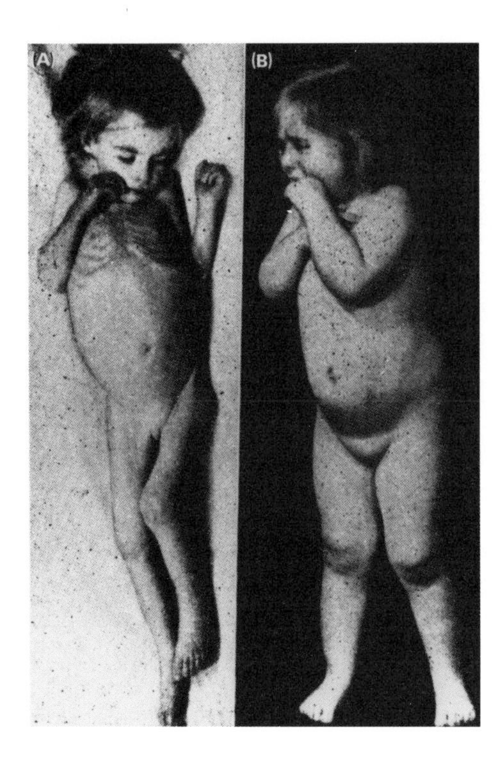

Fig. 1.3 Judith, the first coeliac child treated with a wheat-free diet in Birmingham, 1950–1951. (A) before treatment and (B) after dietary restriction of wheat-containing foods.

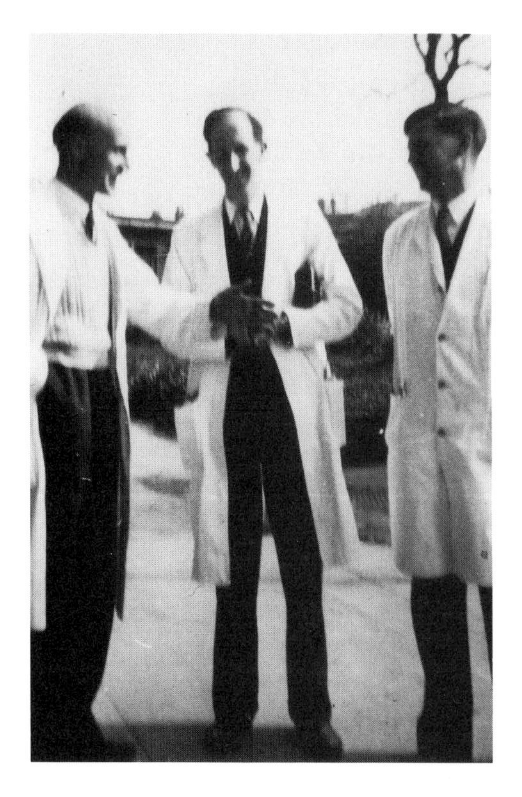

Fig. 1.4 John Gerrard (in characteristic pose), 1952, with Professor Parsons on the left of photograph.

Parsons was probably turning in his recent grave). French had to persuade a doubtful Gerrard to give the wheat-free diet a trial but now, after Judith's maintenance of good health and nutrition for some months, they were negotiating with their respective chiefs, Professors Frazer and Smellie, to set up a more comprehensive, cooperative study between the two departments. This study was to confirm and extend the Dutch work and identify, if possible, the offending constituent of wheat flour; at that stage 'gluten' had never been mentioned. Before I returned to London it was suggested that I might be interested in taking part in this project as a research fellow linking the two departments. Of course I agreed to this proposal and so in 1951 when a grant was obtained, my long and fascinating career in what came to be the new speciality of paediatric gastroenterology began.

Now a few comments on the members of our team. Alistair Frazer was an enthusiastic and stimulating boss who was adept at passing on this enthusiasm to all members of the team in both departments, even to the nursing staff, whose goodwill was vital to the success of the project. He was a man of great bonhomie but somewhat overweight, resulting from his enjoyment of good nutrition which contributed towards his nickname of 'Fats Frazer' (Fig. 1.5). Nevertheless, 'Fats' was also a very hard worker, a good organizer and publicist, who kept

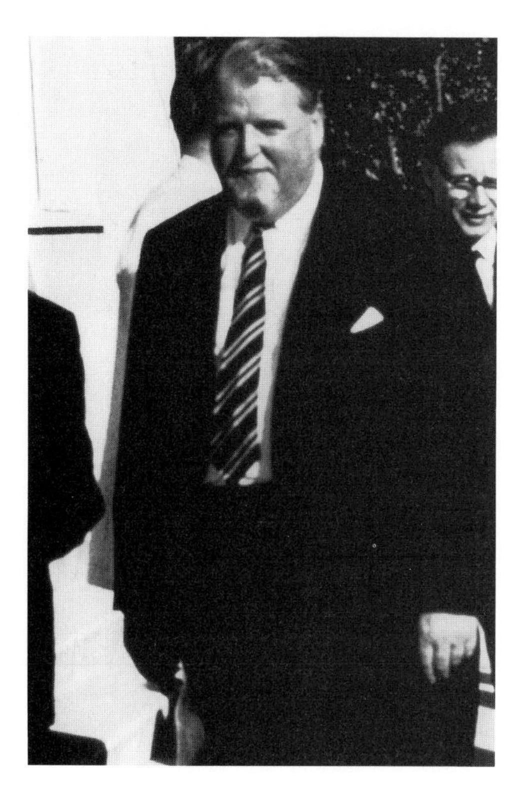

Fig. 1.5 Professor Alistair Frazer. From a photograph taken at the Ciba Foundation meeting on 'Intestinal biopsy', Madrid, 1962.

CENTRAAL INSTITUUT VOOR VOEDINGSONDERZOEK 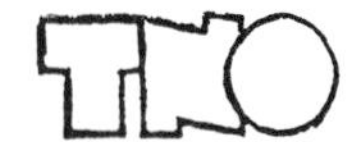

CENTRAL INSTITUTE FOR NUTRITION AND FOOD RESEARCH
INSTITUT CENTRAL DE LA NUTRITION ET DE L'ALIMENTATION
ZENTRALINSTITUT FÜR ERNÄHRUNGSFORSCHUNG

Utrechtseweg 48
Ziest
Tel.(03404) 18411
Giro 271906

Professor Charlotte M. Anderson
Institute of Child Health
The Nuffield Building
Francis Road
Birmingham 16
ENGLAND

UW REF:	UW DATUM:	ONZE REF:	DATUM
CMA/AMD	23rd June, 1969	5985 Ka/LN	7th July, 1969

Dear Charlotte,

Dolf asked me to answer your letter to him about Wim Dicke's "wheat-story", since Dolf is on holiday during the month of July. Before he left, however, we had a few minutes to recapitulate what we know about it from Dicke himself.

First the questions of ex-Professor Sir Lorimer Dods of Sydney:

We do not know in detail how Dicke made his first clinical observations in coeliacs about wheat sensitivity. Hence I cannot answer the questions about aggravation after "feast days". Neither did Dicke tell us about the consumption of special "biscuits". He observed that introduction of bread or normal biscuits lead to aggravation of the syndrome. Indeed he submitted this slender evidence during the International Congress of Paediatrics in New York in 1947 (?). As a matter of fact he did not read a paper about it but he told about his observations several times in personal discussions. However, nobody believed him and he came back from the States very disappointed but unshocked in his opinion. Shortly afterwards he told his "story" again, this time to Prof. ten Bokkel Huinink in Utrecht (the name ten Bokkel Huinink is also mentioned as one of my co-workers setting up the determination of fat in faeces - Rapid method for the determination of fat in faeces by J.H.van der Kamer, H. ten Bokkel Huinink and H.A. Weijers in J. Biol. Chem. 177 347 (1949). This ten Bokkel Huinink, a physician, was a son of the old Professor). He did not believe him either, but since Dolf and I had already been working for some years about the coeliac syndrome - just before the wheat period resulting in the thesis of W.Tegelaers, nowadays professor of paediatrics in Amsterdam - Prof. ten Bokkel Huinink asked us to test the idea of Dicke. As a matter of fact we - i.e. Dolf, Dicke and I - set up some experiments and after some months it was proved that administration of wheat to the coeliacs resulted in an increasing amount of steatorrhoea.

In close co-operation the search for the toxic component in wheat followed these initial experiments. The work resulted in the theses of Dicke and Weijers, three weeks after each other, Professor ten Bokkel Huinink presenting them both. Further the work was embodied in 4 papers and presented to a well-known American paediatric journal. We got it back without any comments as not acceptable. We felt, however, absolutely sure of our experiments, hence we presented it unchanged to the Acta Paediatrica Scandinavica. It was accepted and it appeared as Coeliac Disease I. Criticism of the various methods of investigation by H.A. Weijers and J.H. van de Kamer; Coeliac Disease II. The presence of wheat of a factor having a deleterious effect in cases of coeliac disease by W.K. Dicke, H.A. Weijers and J.H. van de

Fig. 1.6 Letter from Jan van de Kamer, 1969, in answer to a letter from the author of this chapter requesting information for an Australian colleague about Dicke's reason for suspecting the harmful effect of wheat in coeliac disease.

Kamer; Coeliac Disease III. Excretion of unsaturated and saturated fatty acids by patients with Coeliac Disease by H.A. Weijers and J.H. van de Kamer; Coeliac Disease IV. An investigation into the injurious constituents of wheat in connection with their action on patients with coeliac disease by J.H. van de Kamer, H.A. Weijers and W.K. Dicke, published resp. in Acta Paediatrica

42 (1953) 24 - 33 | 42 (1953) 97 - 112
42 (1953) 34 - 42 | 42 (1953) 223 - 231

Afterwards this series was extended with Coeliac Disease V. Some experiments on the cause of the harmful effect of wheat gliadin by J.H. van de Kamer and H.A. Weijers (Acta Paediatrica 44 (1955) 465 - 469); Coeliac Disease VI. A rapid method to test wheat sensitivity by H.A. Weijers and J.H. van de Kamer Acta Paediatrica 44 (1955) 536 - 540; Coeliac Disease VII Application and interpretation of the gliadin tolerance curve by H.A. Weijers - J.H. van de Kamer (Acta Paediatrica 48 (1959) 17 - 24).

Picking up again the letter of Sir Lorimer Dods: a significant diminution in the manifestations of coeliac disease during the period of starvation in Holland was neither reported nor observed.

I do hope this is clear cut enough. I do not know any one who could tell you more about it.

We do look forward very much indeed to meeting you in Interlaken in September and again in London in November.

Also on behalf of Dolf,

Best regards,
Yours sincerely,

Fig. 1.6 *continued.*

us all 'on the move'. I was to be in charge of the details of the feeding trials of the coeliac children under the supervision of Professor Smellie and John Gerrard, as well as to carry out the laboratory work involved in daily faecal fat estimations, chyomicron counts and pancreatic function studies under the supervision of Dr Sammons (Sammy), a biochemist in Frazer's department. Jack French, who was also attached to the Department of Medicine, was working with 'tropical sprue' patients (soldiers returned from Hong Kong) and adult coeliac patients, carrying out similar dietary trials and laboratory tests. We had no technicians until much later.

Frazer immediately arranged a visit to Holland for me and our ward sister, the late Nellie Howells, so that we could study the work of Dicke and his Utrecht colleagues first hand. I spent a day with Dicke, seeing coeliac patients then in hospital and discussing what had led up to his realization that wheat flour was the noxious dietary agent. As can be seen from Fig. 1.6, in a letter I received from Jan van de Kamer many years later and after Dicke's unfortunate early death there was, and probably always will be, uncertainty about this aspect of coeliac disease.

I can only refer here to what Dicke told me during my visit. During our ward round, his coeliac toddler patients were having lunch which seemed to consist in large measure of a bowl of what would then be called 'gruel', this being of porridge consistency and perhaps more familiar to the Dutch than to the English as a meal. Dicke told me that he had observed considerable variations in the well-being of individual patients at different times during their stay in hospital, for instance, sometimes they would seem to be clinically improving, in a happier mood and more active and then would revert to being miserable, depressed and inactive. These changes seemed to correlate with variations in weight and stool frequency. Their diet was similar during both phases but *on enquiry from the food preparation staff* he discovered that the 'gruel' feed at times had wheat flour as its basis, whereas at other times rice or potato flour was used. This had occurred in the late 1940s when a constant supply of individual flours was not always possible in Holland.

Dicke was a general paediatrician but a very observant clinician, modest and reticent, so that he waited until he was sure of his clinical findings before talking to other paediatricians about them. As can be seen from a perusal of the letter in Fig. 1.6, when he did discuss his ideas during a visit to the USA, they were not received with any enthusiasm. However, he was tenacious, and finally gained the cooperation of his Utrecht colleagues, Professor Dolf Weijers and Jan van de Kamer, biochemists from the Central Institute of Nutrition, Utrecht, who had already developed laboratory methods for studying malabsorption in children. In particular, van de Kamer and colleagues [9] had perfected a simple, quick method for the estimation of faecal fat output and the results of long-term fat excretion studies [6] became the vital laboratory evidence which was to confirm Dicke's clinical observations.

The group then tested a wide range of cereals, but out of the wheat, rice, oats, potato, corn, or rye flour tested, only wheat and rye flours were found to be deleterious. Faecal fat increased when they were fed, accompanied by worsening clinical signs but there were no ill-effects when the other foods were fed [6]. A paper containing these results was sent to an august paediatric medical journal in the USA in 1950 (Fig. 1.6) but was rejected and returned without comment, apparently indicating continuing scepticism and possible bias by some paediatricians in that country. This scepticism continued for several years, as I discovered in 1953 when travelling through the USA.

The Dutch paper was promptly accepted by the *Acta Paediatr Scand*, Stockholm, but not published until 1953 [6], followed by further papers (listed in Fig. 1.6). Unfortunately, this delay meant that an English language version of the Dutch work was not widely available until after the report of the Birmingham Study had appeared in the *Lancet* in 1952 [7]; this journal having a policy of quick publication for significant advances in medical knowledge. Both Dicke [5] and Weijers had presented theses in 1950 to the University of Utrecht but only, of course, in Dutch and not widely distributed.

A small anecdote of my visit to Dicke illustrates his old-world gentility. In the evening when we attended the weekly meeting of junior clinical staff of the hospital, he asked them, with no prior warning, to present all their reports in the English language for my benefit. I felt duly humbled both because of my ignorance and junior status.

Our Birmingham study was organized along similar lines to that of the Dutch group. On suspicion of coeliac disease, the children, usually aged between 1.5 and 2.5 years, were admitted on to the professorial ward in order to establish the diagnosis. At that time, a diagnosis had to be made from the clinical history, demonstration of steatorrhoea, exclusion of chronic bowel infection or infestation and cystic fibrosis in which steatorrhoea was due to pancreatic enzyme deficiency. The study was allotted four beds in the professorial ward at the Birmingham Children's Hospital, but the patients were considered to be under the care of Professor Smellie. Everything we wished to do with the patients was discussed with him on ward rounds while the beds could not be used for patients other than those in the study. These arrangements were very satisfactory. Care of these children involved considerable extra work for the nursing staff as they were responsible for collecting *in toto*, as far as possible, all stools passed each 24 hours, as well as supervising the consumption of specially prepared meals of calculated fat content, and saving what was refused for the dieticians' attention. Sister Nellie Howells was an ideal person for this study as she gave the right mixture of authority and kindness to her staff and patients. We rarely lost a stool during 18 months of our study and we had happy children (Fig. 1.7).

As well as certain routine tests, we made estimates of faecal fat, intermittent glucose tolerance tests, chylomicron counts after measured fatty meals and pancreatic function studies. Dr Sammons had further simplified the van de Kamer method of estimating faecal fat [7]. This was estimated daily, and recorded as such, but also as a percentage of intake, giving an estimate of absorption. The daily results were converted to 3-day running means to iron out irregularities in stool habit and varying appetite. Fig. 1.8 shows one of the original charts with faecal fat measurements going on for months on various dietary regimens such as exclusion and reintroduction of wheat products, and replacement of wheat by cornflour, oat porridge, or wheat starch washed free of its

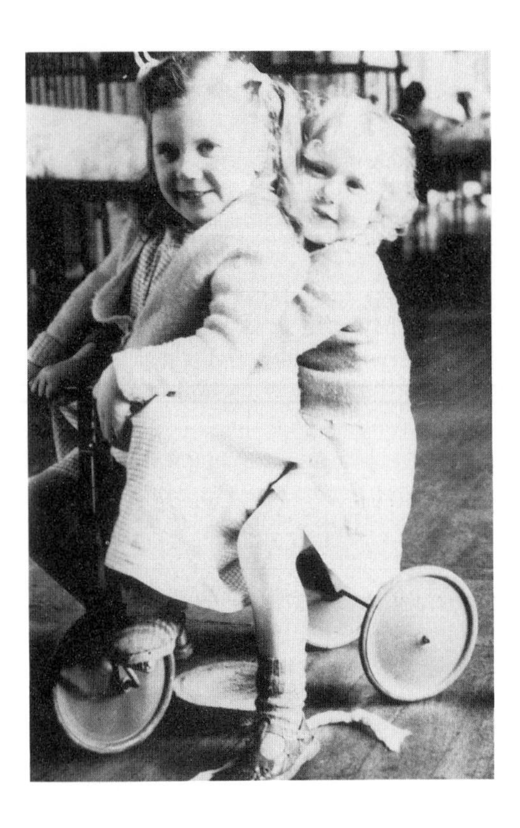

Fig. 1.7 Two of our treated coeliac patients taking exercise on a tricycle in 1951, after treatment with wheat- and rye-free diets for some months.

protein fraction. Rye flour was not a usual constituent of English children's diets at that time.

During the early part of the study, we confirmed in several other children the response of the first child, Judith (Fig. 1.3), to a wheat-flour-free diet; then we demonstrated that the addition of dietary corn flour did not produce symptoms or any increase in faecal fat, nor did wheat starch. The latter was obtained by mixing flour with water and then filtering it through fine muslin. The white starch came through, leaving a sticky residue which is the protein fraction, a mixture of proteins known as gluten. This is the component of flour which is necessary to achieve the production of a light aerated bread loaf. As the starch component did not increase faecal fat, a powdered preparation of gluten was then added to the diet, the amount given calculated to be roughly equivalent to the gluten content of what would be considered a normal daily bread intake for the child. Fig. 1.9 illustrates Pamela, before and after treatment on a wheat-flour-free diet and Fig. 1.10, her fat excretion graph, showing reappearance of steatorrhoea and weight loss when gluten was fed [7], an observation confirmed in several other children. The Dutch workers also tested the effect of gluten in parallel with us and obtained identical results.

Concurrent with the studies in children, Jack French carried out

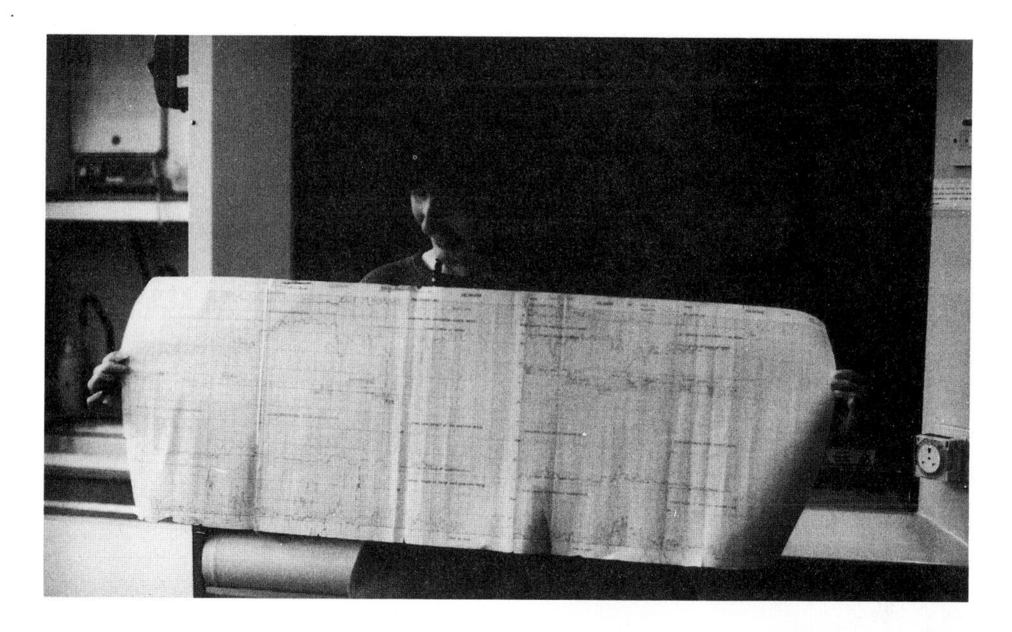

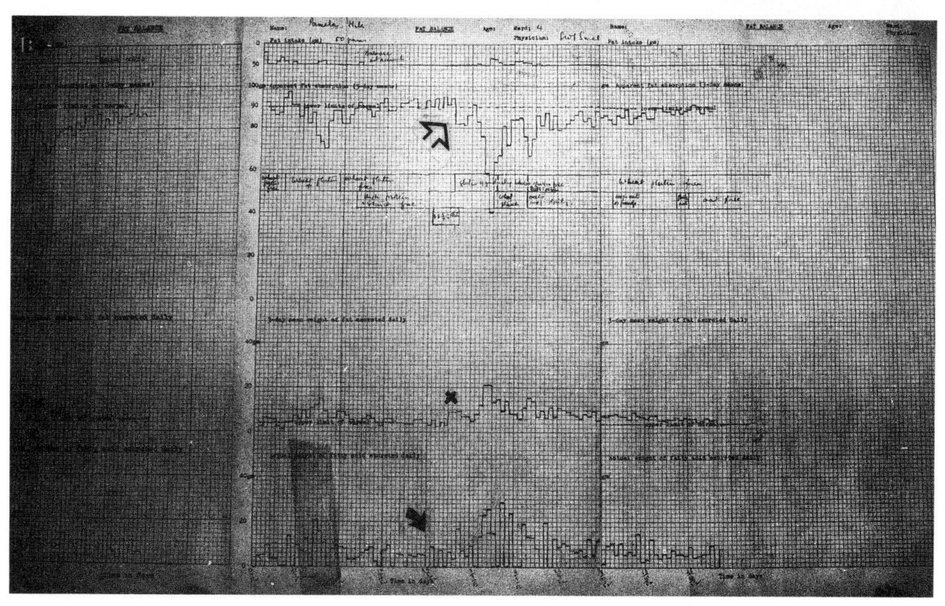

Fig. 1.8 Extract from one of our original working fat excretion and absorption sheets, Birmingham, 1951–1952. (A) shows one of the original charts for Judith and emphasizes the enormous size, and the immense quantity of data recorded, as the daily running totals were accumulated. (B) is a close-up, illustrating percentage fat absorption (upper graph) and 3-day running means for faecal fat (lower graph). In the middle panel, the reciprocal changes in fat absorption (open arrow) and excretion (closed arrow) in response to gluten challenge can be seen. In between the actual weight of fatty acid excreted per day is tabulated (X).

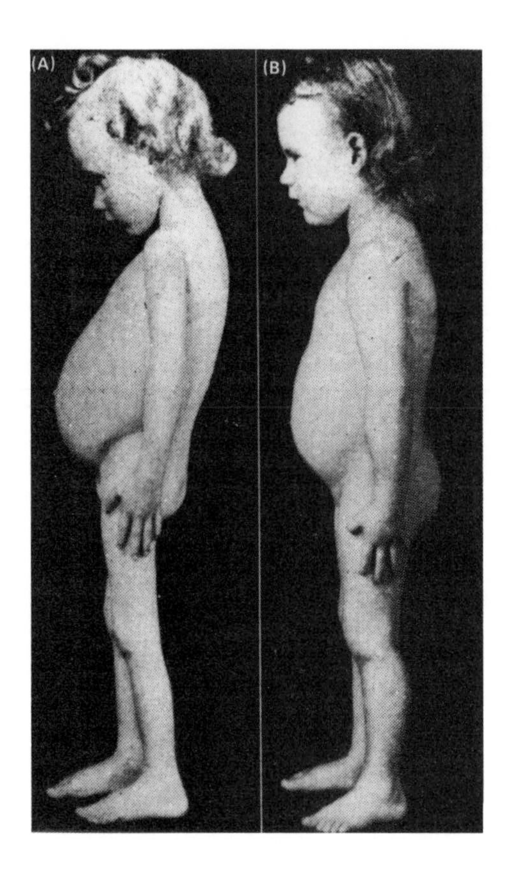

Fig. 1.9 Pamela: our second child at Birmingham to be treated on a wheat-free diet. Clinical appearance before (A) and after (B) dietary exclusion of wheat and rye products.

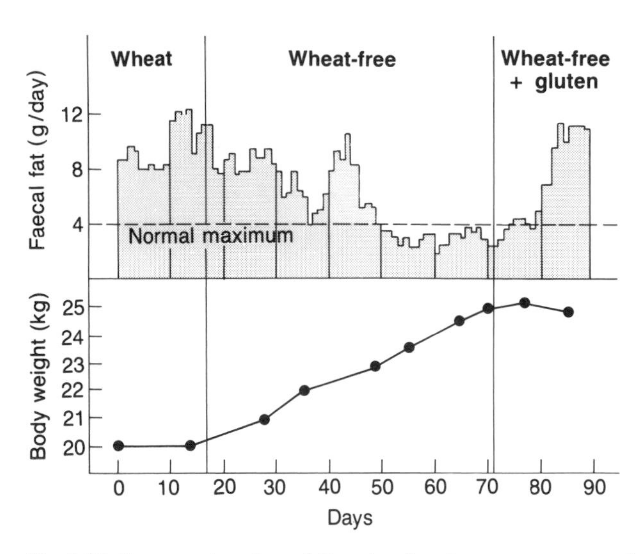

Fig. 1.10 Fat excretion data of Pamela, showing reappearance of excess stool fat and fall-off in body weight when gluten was added to a diet consisting of wheat starch.

similar feeding regimens in adult coeliac patients and was the first to publish [10] documentation of their favourable response to a wheat-gluten-free diet, although the response was not always as speedy as in the young coeliacs. His demonstration of the benefit of extended periods of antibiotic administration in cases of tropical sprue was also a first [11].

During the second year of our study, a small room at the entrance to the ward was made into a laboratory which relieved me of a daily 2-mile journey to the Medical School with the boot of my Morris minor estate car filled with billy cans containing 'you know what'! I wonder if anyone would now agree to carrying out long-term faecal collections and estimating daily faecal fats. Long-term hospitalization would certainly not be tolerated nowadays even to permit such data to be obtained. Our patients did have schooling during their stay, outdoor exercise, frequent family visiting and seemed happy (Fig. 1.7) except when consuming wheat products. Our four beds were the first in the ward as one entered, and when Frazer visited, we played a sort of game with him to see whether he could detect which patient was taking wheat or gluten. He was mostly right, to his gratification, picking the ones sitting inactive in bed with doleful expressions.

We published our results in the *Lancet* in late 1952 [7]. By this time many paediatricians in England were using the wheat- and rye-free diet, as papers had been given at meetings by us, and the Dutch work had become known, especially following a paper they had given at the International Paediatric Society Meeting in Zurich. However, even by early 1953, their work was largely unrecognized in the USA, as I was to discover later.

Frazer had a rule in his department that all publications should have the authors' names in alphabetical order which, of course, proved an advantage to me but poor Jack French always came after Frazer, even when his ideas and work were predominant. This eventually led to French transferring to the Department of Medicine altogether. Our Anderson *et al.* paper [7] in the *Lancet* found its way to Melbourne and apparently impressed the Research Committee, with the result that I was offered a more senior post in the Clinical Research Unit at the Royal Children's Hospital and also the funds to spend some weeks in various USA centres on my way home. This was an opportunity which had not so far been readily available and I was very pleased, as was Frazer. As I mentioned earlier, he was a great publicist and early in 1953, arranged for me to undertake a kind of whistle-stop tour across the USA giving a paper on our work at a number of hospital centres, both paediatric and adult. The data shown was so clear-cut that the doubters were convinced. The adult gastroenterologists seemed to be more accepting than the paediatricians whose low complex carbohydrate diets had been lacking in gluten anyway.

My visit to Dr Dorothy Anderson at the Babies' Hospital in New York was especially interesting. Her colleagues, Darling and Di Sant' Agnese, presented for the first time their finding of increased sodium and chloride in the sweat of cystic fibrosis patients. My interest in that condition was greatly stimulated, and I had therefore much to develop on my return to Melbourne where, at the Royal Children's Hospital, I was given the opportunity to build up a research unit to study gastroenterological problems. At first we concentrated on small intestinal absorptive problems.

Although the treatment of coeliac disease has remained unchanged apart from refinements of the diet to increase its palatability and acceptability, the demonstration by Dicke and others of the deleterious effect of dietary wheat and rye gluten stimulated an enormous amount of research in succeeding years, in many countries, in the attempt to discover the mechanisms by which this protein brings about malabsorption.

The next significant discovery followed the advent of equipment enabling specimens of the living intestinal mucosa to be obtained by the oral route. By 1958, the use of this technique had allowed the demonstration, both in England and the USA almost simultaneously, of the 'flat mucosa' in the small intestine in untreated adults and children with coeliac disease. I was visiting the USA that year for further study and was fortunate to be able to attend a meeting in Atlantic City where Cyrus Rubin of Seattle (Fig. 1.2) showed his exciting pictures of the abnormal villous structure of the upper small intestinal mucosa in adult coeliac patients. I then visited his unit in Seattle, learned how to process biopsy material, acquired the first commercially produced 'Rubin tube', and back in Australia proceeded to confirm his findings and those of others in untreated child patients, and to show regeneration of normal villi after exclusion of wheat and rye products from their diets.

The investigational methods that had largely been developed to study coeliac disease eventually enabled the study of many other small intestinal problems, and in the early 1960s our relatively small band of early paediatric gastroenterologists was busily studying problems of carbohydrate digestion and absorption. Again Weijers and van de Kamer were to the fore in identifying that in some infants, dietary sucrose produced fluid diarrhoea which was of an acid pH. They then developed a method for estimating the lactic acid content of the faeces [12]. Other workers, particularly in Switzerland and Sweden, and in our own unit went further in opening up this field. Intestinal biopsy material was used to estimate disaccharidases and various deficiencies of such enzymes were demonstrated. Thus paediatric gastroenterology was on the move.

In 1968, shortly after I had returned to Birmingham University to

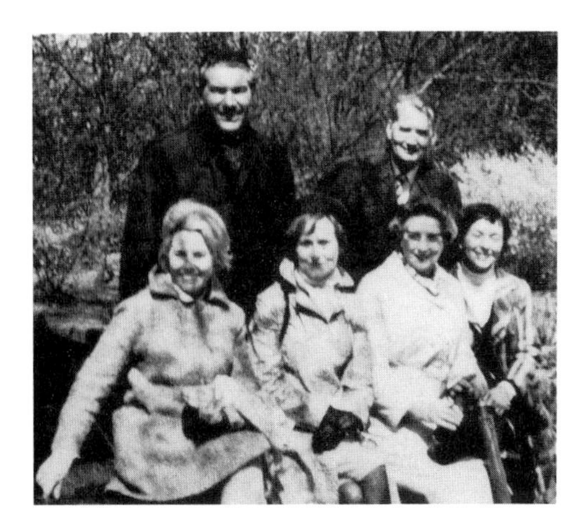

Fig. 1.11 This photograph (taken shortly before his fatal heart attack) shows Dolf Weijers (back row, left of photograph) in jolly mood in a Dutch tulip garden during a leisure period from a Council meeting of the European Society for Paediatric Gastroenterology. (The author of this chapter, Professor Anderson, is seated third from left in front row — Ed.)

take up the post of Head of Paediatrics and Child Health, a group of 14 paediatricians involved in researching gastroenterological problems in children met in Paris and formed the European Society for Paediatric Gastroenterology (later Nutrition was added to the title). Dolf Weijers was elected the first president and I joined the council (Fig. 1.11). This society has met each year since then in a European city and on one occasion in the USA with their paediatric gastroenterologists, but the membership has grown to several hundreds.

One of the first projects carried out by the Society was to seek unanimity amongst its members of the definition of coeliac disease and the criteria for its diagnosis, particularly for scientific study [13].

There is no doubt that we owe a debt to Wim Dicke for his astute observation regarding the deleterious effect of wheat cereal to coeliac children and to his colleagues Dolf Weijers and Jan van de Kamer for its scientific confirmation and to them all for the stimulus their work gave to the subsequent study and clarification of many other malabsorptive problems.

References

1 Gee SJ. On the coeliac affection. *St Bartholomew's Hosp Rep* 1888;24:17–20.

2 Herter CA. *On Infantilism from Chronic Intestinal Infection*. New York: MacMillan, 1908.

3 Parsons LG. Coeliac disease. *Am J Dis Child* 1932;43:1293–346.

4 Howland DJ. Prolonged intolerance of carbohydrates. *Trans Am Pediatr Soc* 1921;33: 11–9.

5 Dicke WK. *Coeliakie: een onderzoek naar de nadelige invloed van sommige graansoorten op de lijder aan coeliakie*. MD Thesis, University of Utrecht: 1950.

6 Dicke WK, Weijers HA, van de Kamer JH. Coeliac disease: II. The presence in wheat of a factor having a deleterious effect in cases of coeliac disease. *Acta Paediatr Scand* 1953;42:34–42.

7 Anderson CM, Frazer AC, French JM, Gerrard JW, Sammons HG, Smellie JM. Coeliac disease. Gastrointestinal studies and the effect

of dietary wheat flour. *Lancet* 1952;i:836–42.
8 Haas SV. Beriberi in late infancy: the result of coeliac disease. *Am J Dis Child* 1929;37: 1111.
9 van de Kamer JH, ten Bokkell Huinink H, Weijers HA. Rapid method for the determination of fat in faeces. *J Biol Chem* 1949; 177:347–55.
10 French JM, Hawkins CF, Smith NM. The effect of wheat-gluten-free diet in adult idiopathic steatorrhoea. A study of 22 cases. *Q J Med* 1957;26:481–99.
11 French JM, Gaddie R, Smith NM. Tropical sprue: a study of seven cases and their response to combined chemotherapy. *Q J Med* 1956;25:333–51.
12 Weijers HA, van de Kamer JH, Dicke WK, Isseling J. Diarrhoea caused by deficiency of sugar-splitting enzymes. *Acta Paediatr Scand* 1961;50:55–71.
13 Meeuwisse GW. Diagnostic criteria in coeliac disease (European Society of Paediatric Gastroenterology). *Acta Paediatr Scand* 1970;59:461–3.

Chapter 2/Coeliac disease in childhood

JACQUES SCHMITZ

In 1888, in the first accurate clinical description of coeliac disease (CD), Samuel Gee stated that 'it is especially apt to affect children between one and five years old' although he recognized that it could also be observed in 'persons of all ages' [1]. Later, the term 'coeliac disease' came into general use among paediatricians earlier than among adult gastroenterologists [2,3] and it was in children that, in the 1950s Dicke, Weijers and van de Kamer demonstrated the toxicity of a protein fraction in wheat flour [4]. As a consequence of the continuing concern of paediatricians for a condition which was estimated to be more frequent in children than in adults [5], which was still sometimes fatal 30–40 years ago and which could not be characterized unequivocally by its intestinal lesion, the European Society for Paediatric Gastroenterology and Nutrition (ESPGAN) finally issued in 1970 the most rigorous criteria of the disease, which was characterized by the following sequence:

1 a state of malabsorption with total or subtotal 'villous atrophy' of the intestinal mucosa observed while the diet contains gluten;

2 cure of the clinical disorder and histological lesions after gluten withdrawal, and

3 relapse of the clinical symptoms and/or the intestinal lesions after reintroduction of gluten into the diet (challenge) [6].

The latter criterion was instituted as a means of differentiating CD from other transient causes of villous effacement. This criterion demonstrates the long-lasting, 'permanent' sensitivity of the intestinal mucosa to gluten which establishes the identity of the disease observed in children to the identity of the disease observed in adults in whom a relapse is not required.

Since then, the widespread practice of gluten challenge has allowed the observation that clinical and mucosal sensitivity to gluten may decrease during childhood and adolescence. Together with the clinical presentation of the disease and the fact that it occurs at an age when other food proteins may trigger similar but transient enteropathies, this heterogeneity in long-term evolution is a major feature which individualizes CD in children in comparison to that observed in adults.

Clinical presentation

Age at onset

In general, the first symptoms appear in the months following introduction of gluten in the diet [7–9]. The interval between the first symptoms and the first ingestion of gluten is less than 1 month in 5–25% of patients, less than 9 months in most cases and longer than 1 year in only a few per cent of cases (2/60 [8]; 5/63 [9]). In the largest published series of children, this time interval seemed to follow a bimodal distribution with a large group of children (47/60; 78%) presenting within 1–6 months (average 3.7 months) and a small group (13/60; 22%) within 8–12 months [9]. It has been shown that the sooner gluten is introduced into the diet, the shorter is the interval between introduction and occurrence of the first symptoms [10]; the interval averages 2 months when gluten is introduced at the age of 2 months, and 4 months when introduction occurs at 6 months [11]. This relationship, however, seems to be linked to the duration of breast feeding since, when the latter is taken into account, the onset of symptoms appears unrelated to age at gluten introduction [12].

The first symptoms of CD, therefore, traditionally occur between 6 months and 2 years of age [7–10]. This is still the case in Sweden [13] and in southern Europe; in a large cohort of 463 cases diagnosed after 1973 in the Naples area, diagnosis of CD was made before the end of the second year of life in the vast majority of cases (80%) [14]. In Finland, however, age at diagnosis seems delayed; thus, since 1973 in the area of Tampere no case of CD was diagnosed under the age of 1 year, while 43% of children were 6 years old or more at diagnosis [15]. In this group of older coeliac children, there is a significant correlation between the age at diagnosis and the duration of breast feeding [15]. Indeed, several retrospective [16] case-control studies of healthy siblings [17] or children from the general population [18] have shown that breast feeding is associated with a decreased risk and/or delayed onset of the disease.

In a small proportion of children, diagnosis is not made by the age of 2 years, therefore CD can be diagnosed at any time up to adulthood, either because symptoms have been ignored or misinterpreted (i.e. short stature [15]) or because the disease is truly symptomless. In the latter case an intercurrent gastrointestinal episode may trigger the symptoms which will reveal the disease (personal observation). Increased gluten ingestion might have the same triggering effect; yet it has been shown that increasing gluten load in healthy siblings with human leucocyte antigen (HLA) haplotypes indentical to those of the patients does not induce mucosal damage [19].

Clinical features: early presentation

Clinical symptoms depend on the age at presentation. The characteristic features of the disease are most often encountered in infants 9–18 months of age. Within weeks or months of gluten introduction there occurs the classical syndrome of chronic diarrhoea, failure to thrive and abdominal distension [7–10,20–22]. Stools become looser, more bulky, frequent and offensive, but seldom grossly greasy. Stools may be liquid and responsible for dehydration during exacerbation of the disease ('coeliac crisis'). On the contrary, stools are normal or even constipated in a few per cent of cases [21–23]. Anorexia is common and may precede digestive symptoms; it may be prominent and hence wrongly attributed to psychological factors. Vomiting is noted in one-third to one-half of cases [20–22].

The general condition of the child is severely impaired. He or she is pale, looks miserable, and depressed. At an age of rapid psychomotor development, the latter ceases to progress; walking, just acquired, may be lost. Weight gain is more affected than height (Fig. 2.1A). Subcutaneous fat has disappeared, the skin is dry, the hair is crisp and thin, and colourless at the roots when malnutrition is severe. Muscle wasting, affecting mostly the buttocks, thighs and shoulders, contrasts markedly with the prominent, virtually constant abdominal distension that is best seen in the standing position, with dilated intestinal loops under a thin parietal wall [20] (Fig. 2.2). This distension may be so marked as to suggest Hirschsprung's disease. Rectal prolapse is sometimes observed, linked both to the abnormal stools and to muscle wasting [21].

Besides this classical presentation, a variety of symptoms have been noted in CD [21]. Oedema due to hypoalbuminaemia, rickets (rare in Caucasian children [7,20]), haematomas indicative of vitamin K malabsorption, mild finger clubbing and long eye lashes have been reported in some instances [21]. In addition, dental enamel hypoplasia has been shown recently to be a frequent finding in untreated CD [24].

In the last 10–15 years, however, because of greater awareness, diagnosis of CD tends to be suspected when clinical symptoms are less prominent, such as altered bowel habit, reduced appetite, a change in behaviour or reduced gain in weight [13].

Clinical features: late presentation

Diagnosis of CD may be made in later childhood in 10–20% of cases [9,14,21]. Decreased appetite and abnormal stools are then often revealed only on direct questioning, the child and his or her family taking as normal a digestive status that had existed for years. Constipation is more frequent at that age than in infants. In early school years,

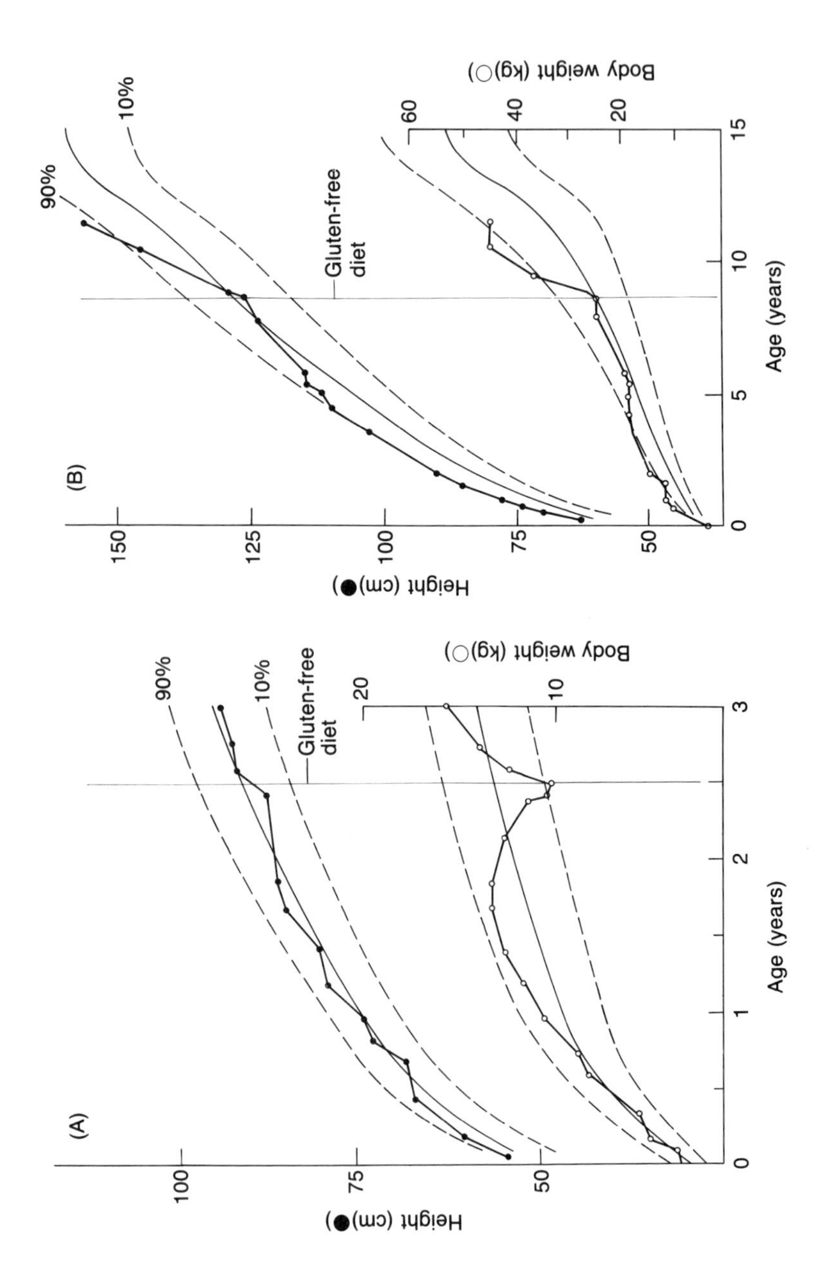
(A)
Height (cm●)
Body weight (kg○)
Age (years)
90%
10%
Gluten-free diet
100
75
50
20
10
0
1
2
3
(B)
Height (cm●)
Body weight (kg○)
Age (years)
90%
10%
Gluten-free diet
150
125
100
75
50
60
40
20
0
5
10
15

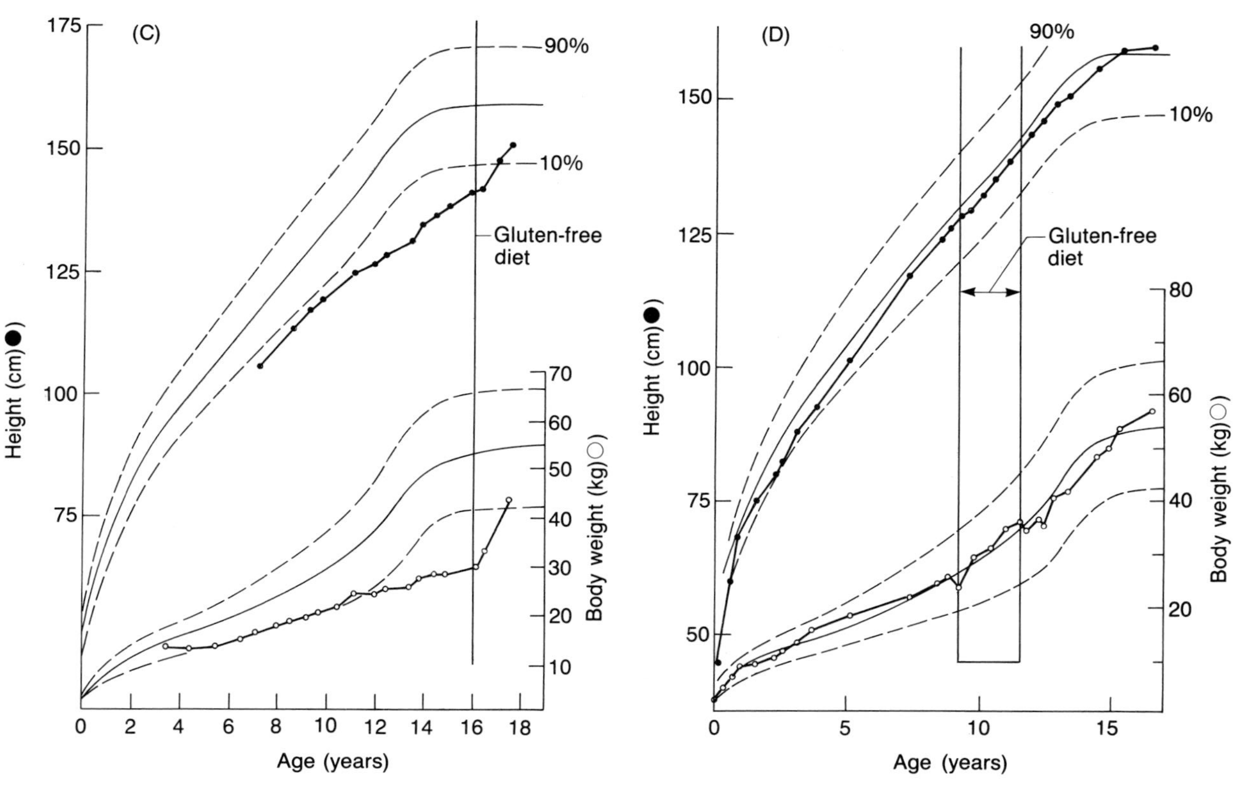

Fig. 2.1 These charts illustrate the variable effect of active CD on growth. (A) in a boy, 2.5 years of age, loss of weight is more pronounced than growth retardation. (B) growth failure may occur late in childhood; here it starts at 5 years of age in a girl with previously normal growth. (C) ignored CD induces both a short stature and infantilism as in this 16-year-old girl. (D) CD may be discovered following an acute diarrhoeal episode in a child with normal growth; in that case, CD is diagnosed by 'chance' as in this 9-year-old girl with previously normal growth. (A) to (D) vertical line illustrates point at which treatment was started with a gluten-free diet.

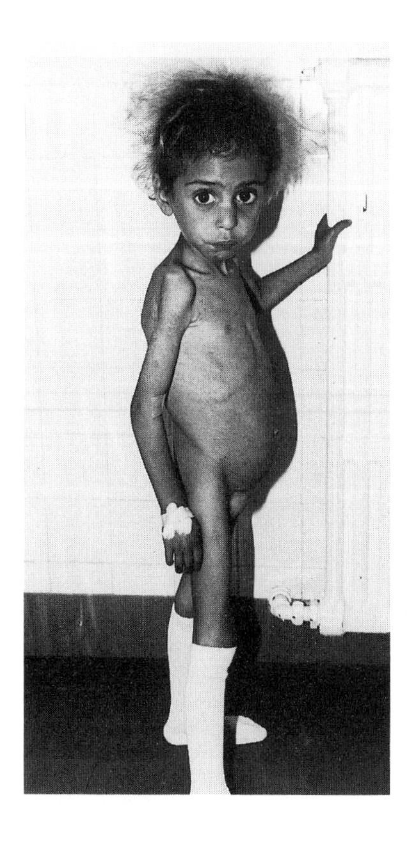

Fig. 2.2 A typical 3-year-old coeliac of north African descent with active disease. Note her sad look, distended and prominent abdomen, muscle wasting and discoloured hair.

apparently isolated short stature is a frequent presentation, sometimes being associated with infantilism in the older children [20] (Fig. 2.1B–D). A mild degree of abdominal distension, a microcytic anaemia, or osteoporosis may lead to the diagnosis. Such children may be first referred to an endocrinologist. The prevalence of these cases depends probably on many factors; awareness of the diagnosis, amount of gluten ingested [13] and average height of the general population.

CD has been estimated to account for 8–20% [25–27] of cases of children with retarded growth. In these children plasma growth hormone levels are low or normal whereas circulating insulin-like growth factor (IGF1) activity is constantly decreased [28].

Clinical features: atypical presentations

Finally, CD may be symptomless and discovered only because of a systematic search for it in family studies, or in children affected with conditions associated with CD (insulin-dependent diabetes [29], arthritis [30], for example). A recent study, indeed, indicated that in Finland, CD is now mostly diagnosed in school-age children with few, or atypical symptoms such as arthritis, arthralgia or isolated megaloblastic anaemia due to folic acid deficiency [15].

In subtropical countries, CD is traditionally considered to be rare. Small series have nonetheless been published from India [31–33], Kuwait [34], Cuba [35] and Sudan [36] where onset of the disease is retarded to the second or third year of life probably because of prolonged breast feeding and later gluten introduction. Presentation is more severe than is actually the case in Europe and northern America. However, symptoms, dominated by chronic diarrhoea and malnutrition, are the same, other than a high prevalence of rickets that has been linked to dietary deficiencies as well as insufficient sunshine [32].

Laboratory features

Although ultimately the diagnosis of CD depends on the demonstration of a flat intestinal mucosa, the intestinal peroral biopsy is usually performed after biological signs of malnutrition and malabsorption have been gathered.

Nutritional consequences of CD

Anaemia, defined by a haemoglobin level below 10 g/100 ml, is observed in more than one-third of affected children. It is usually microcytic, due to iron deficiency in more than one-half of the cases [8,21,22]. Seldom is anaemia macrocytic because of folate deficiency, although the latter is nearly constant at the florid phase of the disease [37]; whole blood folate level is thus usually considered a useful screening test [38]. It is, however, less reliable in adolescents, when the disease is clinically silent [39]. Vitamin B_{12} deficiency, well-documented in adults, is extremely rare in infants and children [21], probably because of the stores constituted *in utero*; it may, however, be observed in adolescents [40].

Hypoproteinaemia occurs in about 50% of children; it is usually moderate and has no clinical consequences. It is probably more the result of decreased intake, and of protein-losing enteropathy, which have both been documented in CD [41], rather than of malabsorption (see p. 24). It is thus mainly secondary to hypoalbuminaemia, intestinal loss of IgG occurring only when protein-losing enteropathy is severe. Hypocholesterolaemia (plasma cholesterol <150 mg/dl), essentially secondary to intestinal fat malabsorption, occurs in 30–60% of cases at the initial phase of the disease [7,22]. It is usually associated with decreased plasma levels of lipid soluble vitamins. A fall of plasma vitamin-K-dependent coagulation factors (prothrombin, proconvertin) has been noted in 10–40% of cases [8,21,22]. It is rarely symptomatic [21] and is corrected in 24–48 hours by an intramuscular injection of vitamin K. Thus, prothrombin levels should be checked before an intestinal biopsy is performed. Plasma levels of vitamin A and E have also been found lowered in 50–60% of cases [37].

Malabsorption of vitamin D and Ca^{2+} is responsible for the abnormalities of phosphorus and calcium metabolism seen in the florid phase of the disease. Plasma calcium concentration is decreased to 2.0–2.25 mmol/l in almost half of the cases, while plasma phosphate levels are more often normal. Alkaline phosphatase activity in the plasma is normal or raised. Calciuria is often decreased below 0.05 mmol/kg per day. On X-ray films, bone appears osteroporotic in most cases; the cortical bone is abnormally thin with a cortex : diaphysis ratio <0.5, bone texture is abnormally visible with a latticed appearance and striae in the metaphyseal areas [7,21,22,37]. Osteomalacia is uncommon, calcium malabsorption being associated with protein deficiency. Rickets is even rarer in European children, protein deficiency being proportionately more severe in infants than in older children and growth being slowed [7,21,32]. In contrast, rickets is a major feature of severe forms of CD in subtropical countries [32]. Bone age is retarded to an extent which is roughly the same as growth [22].

Many other deficiencies may be observed in CD. Well-documented are: (1) Zn^{2+} deficiency; this in fact occurs in most cases, which could be partially responsible for anorexia (because of the dulling of taste it causes) and of retarded growth [42]; (2) Mg^{2+} deficiency which may account for calcium resistant tetany [21]; and (3) Cu^{2+} deficiency associated with neutropenia [43]. Vitamin B_6 deficiency, witnessed by anomalies of tryptophan metabolism [44], has also been observed in CD. All these abnormalities disappear within a few weeks or months once a gluten-free diet has been started.

Intestinal malabsorption

Malabsorption is best demonstrated by balance studies performed during periods of 3–6 days of stool collection with daily records of dietary intakes. It is, in fact, by using this technique for more prolonged periods that Weijers and colleagues were able to demonstrate the 'toxicity' of gliadin [4]. In childhood, CD malabsorption is usually not extremely severe (Table 2.1). Fresh weight of stools is increased but to a variable extent, while nitrogen excretion is increased >0.5 g/day. Steatorrhoea is usually moderate, typically between 5 and 10 g/day, with a lowered coefficient of fat absorption between 75 and 85%, so that stools are rarely grossly greasy [7,21]. Although steatorrhoea is almost constant in infants and young children, it may be minimal or even absent in older children, especially in those presenting with short stature (Table 2.1). Volatile short-chain fatty acids, produced in the colon by the bacterial fermentation of non-absorbed carbohydrates are

Table 2.1 Balance studies in children with CD

Group studied	Fresh stool weight (g/day)	Nitrogen (g/day)	Fat (g/day) [coeff. of absorption (%)]	Volatile fatty acids (mmol/day)	Lactic acid (mmol/day)
Coeliacs (n = 28) (<3 years of age)	118 ± 75*	0.9 ± 0.3	6.7 ± 2.0 [75 ± 8]	16.6 ± 11.3	4.4 ± 5.8
Controls† (n = 17)	61 ± 20	0.5 ± 0.2	2.0 ± 0.5 [94 ± 2]	10.1 ± 3.7	—
Coeliacs (n = 22) (>3 years of age)	161 ± 88	1.5 ± 0.4	7.3 ± 3.2 [85 ± 7]	24.9 ± 11.5	2.1 ± 2.8
Controls‡ (n = 48)	79 ± 32	0.7 ± 0.3	2.0 ± 0.6 [95 ± 2]	13.7 ± 5.4	—

* Mean ± 1 SD (personal data).
† Children between 1 and 2 years of age.
‡ Children between 2 and 6 years of age.

also excreted in abnormally high quantities, in cases with most severe carbohydrate malabsorption, together with lactic acid. Stool pH is then acid, below 5.5. The increased excretion of these short-chain acids is a major factor determining the volume of diarrhoea. There is a significant linear relationship between stool weight and the quantity of short-chain acids (volatile acids + lactic acid) excreted in the stools. Carbohydrate malabsorption thus appears to be a major factor determining the severity of diarrhoea in CD [7]. Finally, although in most cases malabsorption, at least in part, may be the cause of malnutrition in CD, in other instances it is too moderate to account for growth retardation; anorexia may then be an important factor to consider.

Tests of carbohydrate malabsorption

Many oral tolerance tests have been proposed to assess carbohydrate absorption. The 1-hour blood xylose test is the simplest and most reliable as D-xylose, rapidly absorbed in the proximal jejunum [45], is not metabolized. One hour after an oral load of 10 g/m^2 (never less than 5 g) xylosaemia separates almost completely untreated coeliac from non-coeliac children, the discriminating concentration being 20 mg/100 ml [46]. Although the test is not as discriminating in older children as in infants (for whom it was originally set up), or in relapsing patients rather than in newly diagnosed ones [47], it is still considered [48,49] a useful screening test. It has been used more or less successfully in gluten challenges planned to confirm the diagnosis [50]. It must be kept in mind, however, that impaired xylose absorption only indicates altered mucosal integrity, so that in children a decreased 1-hour xylosaemia is also observed, for example, in cow's milk protein sensitive enteropathy or viral gastroenteritis.

Permeability tests

More recently, and following studies in adult patients, tests assessing the differential permeability of the small intestinal mucosa to non-metabolized carbohydrates (lactulose : mannitol; lactulose : rhamnose; cellobiose : mannitol) have been devised. The sensitivity of these tests is excellent since in all studies there is no overlap between coeliac and normal children [51,52]. Other molecules have been used with equal success: polyethylene glycol (PEG) of 200–1000 Da [47,53], ^{51}Cr-ethylenediaminetetra-acetic acid (EDTA) [54]. These tests are poorly specific, however, only indicating an altered mucosa as in Crohn's disease [51], cow's milk protein sensitive enteropathy [52], atopy [55], etc. Whereas these permeability tests seem extremely useful in the active phase of the disease, their sensitivity in assessing relapse at challenge remains debatable [47].

Fat absorption tests

Since fat balance studies can only be carried out reliably in metabolic wards with special laboratory facilities and are regarded as unpleasant, other methods have been devised to assess fat malabsorption. Increased levels of plasma triglycerides or of chylomicrons can be estimated by enzymatic methods or turbidity measurements after an oral fat load [56] or after a fatty meal [57]. Although these tests may rather satisfactorily discriminate between children with and without steatorrhoea, they cannot separate children with intestinal malabsorption from those with exocrine pancreatic insufficiency [56,57]. A combination of ^{13}C-triolein and ^{13}C-trioctanoin or ^{13}C-palmitic acid breath tests may achieve this discrimination [58]. These breath tests, however, are extremely difficult and expensive to set up and their use remains confined to a few centres only. Thus, fat absorption tests are less useful than tests of carbohydrate absorption in suggesting an intestinal lesion and therefore indicating an intestinal biopsy.

Immunological tests for CD

In the active phase of the disease, serum IgA is markedly increased whereas IgM remains stable; IgG may decrease probably because of protein-losing enteropathy. These variations revert to normal within a few months of starting a gluten-free diet, in parallel with mucosal lesions [59]. Simultaneously, antibodies directed against a number of alimentary antigens, in particular against proteins of other cereals, of milk and of egg can be demonstrated in the circulation with frequencies and titres greater than in healthy children [60,61].

Only recently have newer methods of detection (indirect immunofluorescence, enzyme-linked immunoassay (ELISA), antigens of greater purity and characterization of antibodies to their isotypes) allowed the extensive use of antigliadin antibodies as a sensitive non-invasive screening test. Thus, in young children with active CD IgG antigliadin antibodies are found in 90–100% of cases while sensitivity of IgA antibodies is somewhat lower (60–100%). On the contrary, IgA antigliadin antibodies are more specific (86–100%) than IgG antibodies (60–95%) [49,60,62–69]. IgA antigliadin antibodies are mainly polymeric IgA [70]. Titres, and the overall sensitivity of both IgA and IgG antigliadin antibodies tend to decrease with age to 50–60% in children >3 years of age, or adolescents [60,63,69] (Table 2.2A).

Antibodies to other antigens have also been found at a high level in sera of coeliacs. IgG as well as IgA antireticulin antibodies are extremely specific, being almost never found in children with enteropathies other than CD. However, their sensitivities have often been found to be too low (50–60%), except for IgA antibodies in an isolated report (Table 2.2B) [64,65,71–74]. The specificity and sensitivity of IgA anti-endomysium antibodies have been found respectively to be as high or higher than those of antireticulin antibodies in certain series where they reach 100% (Table 2.2B). These antibodies react with yet unknown antigens from smooth muscle. Similarly, antibodies reacting with a mannose rich, 90 kDa glycoprotein, found in skin and intestinal wall, have been demonstrated in the sera of children with untreated CD [78]. These antibodies behave somewhat differently from antireticulin antibodies, decreasing after gluten withdrawal or increasing after

Table 2.2A Sensitivity and specificity of serum antigliadin antibodies for the diagnosis of CD in children

Authors	Number of children	IgG		IgA	
		Sensitivity	Specificity	Sensitivity	Specificity
Unsworth *et al.* [62]	11	100	68	91	96
Savilahti *et al.* [63]	19 (<2 years)	100	—	100	—
	13 (>2 years)	55	—	64	—
Bürgin-Wolff *et al.* [60]	72	100	84	—	—
Stenhammar *et al.* [64]	14	93	96	93	98
Volta *et al.* [65]	24	100	95	79	100
Ribes Koninckx *et al.* [67]	19	—	—	100	95
Arranz *et al.* [68]	35	91	77	61	88
Stählberg *et al.* [66]	31	94	66	90	86
Bürgin-Wolff *et al.* [69]	331	100	80	89	96.5
Rich *et al.* [49]	15	100	58	53	93

Table 2.2B Sensitivity and specificity of serum antireticulin and anti-endomysium antibodies for the diagnosis of CD in children

		Antireticulin antibodies				Anti-endomysium antibodies	
		IgG		IgA		IgA	
Authors	Number of children	Sensitivity	Specificity	Sensitivity	Specificity	Sensitivity	Specificity
Mäki *et al.* [71]	29	59	97	97	98	—	—
Volta *et al.* [65]	24	50	100*	—	—	—	—
Lazzari *et al.* [72]	24	67	100*	—	—	—	—
Kapuscinska *et al.* [75]	11	—	—	—	—	—	100
Rossi *et al.* [76]	11	—	—	—	—	91	100
Khoshoo *et al.* [74]	12	83	100	—	—	—	—
Hällström [77]	18	50	100	100	100	100	100

* For IgG and IgA.

challenge with a longer delay of several months [78]. Elevated titres of anti-endomysium and anti-90 kDa protein would seem to reflect, then, the degree of mucosal damage [76,78].

For screening purposes, the combined use of IgG and IgA antigliadin antibodies and of antireticulin or anti-endomysium antibodies has been proposed, thereby permitting the diagnosis of active CD in young children in more than 95% of cases [69] and avoiding in the most typical cases, the necessary sequence of two or three biopsies. However, antireticulin and anti-endomysium antibodies detected by immunofluorescence on sections of rat tissue (kidney, liver) or on monkey oesophagus are not yet used routinely. Similarly, several groups have recently advocated a combination of several of the above cited tests: antigliadin antibodies, 1-hour xylosaemia, permeability tests [47,49, 50,79] in order to best predict when to perform a biopsy, or when to avoid it [80].

Although mucosal cell-mediated immunity is altered in CD and plays an important role in the development of intestinal lesions (see Chapter 6), tests based on peripheral alterations of cell-mediated immunity are few [81] and have not gained a wide audience, mainly because of their lack of specificity and sensitivity.

Intestinal biopsy

Intestinal biopsy is essential to the diagnosis of CD since it enables the histological lesions to be demonstrated. Biopsies are more and more often obtained through a fibre endoscope from the second or third parts of duodenum, at least in older children. Thus, fragments of mucosa are usually smaller and oriented with more difficulty than was the case when biopsies were performed by means of a paediatric suction capsule at the angle of Treitz. This is why, recently, an ESPGAN Working Group on CD recommended that biopsies should be taken with a suction capsule [82].

Lesions are already visible under a dissecting microscope; the intestinal mucosa has lost its leaf-like or, less often in children, its finger-like appearance and its surface has the classical mosaic pattern [20]. On conventional histological examination, the characteristic, though non-specific changes identical to those seen in adults, are found; crypts are hyperplastic with numerous mitotic figures and villi are flattened or have disappeared, being replaced by surface plateaux. There is a considerable increase in lamina propria cellularity (see p. 30). Surface epithelium is extensively deteriorated; it is densely infiltrated with small lymphocytes (see p. 30) and enterocytes appear cuboidal or even flattened with scarcely discernible brush borders, vacuolated cytoplasm and sometimes pyknotic nuclei [83,84]. By electron microscopy microvilli appear shortened, widened and irregularly arranged; lysosomes and phagolysosomes are increased as are free ribosomes. Abnormal lipid droplets are often visualized, suggesting impaired chylomicron formation [85,86]. Recent studies performed in children with the scanning electron microscope have confirmed the above data. Shortened and irregularly spaced microvilli of surface enterocytes were easily observed because of a poor glycocalyx [87]. Using freeze-fracture electron microscopy, tight junctions of coeliac children, as in coeliac adults, were found to be of reduced depth with a decreased number of strands, microvillus membrane having also a reduced density of intramembrane particles [88]. These findings may, at least in part, explain the increased mucosal permeability to disaccharides noted above.

Immunohistochemical techniques have permitted a better description of the cell populations involved in the inflammation of the intestinal mucosa characteristic of CD. In children, as in adults, the epithelium has an increased density of T ($CD3^+$) lymphocytes. Fifty, to more than 100, may be counted per 100 surface enterocytes, instead of 10–40 in a normal epithelium; most of them bear the α/β T cell receptor (TCR) for antigen and are of the suppressor–cytotoxic phenotype ($CD8^+$) [89,90]. The number of T cells bearing the γ/δ TCR is also increased to 5–40 per 100 enterocytes (normal 3 ± 2) [90,91]. In the lamina propria there is also an increased number of T cells, mainly of the helper phenotype ($CD4^+$), especially around the bottom of the crypts [89,90], together with numerous activated ($CD25^+$) macrophages. These cells are probably responsible for the expression of DR antigens by enterocytes in the crypts [90,92]. Besides the lymphocytes and macrophages, the lamina propria is densely filled with plasmocytes synthesizing mainly IgA, but also IgM and IgG immunoglobulins [59,93].

Specific activities of brush border hydrolases are decreased in proportion to the degree of villous atrophy. Among the disaccharidases, lactase is the most affected [94] as is its synthesis in organ culture [95]. Lactose is indeed the carbohydrate whose malabsorption is the most noteworthy at the active phase of the disease [96]. The dissacharidase deficiency secondary to microvillous lesions accounts for the fermentative aspect of diarrhoea in CD. Peptidase activities are also diminished [95,97]. Enterokinase activity is little impaired perhaps because it is not solely localized in the brush border [98]. All brush border activities return to normal when the normal architecture of the mucosa is restored after gluten is withdrawn from the diet.

Evolution

Effect of gluten-free diet

The effects of the gluten-free diet are most often spectacular, particularly in toddlers. Behavioural disorders are the first to subside; after a few days the child is smiling again and recovers his or her appetite which later may seem excessive. During the subsequent weeks, the child's activity recovers and after 1 or 2 months, rarely longer, the delay in psychomotor development is corrected [7,20].

The stools return to normal in a few days or weeks. However, their volume and consistency sometimes remain variable for months. Months are also necessary for abdominal distension to subside. In parallel with stool appearance, steatorrhoea decreases and fat excretion becomes normal 2–4 weeks after gluten withdrawal [7]. One-hour xylosaemia returns to normal within the same period [46].

Weight gain begins in a few days, always within the first 3 weeks after gluten exclusion. If the delay is longer, intolerance to an associated food antigen should be suspected. The toddler usually reaches his or her ideal body weight in 6 months to 1 year. Catching up of growth starts 1–3 months after catch-up of weight. Thus, a transient overweight may occur during the first year of gluten-free diet [99,100]. In teenagers, growth velocity may reach 1 cm/month when puberty is triggered by gluten exclusion; to catch-up growth is then added the growth spurt of puberty. The bone age varies simultaneously. Even in teenagers the final height achieved is, in general, that predictable from the parents' heights.

Spontaneously, the nutritional consequences of malabsorption resolve over several months. After 1 year on a gluten-free diet, the major biochemical parameters are normal. Only osteoporosis may take years to be corrected in the most severe cases [99].

Normal villous architecture is restored within several months to 1 year when the diet is strictly observed. Epithelial lesions are repaired first, enterocytes recovering their columnar shape within a few weeks while the density of intraepithelial lymphocytes falls. The cellularity of the lamina propria decreases as villi reappear. Villi are usually still too wide and too short after 2–3 months, becoming normal only after 1 year of gluten-free diet [7,101]. In rare instances 2 or even 3 years are necessary for lesions to resolve. In these cases the possibility of non-compliance to the diet, even if non-intentional, should always be raised before associated intolerances to other food proteins (primarily cow's milk, rice, soya proteins) are considered likely.

As mucosal morphology improves, there is a return to a more normal distribution of local immunocompetent cells; the number of intraepithelial lymphocytes expressing the α/β TCR and of the $CD8^+$ phenotype decreases steadily, whereas lymphocytes expressing the γ/δ TCR remain too numerous, so that this immunohistochemical feature has been proposed as a marker of CD [90,91]. Expression of DR antigens by crypt enterocytes progressively (1 year or more) fades, seldom disappearing completely. In the lamina propria macrophages are no more activated and numbers of plasma cells return to normal [59]. IgA antigliadin antibodies levels fall to normal in 2–3 months whereas IgG antigliadin antibodies levels decrease more slowly (2–6 months) and may not be normal after more than 6 months of gluten exclusion [63,69]. IgA antireticulin and anti-endomysium antibody levels decrease and return to normal in parallel to IgA antigliadin antibodies [71,77], whereas IgA anti-90 kDa glycoprotein do so in more than 4 months [78].

The provocation test or gluten challenge

A gluten challenge is performed in order to confirm the lasting nature of the sensitivity of the intestinal mucosa to gluten. This distinguishes CD which is supposed to be a permanent condition, from transient food, and especially gluten intolerance, which may induce histological lesions similar to those of CD. Its necessity has recently been discussed in children >2 years of age [82].

Gluten is reintroduced in the diet once the child's clinical state, mainly growth, and intestinal mucosa have returned to normal and usually when growth velocity is linear (between 4 and 10 years of age). In our department gluten challenge is performed after 2–4 years of exclusion diet and never before the age of 4 years. In other groups, gluten challenge is performed in younger [102] or older children after the age of 6 or 7 years, once the dental enamel of permanent teeth is formed [103]. The test may be performed either by adding to the gluten-free diet powdered gluten or biscuits which allows an accurate estimation of gluten ingested (usually 5–10 g/day or two slices of bread) or by allowing the child to resume a normal diet [102–105]. Although daily gluten intake, then, may vary widely from 1 to 10 g or more, this way of challenging is less constraining for the child. The duration of the challenge varies from 1 or 2 months (with known amounts, usually 10 g, of added gluten to the diet) to 1 year (with a spontaneous normal free diet) when the child remains symptom free [9]. The timing of the biopsy may be monitored and shortened by the use of a 1-hour blood xylose test [104] or determination of antigliadin or antireticulin antibodies [50].

The clinical features of the relapse are variable (Table 2.3). Only in a minority of children, varying from 20 to 40% [106–110], is there a recurrence of clinical symptoms which are more severe the earlier they occur, such as loss of appetite, decreased activity, abdominal pain, bloating, diarrhoea and loss of weight. More often, the clinical relapse is limited to episodes of abdominal pain and to decreased weight gain or even to a decreasing growth velocity with a normal weight : height ratio (Table 2.4). In this group of children, malabsorption also recurs with steatorrhoea, increased loss of nitrogen and of volatile fatty acids in the stools, sideropaenic anaemia and low blood folate

Table 2.3 Different types of relapse (personal data)

	Clinical symptoms	Malabsorption	Severe mucosal lesion on biopsy
Group I (*n* = 24)	+	+	+
Group II (*n* = 11)	—	+	+
Group III (*n* = 34)	—	—	+
Total	24	35	69

Table 2.4 Group I clinical symptoms (personal data)

	Early relapse (*n* = 6)	Late relapse (*n* = 18)	Total (*n* = 24)
Diarrhoea	5 (190 g/day)*	7 (140 g/day)*	12
Abdominal pain	3	4	7
Vomiting	2	—	2
Anorexia, amenorrhoea	—	3	3
Loss of weight	4	9	13
Growth retardation	—	15 (isolated: 10)	15

* Mean daily stool weight.

levels. In a smaller group of children (18% in our experience) malabsorption is only biological; growth is normal, there are no clinical symptoms and stools remain apparently normal. However, balance studies performed after 1 year of a gluten-containing diet reveal a moderate increase of stool wet weight, of steatorrhoea, of faecal loss of nitrogen and volatile acids. Haemoglobin level is normal but iron and folate plasma levels may be decreased in some children. In both groups of children relapse is also histological. Villous flattening is usually severe although in rare cases of very early clinical relapse, mucosal damage may be of intermediate severity.

Finally, the most important group of children concerns those in which gluten reintroduction has neither clinical, nor biological consequences (except, in some instances, for low plasma folate levels). In this group, which comprises some 50–70% of all relapsing patients, the relapse is only histological, characterized by the reappearance of mucosal damage, usually severe (85% in our experience) or sometimes moderate, when the intestinal biopsy is subsequently performed after 1 or 2 years of a gluten-containing diet [106,108,110]. Thus, at this stage of the disease (between 3 and 12 years of age), a severe mucosal lesion may be associated either with an obvious malabsorption syndrome or with an apparently perfectly normal child (Table 2.3). This variability also concerns the time necessary to obtain a histological relapse; it may occur up to 5–7 years with a normal gluten-containing diet [111].

Long-term evolution

Once the persistent character of mucosal sensitivity to gluten has been demonstrated, and thus, a final diagnosis achieved, a gluten-free diet is recommended. The effect is constant; clinical symptoms when present, alleviate, normal growth resumes and villous architecture is restored, within the same timespan as when gluten was withdrawn for the first time. Thereafter, as long as the child adheres to the gluten-free diet, he or she may be considered a 'normal' child. Long-term follow up of such adolescents, however, indicates that a noticeable proportion of them (25–45% [103,112]), in fact, do not adhere strictly to the diet, without substantial problems [103,112–114].

Prolonged observation (for up to 25 years in our experience) of children in whom relapse was purely histological and who were left on a normal diet because it was clinically well-tolerated, has shown that, in these conditions, gluten is not or little deleterious [115,116]. Although puberty may be delayed for less than 1 year, final height attained is that which could be predicted from the parents' height. Indeed, in series of patients seen by adult gastroenterologists as young adults, height is normal in most (>90%) cases [117,118]. In our experience, in two-thirds of these adolescents or young adults, severe mucosal damage persists. However, in the one-third, villous architecture improves; damage is only partial, or in some cases (10%) returns to normal ('transient CD') [116,119]. This improvement is accompanied by a decrease of intraepithelial lymphocytes expressing the α/β TCR, $CD8^+$ phenotype to normal values whereas γ/δ TCR lymphocytes remain elevated [90]. The latter findings are in agreement with the observation of a clinical remission of the disease at puberty and further indicate that, at least in a noticeable fraction of coeliac children, a complete or partial tolerance to gluten develops.

Similar findings have been made by others. In a group of 91 patients having had a planned challenge or a spontaneous diet interruption of up to 15 years, full relapse with a flat mucosa was observed in 71; intermediate lesions were found in 11 subjects, who did not present with any clinical or biological signs of malabsorption; and a normal mucosa was seen in six patients, after more than 2 years of normal diet. In three patients with a normal mucosa the normal diet lasted for less than 2 years. Thus, in 20% of the patients (17 out of 88) there was only either a partial, or no relapse (7%) at all [120]. Interestingly, the latter two groups of patients were older at the time of challenge (median age; 14.8 or 10 years, respectively, for those having a partial or no relapse) compared with those having a full relapse (median age; 5.8 years) [120], as if some degree of tolerance had developed with time. However, only 16 patients had an initial challenge many years before the study was performed so that it is not possible to know whether the patients who did not relapse had either transient gluten intolerance (see p. 39) or 'transient CD'.

In a more recent study from Finland 38 adolescents accepted a late gluten challenge (a second, for many of them) after biopsy. In nine (24%) an altered mucosa (from slight villous changes to a flat mucosa) indicated poor adherence to the diet. Out of the remaining 29, 24 relapsed after a mean challenge of 7 months; in one patient the relapse was dubious (slight alteration in villous height). In these 25 patients the mucosa was flat on 18 occasions, or showed severe (2) or moderate (5) architectural disturbances. In the remaining four patients, the intestinal mucosa stayed normal after more than 2 years exposure to a gluten-containing diet. Twenty of these patients had an earlier positive challenge, including four with a recovered (normal) mucosa. Thus, 11 of 38 patients (29%) showed improvement (7) or complete normalization (four patients = 11%) of their mucosal architecture [103]; these data are very similar to ours [115,116].

The long-term evolution of the intestinal mucosa of children with proven CD is thus rather variable, from the time of the diagnostic challenge up to adolescence and adulthood, with a general trend towards greater tolerance. The latter is first revealed by a reduction in the frequency of clinical symptoms as time passes. It is probable that this decrease in clinical severity is related to a reduction in the length of intestine affected by the immunological conflict [121], although this relationship has never been demonstrated in children, in whom intestinal biopsies are never taken more distally than the duodenojejunal flexure. In adolescence, an even greater tolerance seems to develop in a subgroup of patients whose mucosa is no more, or only moderately, sensitive to gluten. The recent observations that the disease appeared late in a monozygotic twin of a coeliac child [122] and that children or adults with CD may have a normal intestinal mucosa several years before the diagnosis is made [123], provide further strong evidence against the dogma that, in CD, the sensitivity of the intestinal mucosa to gluten is permanent throughout life. The reasons for this variability in time, and from one child to another, remain elusive. It has been proposed that genetic factors could determine the severity of the disease [124]. It is difficult, however, to understand how the same factors could explain the development of tolerance, as well as of sensitization, in a given child kept on the same diet. This variability also implies that gluten cannot be the only factor inducing villous effacement [19,125].

Complications and associated diseases

Complications

CD of children is now a benign illness which may not deserve hospitalization or rarely poses a threat to life. Marasmus has become an unusual presentation. The other main complications of the disease: skeletal (osteoporosis or osteomalacia leading to pathological fractures or bone deformation), haematological (isolated microcytic or rarely macrocytic anaemia, splenic atrophy, cavitation of mesenteric lymph nodes), neurological (peripheral neuropathy), or digestive (ulcerative duodenojejunoileitis) are generally seen in adults and will not be detailed here (see corresponding Chapters 3 and 5).

The risk of malignancy is increased in adults with CD [126] and malignant diseases are the main factor responsible for the fact that the overall mortality of adult coeliac patients is nearly twice that of the general population [127]. However, the occurrence of malignancy in coeliac children is poorly documented. Indeed, to our knowledge, only one such observation has been published. It concerned a 10-year-old north African girl maintained for 6 years on a gluten-free diet. Gluten challenge, performed at 9 years of age, caused relapse both clinical and histological after 7 months; a gluten-free diet was again prescribed. However, within the next month an abdominal malignant lymphoma developed and despite chemotherapy, death occurred 6 months later. As in the vast majority of similar cases reported in adults, the histophenotype of the lymphoma was not characterized [128]. Recently, however, the possibility of studying this unique case again, with antibodies directed against antigens preserved in fixed tissue, arose. Tumour cells strongly expressed antibodies directed against B cells (CD 20) and the final revised diagnosis of a B cell malignant lymphoma of Burkitt type was made (N. Brousse *et al.*, unpublished observation). Thus, this lymphoma was not a direct complication of overstimulation of intraepithelial T cells, as in adults [129]; it appears to have been a fortuitous association.

In fact, in the large series of coeliac patients in which mortality and/or risk of malignancy were evaluated [127,130–133], as in reported series of malignancies in coeliac patients [134–137] no case of lymphoma or of other malignancy was seen in patients less than 28 years of age [114] even in cases with familial involvement [138]; the majority occurred in adults >40 years of age. Furthermore, in a recent report, mortality rates in patients diagnosed as having CD in childhood were similar to those of the general population [127]. It is not known whether this observation is explained by adherence to a gluten-free diet (supposed to be stricter in children than in adults) or to some kind of 'protective' effect of age. The latter possibility seems more likely since it was shown in the same report that in coeliacs with a clinical history suggestive of early disease in childhood but diagnosed late in adult life, mortality from all causes was similar to that of coeliac patients diagnosed later in adult life [127].

Associated diseases

Numerous conditions have been reported in association with CD [139, 140] although their prevalence is much lower in children [141] than in adults [142].

Isolated IgA deficiency is the most frequent condition associated with childhood CD. It represents 25% of associated conditions according to a recent report [141] and has been considered a factor favouring the development of CD.

Diseases linked to HLA-DR3 antigen, in which autoimmune mechanisms are known to be involved, are the second most frequent diseases associated with CD [141]. Dermatitis herpetiformis (DH) may develop after CD in children, or on the contrary, intestinal lesions undistinguishable from those of CD may be discovered on systematic examination of a child with DH. In a recently published series of 57 children with DH, gastrointestinal symptoms were rare (16%), whereas severe (61%) and intermediate (28%) villous lesions were found in nearly 90% of cases [143]. DH may be atypical in childhood and it should be looked for in a coeliac child as soon as itchy lesions appear in areas atypical for eczema (elbows, knees and buttocks) As in adults, a gluten-free diet allows dapsone to be reduced or even stopped [143].

Diabetes mellitus may also develop in children with CD and represented 12% of associated diseases in a recent series [141]. Conversely, CD should be looked for systematically in children with diabetes mellitus thriving unsatisfactorily. Prevalence of CD in diabetic children has been estimated to be near 3.5% [29,144]. Thyroiditis [145,146], chronic juvenile arthritis [30], chronic active hepatitis [147], Budd–Chiari syndrome [148], fibrosing alveolitis [141], pulmonary haemosiderosis [149] and psoriasis [141] have also been observed in coeliac children.

Finally, the associations of childhood CD with genetic conditions, such as Down's syndrome [146,150] and cystic fibrosis [151,152] are rare but well-documented. On the contrary, the association of CD and atopy is less well-documented than in adults and remains a matter of discussion [153,154]. Associations of CD with inflammatory bowel diseases [155], primary biliary cirrhosis [156] have been reported mainly in adults.

Diagnosis

Malabsorption syndromes not due to intolerance to dietary proteins

The typical malabsorption syndrome caused by CD in a 6–18-month-old child is mimicked by few other conditions that can be distinguished only by intestinal biopsy. This is particularly the case for congenital disorders of fat absorption, not so much abetalipoproteinaemia as Anderson's disease in which the clinically isolated malabsorption syndrome is peculiar only because of the unusually low plasma cholesterol and apolipoprotein B levels. The diagnosis of this rare autosomal recessive condition rests on the demonstration of the absorption defect in the intestinal mucosa. In both diseases, villi of normal height appear lined with enterocytes typically heavily loaded with fat droplets, appearing as empty vacuoles with the haematein–eosin stain or as red or black spots with Oil Red or Sudan Black stains [157]. In other instances the intestinal biopsy can reveal massive infestation by *Giardia lamblia*; the mucosal lesion is usually only partial [158] but may be severe in children with hypogammaglobulinaemia. Only rarely does intestinal biopsy reveal lymphangiectasia, often already suspected because of lymphopaenia, hypoalbuminaemia, and a high α_1-antitrypsin clearance [159].

In more severe cases of protracted diarrhoea, not only may the clinical picture evoke CD, although often in children somewhat younger than expected, but the intestinal biopsy usually shows a flat mucosa. A gluten-free diet is without any effect. Total parenteral nutrition is usually the only way of getting these children to survive. In some of these cases, histological signs of mononuclear cell activation are seen in the intestinal mucosa. Association with autoimmune diseases (as insulin-dependent diabetes) and the favourable effect of immunosuppressive treatments raise the possibility that the intestinal mucosa is the site of an 'autoimmune' reaction [160]. The latter possibility is demonstrated when circulating autoantibodies to enterocytes are detected [161].

Malabsorption due to intolerance to other dietary proteins

Intolerance to cow's milk proteins [162,163], or rarely to proteins of rice [164], soya [165] and egg [166] may lead to a form of chronic enteropathy with malabsorption. This enteropathy can usually be distinguished from CD by an earlier age of onset (before 2–3 months of age) and milder biological and histological features. Mucosal changes are typically less severe with numbers of intraepithelial lymphocytes being slightly increased and immunohistochemical expression of DR antigens by crypt enterocytes less prominent than in CD [92,163]. In some cases, however, with a late onset due to very early introduction of gluten in the diet, or because of extreme mucosal flattening, the distinction is not possible. Little help is provided by antigliadin and anticow's milk protein antibodies [61]. It is possible to distinguish between the two conditions only by the sequential exclusion and reintroduction of the suspected protein(s) in the diet in the first years of life, thereby demonstrating the transient nature of food protein (usually cow's milk) induced enteropathy. Distinction between the two conditions may be particularly difficult, however, since they may be associated [162,167].

Malabsorption due to transient gluten intolerance

Like intolerance to other food proteins (in particular to cow's milk proteins), intolerance to gluten may also be transient and present two clinical pictures.

It can present with acute vomiting, diarrhoea or urticarial rash within hour(s) of gluten ingestion [162]; diagnosis is then straightforward. More seldom transient gluten intolerance, on the other hand, causes a typical malabsorption syndrome with villous flattening. In infants aged from a few weeks to a few months, it may also be associated with true cow's milk protein intolerance [162,167]. In infants >6 months of age, only follow-up of the child considered to have CD permits the diagnosis of transient gluten intolerance, by disclosing absence of both clinical symptoms and histological relapse following gluten reintroduction several months or years after its exclusion, usually before the age of 4 years [168]. Such transient intolerance occurs in a few per cent of children (6.6% in our experience) considered, before the gluten challenge, as having CD [169]. Since in such cases intolerance to gluten is proven only by the clinical and histological improvement following gluten exclusion (a sequence of events which could be fortuitous) some authors have proposed limiting the terms 'transient gluten intolerance' to instances when intolerance has been previously confirmed by a relapse at least histological, after the first reintroduction of gluten [170]. Such temporary intolerance, then, clinically differs from 'transient CD', as described above, in which tolerance seems to develop around puberty, only in the time taken for the intestinal mucosa to lose its abnormal sensitivity to gluten. It is probable, however, that this difference in timing is related to immunogenetic differences since cow's milk protein intolerance is not linked to any particular HLA haplotype [171].

Treatment

The gluten-free diet

A diet excluding gluten is the basis of the treatment of CD. All foodstuffs made from wheat flour, such as bread, pastry, pastas, cakes and confectionery and those to which flour has been added, such as delicatessen condiments, and cooked and canned foods, should be eliminated from the diet as should products based on rye and barley flours, and probably oat meal [20,172]. The diet is easy to realize in infants and toddlers; their diet is still rather uniform, they are usually fed by only one or few persons and they do not have the opportunity of discovering the 'forbidden fruit'. If strong agreement exists within the family among parents, older siblings and even the grandparents regarding the necessity of a strict gluten-free diet, and if too frequent temptations are not offered to the child, the diet is acceptable without great difficulty until school age. The latter may be a reasonable period to perform a gluten challenge, if necessary [82].

Indeed, criteria for the diagnosis of CD have been revised recently by an ESPGAN Working Group. According to these new guidelines, gluten challenge remains mandatory only 'when there are doubts about the initial diagnosis and the adequacy of the clinical response to a gluten-free diet', which is more likely to arise the younger the child at time of diagnosis. In all other situations criteria have been simplified and only 'a characteristic small intestinal mucosal abnormality' at the first biopsy and 'a clearcut clinical remission on a gluten-free diet' remain mandatory [82]. Although not mandatory in these conditions, and discussed by some on the ground that it could lead to a loosening of adherence to the diet [80,120], gluten challenge still appears useful to others; it allows a few per cent of children with transient gluten intolerance to avoid the burden of a useless exclusion diet, while for other children, the demonstration of a permanent sensitivity of the intestinal mucosa to gluten may be a motivation to follow their diet (S Auricchio, I Polanco, personal communications).

Whatever the criteria used in making the diagnosis of CD in a child, either the traditional ones implying the sequence of three biopsies [6], or the simplified ones, omitting the gluten challenge in many instances [82], once made, a life-long gluten-free diet is generally recommended. There is not absolute agreement on this point, however. A life-long gluten-free diet is prescribed not so much to avoid clinical relapses (only 30–40% of children would need it) than to prevent malignancies occurring in adulthood. This attitude is based on two assumptions: (1) the permanent, life-long sensitivity of the intestinal mucosa to gluten in all children with CD; and (2) the ability of a gluten-free diet followed during childhood to prevent malignancies in adulthood, as has been possibly shown in adults [173]. The first assumption is seriously challenged (see p. 34); the second one, unproved. We, thus, think that the reasons for systematically prescribing a lifelong gluten-free diet in a child with CD are not yet firmly established.

Observance of the diet should be controlled, especially if its effects are not those that were expected particularly with regard to growth. Similarly, the consequences of the gluten challenge should be appreciated. In addition to biological markers of malnutrition (blood iron, folate), numerous tests have been proposed to achieve these aims: 1-hour xylosaemia [50], permeability tests using saccharides [53], antibody to various antigens, e.g. gliadin [50,64], reticulin [72,78] or endomysium [75,78]. Most of these tests are able to reflect the restoration of normal mucosal architecture after commencement of a gluten-free diet (see above). Few, however, are sensitive enough to reliably detect a flat mucosa in a symptomless adolescent (see pp. 23–29). Until any such test is validated, the intestinal biopsy remains the only reliable way of evaluating adherence to the diet.

Complementary treatments to the gluten-free diet

Simultaneously, with the beginning of the exclusion diet, it may be advisable to supplement the child with Ca^{2+}, iron and vitamins (A, D, E, K, folic acid) for several weeks to 2 months [7,20]. However, iron supplementation has been shown recently to be unnecessary in a group of coeliac children with mild iron deficiency; it corrected itself spontaneously after gluten exclusion [174].

In rare cases the severity of anorexia or of malnutrition and/or diarrhoea justifies the use of constant rate semielemental, nasogastric feeding during the initial days of treatment. It is advisable in such cases to exclude lactose for 10–15 days. It is not necessary, however, to systematically exclude lactose from the diet since it has been shown recently with the H_2 breath test, that half (48%) of untreated coeliac children tolerate a physiological load of lactose (12.5 g) and that all are able to tolerate and absorb loads of between 5–12 g/day [96].

Although, most often, CD is no longer a serious illness in children, it remains a chronic one. As such, it requires continuous management through childhood to adolescence and adulthood. Adequate explanations to, and discussions with, the parents and the growing child about the disease, its possible mechanisms, the reason for the diet, and eventually for gluten challenge, provide the basis for a trustful relationship and the best guarantee that advice will be understood, accepted and effectively followed.

References

1 Gee S. On the coeliac affection. *St Bartholomew's Hosp Rep* 1888;24:17–20.

2 Parsons LG. Celiac disease. *Am J Dis Child* 1932;43:1293–346.

3 Cooke WT. Adult coeliac disease and other disorders associated with steatorrhoea. *Br Med J* 1958;2:261–5.

4 van de Kamer JH, Weijers HA, Dicke WK. An investigation into the injurious constituents of wheat in connection with their action on patients with coeliac disease. *Acta Paediatr* 1953;42:223–31.

5 Hallert C, Gotthard R, Norrby K, Walan A. On the prevalence of adult coeliac disease in Sweden. *Scand J Gastroenterol* 1981;16: 257–61.

6 Weijers HA, Lindquist B, Anderson CM *et al.* Round table discussion. Diagnostic criteria in coeliac disease. *Acta Paediatr Scand* 1970;59:461–3.

7 Lamy M, Frezal J, Rey J, Nezelof C, Fortier-Beaulieu M, Jos J. Les stéatorrhées par troubles de l'absorption intestinale. *Rapports au XIXe Congrès des Pédiatres de langue française.* Paris, 1963:161–267.

8 Shmerling DH, Zimmerli-Haring SM. Die floride Zöliakie. Untersuchungsergebnisse bei 88 Patienten zwischen 1963 und 1969. *Helv Pediatr Acta* 1971;26:565–84.

9 Young WF, Pringle EM. 110 children with coeliac disease, 1950–1969. *Arch Dis Child* 1971;46:421–36.

10 McNeish AS, Anderson CM. Coeliac disease in childhood. *Clin Gastroenterol* 1974;3: 127–44.

11 Rossipal E. On the incidence of coeliac disease in Austria: a study comprising a nine-year period. In: McConnell RB, ed. *The Genetics of Coeliac Disease.* Lancaster: MTP Press, 1981:23–7.

12 Greco L, Mayer M, Grimaldi M, Follo D, de Ritis G, Auricchio S. The effect of early feeding on the onset of symptoms in celiac disease. *J Pediatr Gastroenterol Nutr* 1985; 4:52–5.

13 Ascher H, Krantz I, Kristiansson B. Increasing incidence of celiac disease in Sweden. *Arch Dis Child* 1991;66:608–11.

14 Auricchio S, Greco L, Troncone R. Gluten-sensitive enteropathy in childhood. *Pediatr Clin North Am* 1988;35:157–87.

15 Mäki M, Kallonen K, Lahdeaho M-L, Visakorpi JK. Changing pattern of childhood coeliac disease in Finland. *Acta Paediatr Scand* 1988;77:408–12.

16 Polanco I, Vazquez C. The influence of breast-feeding in coeliac disease. *Pediatr Res* 1981;15:1193 (abstract).

17 Auricchio S, Follo D, de Ritis G *et al.* Does breast feeding protect against the development of clinical symptoms of celiac disease in children? *J Pediatr Gastroenterol Nutr* 1983;2:428–33.

18 Greco L, Auricchio S, Mayer M, Grimaldi M. Case control study on nutritional risk factors in celiac disease. *J Pediatr Gastroenterol Nutr* 1988;7:395–9.

19 Polanco I, Mearin ML, Larrauri J, Biemond I, Wipkink-Bakker A, Pena AS. Effect of gluten supplementation in healthy siblings of children with celiac disease. *Gastroenterology* 1987;92:678–81.

20 Anderson CM. Coeliac disease. In: Anderson CM, Burke V, Gracey M, eds. *Paediatric Gastroenterology.* Oxford: Blackwell Scientific Publications, 1987:375–400.

21 Hamilton JR, Lynch MJ, Reilly BJ. Active coeliac disease in childhood. Clinical and laboratory findings of forty-two cases. *Q J Med* 1969;38:135–58.

22 Visakorpi JK, Kuitunen P, Pelkonen P. Intestinal malabsorption: a clinical study of 22 children over 2 years of age. *Acta Paediatr Scand* 1970;59:273–80.

23 McNicholl B, Egan-Mitchell B. Infancy celiac disease without diarrhea. *Pediatrics* 1972;49:85–91.

24 Aine L. Dental enamel defects and dental maturity in children and adolescents with coeliac disease. *Proc Finn Dent Soc* 1986; 82(Suppl. 3):1–71.

25 Cacciari E, Salardi S, Lazzari R *et al.* Short stature and celiac disease: a relationship to consider even in patients with no gastrointestinal tract symptoms. *J Pediatr* 1983; 103:708–11.

26 Cacciari E, Volta U, Lazzari R *et al.* Can antigliadin antibody detect symptomless coeliac disease in children with short stature? *Lancet* 1985;i:1469–71.

27 Groll A, Candy DCA, Preece MA, Tanner JM, Harries JT. Short stature as the primary manifestation of coeliac disease. *Lancet* 1980;ii:1097–9.

28 Bresson JL, Prevot C, Rappaport R, Czernichow P, Schmitz J, Rey J. Activité somato-

médine circulante et sécrétion d'hormone de croissance. Modifications au cours de la maladie coeliaque à révélation tardive et effets du traitement. *Arch Fr Pediatr* 1979; 36(Suppl.):13–18.
29 Savilahti E, Simell O, Koskimies S, Rilva A, Akerblom HK. Celiac disease in insulin-dependent diabetes mellitus. *J Pediatr* 1986;108:690–3.
30 Mäki M, Hällström O, Verronen P *et al.* Reticulin antibody, arthritis, and coeliac disease in children. *Lancet* 1988;i:479–80.
31 Walia BNS, Sidhu JK, Tandon BN, Ghai OP, Bhargava S. Coeliac disease in north Indian children. *Br Med J* 1966;2:1233–4.
32 Nelson R, McNeish AS, Anderson CM. Coeliac disease in children of Asian immigrants. *Lancet* 1973;i:348–50.
33 Khoshoo V, Bhan MK, Jain R *et al.* Coeliac disease as a cause of protracted diarrhoea in Indian children. *Lancet* 1988;i:126–7.
34 Khuffash FA, Barakat MH, Shaltout AA, Farwana SS, Adnani MS, Tungekar MF. Coeliac disease among children in Kuwait: difficulties in diagnosis and management. *Gut* 1987;28:1595–9.
35 Blanco Rabassa E, Sagaro E, Fragoso T, Castaneda C, Gra B. Coeliac disease in Cuban children. *Arch Dis Child* 1981;56: 128–31.
36 Suliman GI. Coeliac disease in Sudanese children. *Gut* 1978;19:121–5.
37 Polonovski C, Navarro J, Fontaine JL, Laplane R. L'intolérance au gluten chez l'enfant. Critères actuels du diagnostic (à propos de 40 cas suivis par biopsie). *Ann Med Int* 1971;122:911–24.
38 McNeish AS, Willoughby MLN. Whole blood folate as a screening test for coeliac disease in childhood. *Lancet* 1969;i:442–3.
39 Sanderson MC, Davis LR, Mowat AP. Failure of laboratory and radiological studies to predict jejunal mucosal atrophy. *Arch Dis Child* 1975;50:526–31.
40 Kokkonen J, Simila S. Gastric function and absorption of vitamin B12 in children with celiac disease. *Eur J Pediatr* 1979;132:71–5.
41 Magazzu G, Jacono G, Di Pasquale G *et al.* Reliability and usefulness of random fecal α_1-antitrypsin concentration: further simplification of the method. *J Pediatr Gastroenterol Nutr* 1985;4:402–7.
42 Naveh Y, Lightman A, Zinder O. A prospective study of serum zinc concentration in children with celiac disease. *J Pediatr* 1983;102:734–6.
43 Goyens P, Brasseur D, Cadranel S. Copper deficiency in infants with active celiac disease. *J Pediatr Gastroenterol Nutr* 1985;4: 677–80.
44 Reinken L, Zieglauer H, Berger H. Vitamin B6 nutriture of children with acute celiac disease, celiac disease in remission, and of children with normal duodenal mucosa. *Am J Clin Nutr* 1976;29:750–3.
45 Heyman M, Desjeux JF, Grasset E, Dumontier A-M, Lestradet H. Relationship between transport of D-xylose and other monosaccharides in jejunal mucosa of children. *Gastroenterology* 1981;80: 758–62.
46 Rolles CJ, Kendall MJ, Nutter S, Anderson CM. One-hour blood-xylose screening-test for coeliac disease in infants and young children. *Lancet* 1973;ii:1043–5.
47 Lifschitz CH, Polanco I, Lobb K. The urinary excretion of polyethylene glycol as a test for mucosal integrity in children with celiac disease: comparison with other noninvasive tests. *J Pediatr Gastroenterol Nutr* 1989;9: 49–57.
48 Buts JP, Morin CL, Roy CC, Weber A, Bonin A. One-hour xylose test: a reliable index of small bowel function. *J Pediatr* 1978;90: 729–33.
49 Rich EJ, Christie DL. Anti-gliadin antibody panel and xylose absorption test in screening for celiac disease. *J Pediatr Gastroenterol Nutr* 1990;10:174–8.
50 Mayer M, Greco L, Troncone R, Grimaldi M, Pansa G. Early prediction of relapse during gluten challenge in childhood celiac disease. *J Pediatr Gastroenterol Nutr* 1989; 8:474–9.
51 Pearson ADJ, Eastham EJ, Laker MF, Craft AW, Nelson R. Intestinal permeability in children with Crohn's disease and coeliac disease. *Br Med J* 1982;285:20–1.
52 Hamilton I, Hill A, Bose B, Bouchier IAD, Forsyth JS. Small intestinal permeability in pediatric clinical practice. *J Pediatr Gastroenterol Nutr* 1987;6:697–701.
53 Stenhammar L, Falth-Magnusson K, Jansson G, Magnusson KE, Sundqvist T. Intestinal permeability to inert sugars and different-sized polyethyleneglycols in children with celiac disease. *J Pediatr Gastroenterol Nutr* 1989;9:281–9.
54 Turck D, Ythier H, Maquet E *et al.* Intestinal permeability to (^{51}Cr) EDTA in children with Crohn's disease. *J Pediatr Gastroenterol Nutr* 1987;6:535–7.

55 Lifschitz CH, Shulman RJ. Intestinal permeability tests: are they clinically useful? *J Pediatr Gastroenterol Nutr* 1990;10:283–7.
56 Jonas A, Weiser S, Segal P, Katznelson D. Oral fat loading test. A reliable procedure for the study of fat malabsorption in children. *Arch Dis Child* 1979;54:770–2.
57 Goldstein R, Blondheim O, Levy E, Stankiewicz H, Frier S. The fatty meal test: an alternative to stool fat analysis. *Am J Clin Nutr* 1983;38:763–8.
58 Watkins JB, Klein PD, Schoeller DA, Kirschner BS, Park R, Perman JA. Diagnosis and differentiation of fat malabsorption in children using ^{13}C-labeled lipids: trioctanoin, triolein, and palmitic acid breath tests. *Gastroenterology* 1982;82:911–17.
59 Jos J, Rey J, Frezal J. Etude immuno-histochimique de la muqueuse intestinale chez l'enfant. I. Les syndromes de malabsorption. *Arch Fr Pediatr* 1972;29:681–98.
60 Bürgin-Wolff A, Bertele RM, Berger R *et al.* A reliable screening test for childhood celiac disease: Fluorescent immunosorbent test for gliadin antibodies. A prospective multicenter study. *J Pediatr* 1983;102:655–60.
61 Scott H, Ek J, Havnen J, Michalsen H, Brunvand L, Howlid H, Brandtzaeg P. Serum antibodies to dietary antigens: a prospective study of the diagnostic usefulness in celiac disease of children. *J Pediatr Gastroenterol Nutr* 1990;11:215–20.
62 Unsworth DJ, Kieffer M, Holborow EJ, Coombs RRA, Walker-Smith JA. IgA antigliadin antibodies in coeliac disease. *Clin Exp Immunol* 1981;46:286–93.
63 Savilahti E, Viander M, Perkkio M, Vainio E, Kalimo K, Reunala T. IgA antigliadin antibodies: a marker of mucosal damage in childhood coeliac disease. *Lancet* 1983;i:320–2.
64 Stenhammar L, Kilander AF, Nilsson LA, Stromberg L, Tarkowski A. Serum gliadin antibodies for detection and control of childhood coeliac disease. *Acta Paediatr Scand* 1984;73:657–63.
65 Volta U, Lenzi M, Lazzari R *et al.* Antibodies to gliadin detected by immunofluorescence and a micro-ELISA method: markers of active childhood and adult coeliac disease. *Gut* 1985;26:667–71.
66 Ståhlberg MR, Savilahti E, Viander M. Antibodies to gliadin by ELISA as a screening test for childhood celiac disease. *J Pediatr Gastroenterol Nutr* 1986;5:726–9.
67 Ribes Koninckx C, Pereda Perez RA, Ferrer Calvete J, Pena AS. The value of the measurement of IgA antigliadin antibodies in a pediatric unit in Spain. A prospective study. *J Clin Nutr Gastroenterol* 1986;1:26–9.
68 Arranz E, Blanco A, Alonso M *et al.* IgA-1 antigliadin antibodies are the most specific in children with coeliac disease. *J Clin Nutr Gastroenterol* 1986;1:291–5.
69 Bürgin-Wolff A, Berger R, Gaze H, Huber H, Lentze MJ, Nussle D. IgG, IgA and IgE gliadin antibody determinations as screening test for untreated coeliac disease in children, a multicentre study. *Eur J Pediatr* 1989;148:496–502.
70 Mascart-Lemone F, Cadranel S, Van den Broeck J, Dive C, Vaerman JP, Duchateau J. IgA Immune response patterns to gliadin in serum. *Int Arch Allergy Appl Immunol* 1988;86:412–9.
71 Mäki M, Hällström O, Vesikari T, Visakorpi JK. Evaluation of a serum IgA-class reticulin antibody test for the detection of childhood celiac disease. *J Pediatr* 1984;105:901–5.
72 Lazzari R, Volta U, Bianco Bianchi F, Collina A, Pisi E. R_1 reticulin antibodies: markers of celiac disease in children on a normal diet and on gluten challenge. *J Pediatr Gastroenterol Nutr* 1984;3:516–22.
73 Volta U, Bonazzi C, Pisi E, Salardi S, Cacciari E. Antigliadin and antireticulin antibodies in coeliac disease and at onset of diabetes in children. *Lancet* 1987;ii:1034–5.
74 Khoshoo V, Bhan MK, Unsworth DJ, Kumar R, Walker-Smith JA. Anti-reticulin antibodies: useful adjunct to histopathology in diagnosing celiac disease, especially in a developing country. *J Pediatr Gastroenterol Nutr* 1988;7:864–6.
75 Kapuscinska A, Zalewski T, Chorzelski TP *et al.* Disease specificity and dynamics of changes in IgA class anti-endomysial antibodies in celiac disease. *J Pediatr Gastroenterol Nutr* 1987;6:529–34.
76 Rossi TM, Kumar V, Lerner A, Heitlinger LA, Tucker N, Fisher J. Relationship of endomysial antibodies to jejunal mucosal pathology: specificity towards both symptomatic and asymptomatic celiacs. *J Pediatr Gastroenterol Nutr* 1988;7:858–63.
77 Hällström O. Comparison of IgA-class reticulin and endomysium antibodies in coeliac disease and dermatitis herpetiformis. *Gut* 1989;30:1225–32.
78 Teppo AM, Mäki M, Hällström O, Maury CPJ. Antibodies to 90 kilodalton glyco-

protein in childhood and adolescent celiac disease: relationship to reticulin antibodies. *J Pediatr Gastroenterol Nutr* 1987;6: 908–14.

79 Greco L, Troncone R, De Vizia B, Poggi V, Mayer M, Grimaldi M. Discriminant analysis for the diagnosis of childhood celiac disease. *J Pediatr Gastroenterol Nutr* 1987;6: 538–42.

80 Guandalini S, Ventura A, Ansaldi N *et al.* Diagnosis of coeliac disease: time for a change? *Arch Dis Child* 1989;64:1320–5.

81 Ashkenazi A, Levin S, Idar D, Or A, Rosenberg I, Handzel ZT. Immunological assay for the diagnosis of coeliac disease: interaction between purified gluten fractions. *Pediatr Res* 1980;14:776–8.

82 Walker-Smith JA, Guandalini S, Schmitz J, Shmerling DH, Visakorpi JK. Revised criteria for diagnosis of coeliac disease. *Arch Dis Child* 1990;65:909–11.

83 Shiner M, Doniach I. Histopathologic studies in steatorrhea. *Gastroenterology* 1960;38:419–40.

84 Jos J, Rey J, Frezal J, Nezelof C, Lamy M. La biopsie intestinale chez l'enfant. Acquisitions récentes. *Arch Fr Pediatr* 1967;24: 1159–83.

85 Rubin W. Celiac disease. *Am J Clin Nutr* 1971;24:91–111.

86 Shiner M. Cell distribution in the jejunal mucosa in coeliac disease. In: Hekkens WThJM, Pena AS, eds. *Coeliac Disease. Proceedings of the Second International Coeliac Symposium.* Leiden: Stenfert Kroese, 1974:121–35.

87 Carpino F, Ceccamea A, Magliocca FM, Familiari G, Lombardi ME, Bonamico M. Scanning electrón microscopy of jejunal biopsies in patients with untreated and treated coeliac disease. *Acta Paediatr Scand* 1985;74:775–81.

88 Kohl D, Ashkenazi A, Ben-Shaul Y, Bacher A. Tight junctions of jejunal surface and crypt cells in celiac disease: a freeze-fracture study. *J Pediatr Gastroenterol Nutr* 1987; 6:57–65.

89 Dobbins WO III. Human intestinal intraepithelial lymphocytes. *Gut* 1986;27: 972–85.

90 Kutlu T, Brousse N, Rambaud C, Le Deist F, Schmitz J, Cerf-Bensussan N. TCR $\alpha\beta$+ and TCR $\gamma\delta$+ lymphocytes in celiac disease: relationships with diet and villous atrophy. Submitted for publication.

91 Savilahti E, Arato A, Verkasalo M. Intestinal γ/δ receptor-bearing T lymphocytes in celiac disease and inflammatory bowel diseases in children. Constant increase in celiac disease. *Pediatr Res* 1990;28:579–81.

92 Arnaud-Battandier F, Cerf-Bensussan N, Amsellem R, Schmitz J. Increased HLA-DR expression by enterocytes in children with celiac disease. *Gastroenterology* 1986;91: 1206–12.

93 Savilahti E. Intestinal immunoglobulins in children with coeliac disease. *Gut* 1972; 13:958–64.

94 O'Grady JG, Stevens FM, Keane R *et al.* Intestinal lactase, sucrase, and alkaline phosphatase in 373 patients with coeliac disease. *J Clin Pathol* 1984;37:298–301.

95 Lentze MJ, Naim HY, Sterchi EE. Protein structure and function of brush border enzymes in clinical mucosal disorders. In: Lifschitz CH, Nichols B, eds. *Malnutrition in Chronic Diet-associated Infantile Diarrhea. Diagnosis and Management.* San Diego: Academic Press, 1990:39–49.

96 Roggero P, Ceccatelli MP, Volpe C *et al.* Extent of lactose absorption in children with active celiac disease. *J Pediatr Gastroenterol Nutr* 1989;9:290–4.

97 Sjöström H, Norén O, Krasilnikoff PA, Gudmand-Hoyer E. Intestinal peptidases and sucrase in coeliac disease. *Clin Chim Acta* 1981;109:53–8.

98 Woodley JF, Keane R. Enterokinase in normal intestinal biopsies and those from patients with untreated coeliac disease. *Gut* 1972;13:900–2.

99 Rey J, Rey F, Jos J, Amusquivar Lora S. Etude de la croissance dans 50 cas de maladie coeliaque de l'enfant. I. Effets du régime sans gluten. *Arch Fr Pediatr* 1971; 28:37–47.

100 Barr DGD, Shmerling DH, Prader A. Catch-up growth in malnutrition, studied in celiac disease after institution of gluten-free diet. *Pediatr Res* 1972;6:521–7.

101 McNicholl B, Egan-Mitchell B, Stevens F *et al.* Mucosal recovery in treated childhood celiac disease (gluten-sensitive enteropathy). *J Pediatr* 1976;89:418–24.

102 Danielsson L, Stenhammar L, Astrom E. Is gluten challenge necessary for the diagnosis of coeliac disease in young children? *Scand J Gastroenterol* 1990;25:957–60.

103 Mäki M, Lahdeaho M-L, Hällström O, Viander M, Visakorpi JK. Postpubertal gluten challenge in coeliac disease. *Arch Dis Child* 1989;64:1604–7.

104 Rolles CJ, McNeish AS. Standardised approach to gluten challenge in diagnosing childhood coeliac disease. *Br Med J* 1976;1: 1309–11.
105 Packer SM, Charlton V, Keeling JW *et al.* Gluten challenge in treated coeliac disease. *Arch Dis Child* 1978;53:449–55.
106 Sheldon W. Celiac disease. *Pediatrics* 1959; 23:132–45.
107 Shmerling DH. An analysis of controlled relapses in gluten-induced coeliac disease. *Acta Paediatr Scand* 1969;58:311 (abstract).
108 Visakorpi JK, Kuitunen P, Savilahti E. Frequency and nature of relapses in children suffering from the malabsorption syndrome with gluten intolerance. *Acta Pediatr Scand* 1970;59:481–6.
109 Hamilton JR, McNeill LK. Childhood celiac disease: response of treated patients to a small uniform daily dose of wheat gluten. *J Pediatr* 1972;81:885–93.
110 Bresson JL, Schmitz J, Rey J. Characteristics of the relapse in coeliac disease. *Acta Paediatr Belg* 1980;33:270 (abstract).
111 McNicholl B, Egan-Mitchell B, Fottrell PF. Variability of gluten intolerance in treated childhood coeliac disease. *Gut* 1979;20: 126–32.
112 Kumar PJ, Walker-Smith JA, Milla P, Harris G, Colyer J, Halliday R. The teenage coeliac: follow up study of 102 patients. *Arch Dis Child* 1988;63:916–20.
113 Kumar PJ, O'Donoghue DP, Stenson K, Dawson AM. Reintroduction of gluten in adults and children with treated coeliac disease. *Gut* 1979;20:743–9.
114 McCrae WM, Eastwood MA, Martin MR, Sircus W. Neglected coeliac disease. *Lancet* 1975;i:187–90.
115 Schmitz J, Jos J, Rey J. La maladie coeliaque. In: Ribet A, Frexinos J, eds. *Actualités en Hépato-Gastroentérologie.* Paris: Masson, 1979:95–109.
116 Schmitz J, Arnaud-Battandier F, Jos J, Rey J. Long term follow-up of childhood coeliac disease. Is there a natural recovery? *Pediatr Res* 1984;18:1054 (abstract).
117 Mortimer PE, Stewart JS, Norman AP, Booth CC. Follow-up study of coeliac disease. *Br Med J* 1968;2:7–9.
118 Sheldon W. Prognosis in early adult life of coeliac children treated with a gluten-free diet. *Br Med J* 1969;2:401–4.
119 Schmitz J, Jos J, Rey J. Transient mucosal atrophy in confirmed coeliac disease. In: McNicholl B, McCarthy CF, Fottrell PF, eds. *Perspectives in Coeliac Disease.* Lancaster: MTP Press, 1978:259–66.
120 Shmerling DH, Franckx J. Childhood celiac disease: a long-term analysis of relapses in 91 patients. *J Pediatr Gastroenterol Nutr* 1986;5:565–9.
121 Stewart JS, Pollock DJ, Hoffbrand AV, Mollin DL, Booth CC. A study of proximal and distal intestinal structure and absorptive function in idiopathic steatorrhoea. *Q J Med* 1967;36:425–44.
122 Salazar De Sousa JM, Ramos De Almeida JM, Monteiro MV, Magalhaes Ramalho P. Late onset coeliac disease in the monozygotic twin of a coeliac child. *Acta Paediatr Scand* 1987;76:172–4.
123 Mäki M, Holm K, Koskimies S, Hällström O, Visakorpi JK. Normal small bowel biopsy followed by coeliac disease. *Arch Dis Child* 1990;65:1137–41.
124 Demarchi M, Carbonara A, Ansaldi N *et al.* HLA-DR3 and DR7 in coeliac disease: immunogenetic and clinical aspects. *Gut* 1983;24:706–12.
125 Polanco I, Biemond I, Van Leeuwen A *et al.* Gluten sensitive enteropathy in Spain: genetic and environmental factors. In: McConnell RB, ed. *The Genetics of Coeliac Disease.* Lancaster: MTP Press, 1981: 211–31.
126 Swinson CM, Slavin G, Coles EC, Booth CC. Coeliac disease and malignancy. *Lancet* 1983;i:111–5.
127 Logan RFA, Rifkind EA, Turner ID, Ferguson A. Mortality in celiac disease. *Gastroenterology* 1989;97:265–71.
128 Arnaud-Battandier F, Schmitz J, Ricour C, Rey J. Intestinal malignant lymphoma in a child with familial celiac disease. *J Pediatr Gastroenterol Nutr* 1983;2:320–3.
129 Isaacson PG, O'Connor NTJ, Spencer JO *et al.* Malignant histiocytosis of the intestine: a T-cell lymphoma. *Lancet* 1985;ii: 688–91.
130 Harris OD, Cooke WT, Thompson H, Waterhouse JAH. Malignancy in adult coeliac disease and idiopathic steatorrhoea. *Am J Med* 1967;42:899–912.
131 Holmes GKT, Stokes PL, Sorahan TM, Prior P, Waterhouse JAH, Cooke WT. Coeliac disease, gluten-free diet, and malignancy. *Gut* 1976;17:612–19.
132 Selby WS, Gallagher ND. Malignancy in a 19-year experience of adult celiac disease. *Dig Dis Sci* 1979;24:684–8.
133 Haagen Nielsen O, Jacobsen O, Rask

Pedersen E *et al.* Non-tropical sprue. Malignant diseases and mortality rate. *Scand J Gastroenterol* 1985;20:13–18.

134 Austad WI, Cornes JS, Gough KR, McCarthy CF, Read AE. Steatorrhea and malignant lymphoma. The relationship of malignant tumors of lymphoid tissue and celiac disease. *Am J Dig Dis* 1967;12:475–90.

135 Whitehead R. Primary lymphadenopathy complicating idiopathic steatorrhoea. *Gut* 1968;9:569–75.

136 Barry RE, Read AE. Coeliac disease and malignancy. *Q J Med* 1973;42:665–75.

137 O'Farrelly C, Feighery C, O'Briain DS *et al.* Humoral response to wheat protein in patients with coeliac disease and enteropathy associated T cell lymphoma. *Br Med J* 1986;293:908–10.

138 Barry RE, Morris JS, Kenwright S, Read AE. Coeliac disease and malignancy. The possible importance of familial involvement. *Scand J Gastroenterol* 1971;6:205–7.

139 Cooper BT, Holmes GKT, Cooke WT. Coeliac disease and immunological disorders. *Br Med J* 1978;1:537–9.

140 Mulder CJJ, Tytgat GNJ. Coeliac disease and related disorders. *Neth J Med* 1987;31:286–99.

141 Polanco I, Prieto G, Lama RT, Carrasco S, Codoceo R, Larrauri J. Associated diseases in children with coeliac disease. In: Mearin ML, Mulder CJJ, eds. *Coeliac Disease. 40 Years Gluten-Free.* Dordrecht: Kluwer Acad Press, 1991:123–9.

142 Corazza GR, Frisoni M, Treggiari EA, Valentini RA, Filipponi C, Gasbarrini G. Clinical features of adult coeliac disease in Italy. In: Mearin ML, Mulder CJJ, eds. *Coeliac Disease. 40 Years Gluten-Free.* Dordrecht: Kluwer Acad Press, 1991:117–21.

143 Reunala T, Kosnai I, Karpati S, Kuitunen P, Torok E, Savilahti E. Dermatitis herpetiformis: jejunal findings and skin response to gluten free diet. *Arch Dis Child* 1984;59:517–22.

144 Cacciari E, Salardi S, Volta U *et al.* Prevalence and characteristics of coeliac disease in type 1 diabetes mellitus. *Acta Paediatr Scand* 1987;76:671–2.

145 Chambers TL. Coexistent coeliac disease, diabetes mellitus and hyperthyroidism. *Arch Dis Child* 1975;50:162–4.

146 Ruch W, Schurrann K, Gordon P, Bürgin-Wolff A, Girard J. Coexistent coeliac disease, Graves disease and diabetes mellitus type-I in a patient with Down syndrome. *Eur J Pediatr* 1985;144:89–90.

147 Maggiore G, De Giacomo C, Scotta MS, Sessa F. Celiac disease presenting as chronic hepatitis in a girl. *J Pediatr Gastroenterol Nutr* 1986;5:501–3.

148 Gentil-Kocher S, Bernard O, Brunelle F *et al.* Budd–Chiari syndrome in children: report of 22 cases. *J Pediatr* 1988;113:30–8.

149 Reading R, Watson JG, Platt JW, Bird AG. Pulmonary haemosiderosis and gluten. *Arch Dis Child* 1987;62:513–15.

150 Amil Dias J, Walker-Smith JA. Down's syndrome and coeliac disease. *J Pediatr Gastroenterol Nutr* 1990;10:41–3.

151 Goodchild MC, Nelson R, Anderson CM. Cystic fibrosis and coeliac disease: coexistence in two children. *Arch Dis Child* 1973;48:684–91.

152 Valletta EA, Mastella G. Incidence of celiac disease in a cystic fibrosis population. *Acta Paediatr Scand* 1989;78:784–5.

153 Verkasalo M, Tiilikainen A, Kuitunen P, Savilahti E, Backman A. HLA antigens and atopy in children with coeliac disease. *Gut* 1983;24:306–10.

154 Greco L, De Seta L, D'Adamo G *et al.* Atopy and coeliac disease: bias or true relation? *Acta Paediatr Scand* 1990;79:670–4.

155 Kitis G, Holmes GKT, Cooper BT, Thompson H, Allan RN. Association of coeliac disease and inflammatory bowel disease. *Gut* 1980;21:636–41.

156 Iliffe GD, Owen DA. An association between primary biliary cirrhosis and jejunal villous atrophy resembling celiac disease. *Dig Dis Sci* 1979;24:802–6.

157 Bouma ME, Beucler I, Aggerbeck LP, Infante R, Schmitz J. Hypobetalipoproteinemia with accumulation of an apoprotein B-like protein in intestinal cells. *J Clin Invest* 1986;78:398–410.

158 Welsh JD, Poley JR, Hensley J, Bhatia M. Intestinal disaccharidase and alkaline phosphatase activity in giardiasis. *J Pediatr Gastroenterol Nutr* 1984;3:37–40.

159 Schmitz J. Protein-losing enteropathies. In: Milla PJ, Muller DPR, eds. *Harries Paediatric Gastroenterology.* Edinburgh: Churchill Livingstone, 1988:260–71.

160 Cuenod B, Brousse N, Goulet O *et al.* Classification of intractable diarrhea in infancy using clinical and immunohistological criteria. *Gastroenterology* 1990;99:1037–43.

161 Mirakian R, Richardson A, Milla PJ *et al.*

Protracted diarrhoea of infancy: evidence in support of an autoimmune variant. *Br Med J* 1986;293:1132–6.
162 Visakorpi JK, Immonen P. Intolerance to cow's milk and wheat gluten in the primary malabsorption syndrome in infancy. *Acta Paediatr Scand* 1967;56:49–56.
163 Walker-Smith JA. Food sensitive enteropathies. *Clin Gastroenterol* 1986;15:55–69.
164 Vitoria JC, Camarero C, Sojo A, Ruiz A, Rodriguez-Soriano J. Enteropathy related to fish, rice, and chicken. *Arch Dis Child* 1982;57:44–8.
165 Perkkiö M, Savilahti E, Kuitunen P. Morphometric and immunohistochemical study of jejunal biopsies from children with intestinal soy allergy. *Eur J Pediatr* 1981;137:63–9.
166 Iyngkaran N, Abidin Z, Lai Meng L, Yadav M. Egg-protein-induced villous atrophy. *J Pediatr Gastroenterol Nutr* 1982;1:29–33.
167 Watt J, Pincott JR, Harries JT. Combined cow's milk protein and gluten-induced enteropathy: common or rare? *Gut* 1983;24:165–70.
168 Walker-Smith JA. Transient gluten intolerance. *Arch Dis Child* 1970;45:523–6.
169 McNeish AS, Harms HK, Rey J, Shmerling DH, Visakorpi JK, Walker-Smith JA. The diagnosis of coeliac disease. A commentary on the current practices of members of the European Society for Paediatric Gastroenterology and Nutrition (ESPGAN). *Arch Dis Child* 1979;54:783–6.
170 McNeish AS, Rolles CJ, Arthur LJH. Criteria for diagnosis of temporary gluten intolerance. *Arch Dis Child* 1976;51:275–8.
171 Verkasalo M, Kuitunen P, Tiilikainen A, Savilahti E. HLA antigens in intestinal cow's milk allergy. *Acta Paediatr Scand* 1983;72:19–22.
172 Dissanayake AS, Truelove SC, Whitehead R. Lack of harmful effect of oats on small intestinal mucosa in coeliac disease. *Br Med J* 1974;4:189–91.
173 Holmes GKT, Prior P, Lane MR, Pope D, Allan RN. Malignancy in coeliac disease — effect of a gluten free diet. *Gut* 1989;30:333–8.
174 Stählberg MR, Savilahti E, Siimes MA. Iron deficiency is coeliac disease is mild and it is detected and corrected by gluten-free diet. *Acta Paediatr Scand* 1991;80:190–3.

Chapter 3/Coeliac disease in adults

PETER D. HOWDLE AND MONTY S. LOSOWSKY

Clinical aspects

Definition

Aetiologically, coeliac disease (CD) can be defined as that condition in which an abnormality of the small intestinal mucosa is caused by gluten. In this context, 'gluten' collectively refers to prolamins of wheat, rye, barley and oats.

Diagnostically, there is universal agreement that a mucosal abnormality must be demonstrable in CD while proof of its aetiological relationship to gluten must, logically, require evidence of improvement in that mucosal abnormality with a gluten-free diet. In certain circumstances a gluten challenge may also be necessary to confirm the diagnosis.

Background to the disease

The clinical manifestations of CD are protean and no single group of symptoms or signs can be regarded as characteristic [1–5]. The wide variety of presentations frequently contributes to delay in diagnosis [2], although nearly one-third of adult patients, on close investigation, give a history of illness in childhood [2,3] including failure to thrive after weaning, gastrointestinal symptoms, especially diarrhoea, prolonged periods of ill-health or failure to achieve normal height and weight. The latter should always alert the clinician to the possibility of underlying gluten sensitivity.

Although Gee's account detailed many of the 'classic' features that are regarded as synonymous with CD [6], it has become evident that presentation is now often concerned with minor, or non-specific complaints or, alternatively, involves an apparently normal person found, on routine screening, to have haematological or biochemical abnormalities consistent with the disorder [7,8]. Others may present, or be discovered through screening of a family in whom a coeliac patient has recently been diagnosed, or is known to be present. In addition, the increased availability of endoscopy has contributed to the diagnosis, either by virtue of the larger number of mucosal specimens generated and submitted to routine histology, or specifically through the recognition of loss of duodenal folds [9].

Despite 25–30% of adult patients giving a history of childhood disorders [2,3], the wide variety of modes of presentation is often the reason [2,10] for delayed diagnosis or misdiagnosis which, initially, is said to be as high as 60%. Indeed, a feature repeatedly stressed by individuals in this category is the chronicity of vague ill-health and their resignation in accepting this state of affairs as normal [11]. Conversely, once success in treatment has been achieved, these patients are invariably astonished by their remarkable improvement in well-being. The condition is also characterized by periods of exacerbation and remission [6,12], and it is particularly noteworthy that teenage coeliac patients frequently experience remission even while taking a normal diet [2,13].

Presenting features

Adult patients can present at any age, although there appears to be a bimodal peak, comprising women (fourth to fifth decades) and men (fifth to sixth decades) (Fig. 3.1) [7]. The age of onset of symptoms bears

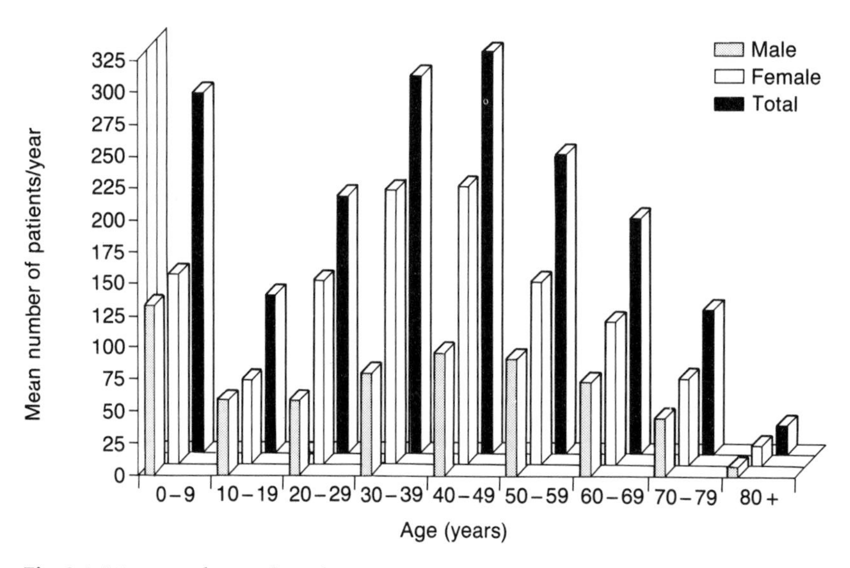

Fig. 3.1 Mean yearly number of new patients joining the Coeliac Society of the UK between 1980 and 1990 in different age groups. The age incidence shows two peaks: in childhood and in adult life. The sex incidence is equal in childhood, but more adult females join the Society than males (2 : 1) thus, perhaps reflecting the sex incidence in adults. The age distribution of the sexes shows a bimodal distribution in adults, suggesting females present a decade earlier than males, although this may reflect varying patterns of joining the Coeliac Society. (From the Coeliac Society of the UK.)

little relationship to the time at which the patient presents, or is diagnosed. In general, patients present either with: (1) constitutional symptoms; (2) gastrointestinal complaints; or (3) metabolic, neurological, psychological or other disturbances [14] (see Table 3.1).

Lassitude, malaise or weakness are probably the commonest complaints [14], while the frequency of weight loss is more variable [2,3,5, 15]; nevertheless, a normal weight, or even obesity, does not contradict the diagnosis [12,15]. Occasionally, there is mild fever [5,12] although severe pyrexia suggests other associated diseases [16]. Low blood pressure [5,12,14,17] that is unrelated to the severity of illness, and occurring in the absence of anaemia or electrolyte disturbance, has been reported. The constellation of lassitude, skin pigmentation and hypotension might be mistaken for Addison's disease.

Diarrhoea is the commonest intestinal symptom of CD [3,18] and may be continuous, intermittent or even alternate with periods of constipation. The diarrhoea may be acute, although is usually mild, the patient passing pale, mushy or watery stools three to four times daily, accompanied by high smell and difficulty in flushing away.

Table 3.1 Presenting symptoms

General	Lassitude, malaise, weakness, weight loss
Gastrointestinal	Diarrhoea (± features of steatorrhoea) Anorexia Nausea and vomiting Flatulence and abdominal distension Abdominal pain Constipation Glossitis/aphthous ulcers
Metabolic	Features of anaemia Bleeding tendency Oedema Cramps/tetany Paraesthesiae Noctural diuresis
Musculoskeletal	Bone pain Rickets Proximal myopathy
Neuropsychiatric	Peripheral neuropathy Cerebrospinal degenerations Anxiety/depression
Reproductive	Menstrual irregularities Reduced fertility (male and female) Relapse associated with pregnancy
Skin	Variety of rashes Dermatitis herpetiformis

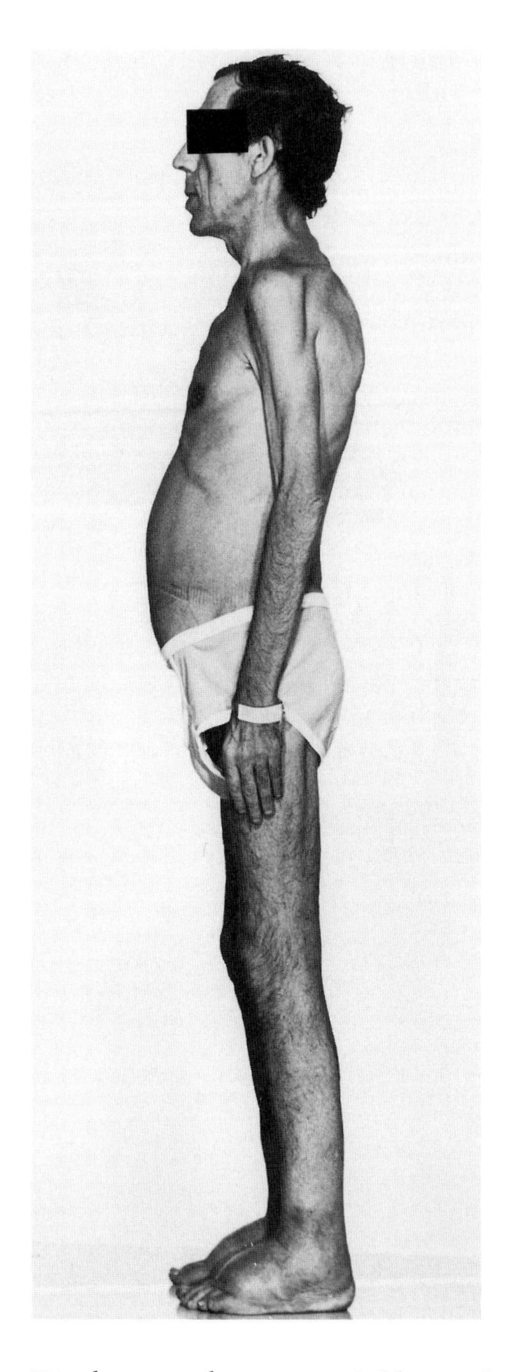

Fig. 3.2 An untreated coeliac patient showing abdominal distension and peripheral oedema.

Diarrhoea may be accompanied by weight loss, anorexia or abdominal distension [3,14] (Fig. 3.2) and even colicky-type pain [12]; nocturnal diarrhoea is also experienced [12,19]. Many authors, since Thaysen onwards [20], have noted that patients with longstanding disease learn to accept their disturbed bowel habit as 'normal'.

The presentation of severe obstructive-type abdominal pain and diarrhoea, even in a well-treated patient, suggests a complication of CD such as lymphoma, carcinoma or stricture and ulceration of the small intestine [16]. Such complications may also cause perforation or haemorrhage [21].

Nausea and vomiting, often related to periods of diarrhoea, may occur in approximately one-third of patients [2,14], while a similar proportion may complain of anorexia [3]. An excessive appetite, despite continued weight loss, has been described [22], thus resembling hyperthyroidism.

Abnormalities of the mouth and tongue, although varying in frequency in different series (10–90%) [2,5], comprise glossitis (a sore, red tongue) or angular stomatitis and are presumably the result of a nutritional deficiency, such as vitamin B, folate or iron. Other body surfaces may be simultaneously involved [14], resulting in perianal excoriation, soreness and even dyspareunia. A smooth, pale tongue, although uncommon in coeliac patients, indicates severe iron deficiency. Aphthous ulceration may also be the sole presenting feature of CD and may respond to treatment with a gluten-free diet [23,24], even without a demonstrable jejunal lesion [25]. However, this would not be the experience of most physicians with a large coeliac practice. There is considerable dispute concerning the incidence of jejunal abnormalities in patients with aphthous ulcers [24,26,27], although the true figure is probably less than 5%.

Anaemia is common in CD [2], although in approximately 50% [3] it does not produce major symptoms and is thus an incidental finding [7,8]. The anaemia is usually due to iron deficiency [2] which may be subclinical [3,28]; such anaemia, unresponsive to oral iron, is highly suggestive of gluten-induced malabsorption. A megaloblastic anaemia may predominate, since folate deficiency is almost universal in untreated CD [29] while vitamin B_{12} malabsorption, although sometimes detectable [30] is hardly ever severe enough to cause symptoms.

Up to one-third of patients [2,3] may present with spontaneous haemorrhage into skin and mucosae, or from bowel, kidney, joints or into deeper tissues [31,32]. This is usually due to vitamin K malabsorption, which may be acutely precipitated following antibiotic therapy. Interestingly, bleeding due to scurvy (vitamin C or ascorbic acid deficiency) is extremely rare [14].

Peripheral oedema is quite frequent, occurring in up to 30% of cases [3,5] and is most likely due to hypoproteinaemia, which might explain the ascites which rarely occurs [31] (Fig. 3.2).

Symptoms referable to the musculoskeletal system are common but are presenting features in only a minority of patients (10%). Others may complain of cramps or display spontaneous tetany. In general, symptoms of rickets or of osteomalacia are insidious in onset and are invariably quite severe before the medical attendant recognizes the true problem. Bone pain, paraesthesiae, latent tetany, proximal myopathy and weakness and pseudofractures are well-described [14,32,33]. In some patients, childhood rickets results in cessation of growth, dwarfism and limb deformities [34–36]. However, in the majority of adults there is no stunting of growth and height is normal or only slightly reduced [3,12].

There may be significant bone pain, which masquerades under such misdiagnoses as 'arthritis' or 'rheumatism'; percussion may reveal actual bone tenderness. The proximal myopathy (of vitamin D deficiency) leads to a waddling gait, difficulty in rising from a chair, climbing stairs, or raising the arms to brush the hair or open overhead cupboards (Fig. 3.3). An important point, made by Cooke and Holmes [14] is the frequent absence of diarrhoea or steatorrhoea in such patients, a point recently reinforced by Molteni *et al.* [37].

Neurological symptoms are not uncommon in patients with severe malabsorption [38,39], although some may be secondary to metabolic disturbances already discussed, such as hypocalcaemia, hypomagnesaemia, B_{12} deficiency, osteomalacia or osteoporosis [11]. In addition, however, evidence has accumulated to suggest that neurological complications may be seen in 5–8% of any larger series [14]; men appear to be involved more frequently than women.

The complaints, deriving from a peripheral neuropathy involving the legs, are numbness, tingling or unsteadiness. Arms are rarely involved, although occasionally fine movements of the hands and fingers may be jeopardized. Importantly, these symptoms may occur while the patient is already on treatment with a gluten-free diet [38]. Central nervous system abnormalities have also been reported in individuals

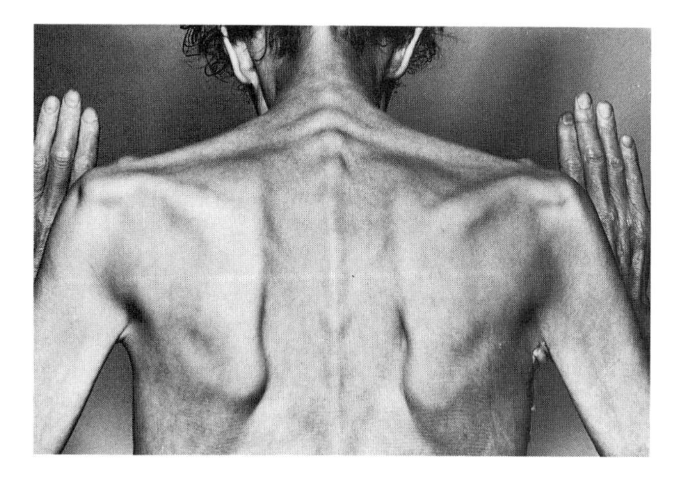

Fig. 3.3 An untreated coeliac patient with weight loss, muscle wasting and a proximal myopathy due to vitamin D deficiency.

or groups of coeliac patients, with involvement of the brain or spinal cord that is progressive and unresponsive to gluten restriction [14,38].

Psychological changes have also been widely investigated [14], but are difficult to quantify. Many patients appear to be depressed [40,41] while others are irritable, morose or difficult to relate to; organic dementia has been recorded but it is difficult to know whether it is a true association. Nevertheless, in some case reports, treatment with a gluten-free diet has resulted in spectacular improvements in mental function [14]. The association with psychoses, although intriguing, is far less certain [42,43].

A reversed diurnal rhythm leading to nocturnal diuresis is well-recognized in coeliac patients [44–46], and may be the complaint that brings them under medical investigation. Although there is delayed absorption of water by the damaged bowel [11] this is an insufficient explanation for the phenomenon, which readily responds to dietary treatment [14].

Disturbances in reproductive function are encountered both in male and female coeliac patients. Menarche may be delayed, menopause advanced, menstrual irregularities present in severe cases and infertility experienced until gluten restriction commences [11,14,47]. It is also well-known that CD may manifest itself, or be subject to relapse, during pregnancy, associated with anaemia, diarrhoea, malnutrition or tetany [12]; this is likely to occur if prenatal care is not optimal. In men there may be tissue resistance to plasma testosterone [48]. Infertility, with oligospermia, may occur, which responds to a gluten-free diet [49].

It is evident that many clinicians have reported unusual complications associated with coeliac patients. In the majority, the association has probably occurred through chance, simply because CD is fairly common, and a life-long condition. Diagnosed patients are also followed-up in hospitals, so that the chances of a second diagnosis being made are increased. If any associations are significant they may be due, in part, to major histocompatibility complex (MHC) similarities, or an activated immune system.

Various pulmonary disorders have been linked to CD, including chronic bronchitis [50], fibrosing alveolitis [51], bird fancier's lung [52,53] and sarcoidosis [54,55], but the relationship is difficult to ascertain, while the effect of tobacco smoking confuses the issue [56].

There has been some considerable interest in the association with bird fancier's lung. Rather than developing antibodies to albumin as is usual in this disease, approximately 30% of coeliac patients have antibodies to avian β-globulin (compared with 1% controls) which probably represents an epiphenomenon. Thus, there is no known mechanism for this apparent association [57,58].

The coexistence of CD and insulin-dependent diabetes mellitus is well-known [15,59–61], but the expected increased incidence in coeliac families has not been identified [62,63]. Although both conditions share the human leucocyte antigen (HLA)-B8, DR3 haplotype, their close association has not yet been explained at the molecular level. On treatment with a gluten-free diet, the diabetes becomes more easily controlled, although insulin requirements may increase [62].

Involvement of the liver is occasionally seen in coeliac patients [12,64–70]. Often there are disturbances of 'liver function tests' [14] which invariably improve spontaneously following gluten restriction [71]. Primary biliary cirrhosis does appear to enjoy a specific relationship to CD [67,72] and probably occurs more often than by chance alone.

Reported associations with thyroid disease continue to appear, such as with hyperthyroidism, myxoedema [14] and non-toxic goitre [12]. Although individual case reports, some bringing in other autoimmune diseases [73], are frequently published, there is little to support an aetiological connection. Similarly, with inflammatory conditions including systemic lupus erythematosus (SLE) [74,75], polymyositis [76], Sjögren's syndrome [77,78] and rheumatoid arthritis, the association could be coincidental. However, the postulated familial relationship between gluten sensitivity and ulcerative colitis [79] invites further study. The association with inflammatory bowel disease is certainly well-described [80–83].

Physical appearances

While some patients may be of short stature, or look thin, weak and wasted, the majority of untreated coeliac patients currently diagnosed are often surprisingly unremarkable in general appearance. It has been said that females have a round, plump face with prominent zygomatic arches [5,33], while males have triangular faces with a widened forehead and narrow jaw [5]. The hair may be fine, with scanty beard and axillary hair; premature greying may occur but baldness is rare [5,14]. There may be a variety of skin lesions and pigmentation [4,11,84,85]. There is no evidence [86,87] that atrophy of dermal ridges [88,89] ('finger-prints') is specific [14] for CD. Brittle nails and koilonychia suggest iron deficiency. Clubbing is seen in about one-fifth of patients [3,5,12] (Fig. 3.4) but may respond to treatment [14]. Abnormalities of the mouth and tongue are common, as described above.

Some of the major presenting features are given in Table 3.2. Note that limb oedema may suggest hypoproteinaemia; purpura or ecchymosesa prothrombin deficiency; and girdle weakness, proximal muscle wasting and a waddling gait, deficiency of vitamin D.

As suggested above, the majority of patients with CD probably now present with mild symptoms and signs, presumably due to earlier diagnosis. The presenting features have therefore been changing over the last four decades (Fig. 3.5).

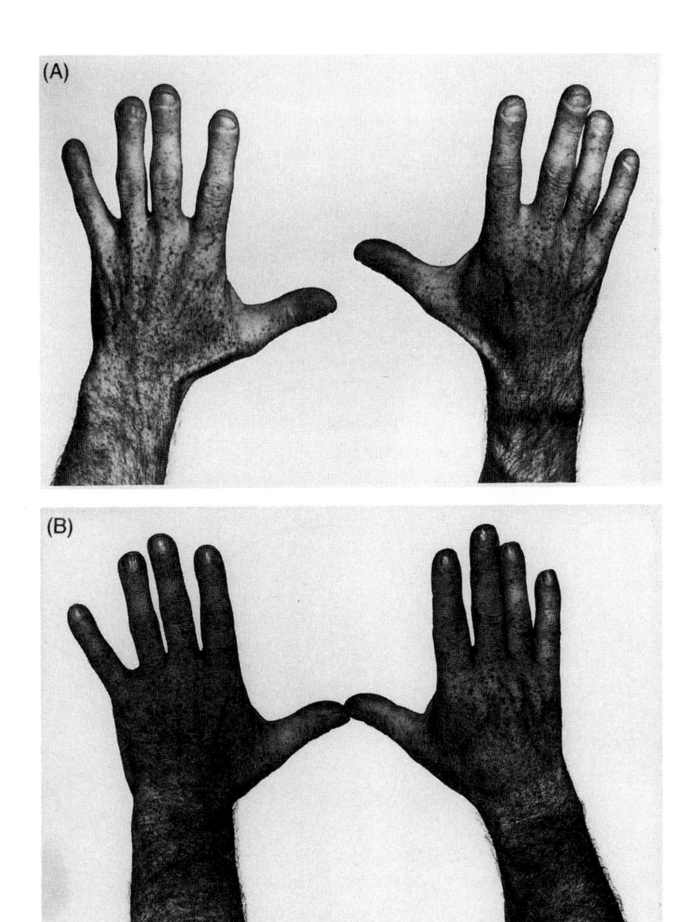

Fig. 3.4 (A) an untreated coeliac patient with finger clubbing and muscle wasting. (B) the same patient after 10 years on a gluten-free diet, showing modest improvement in the degree of clubbing.

Table 3.2 Major physical findings

General	Short stature, slight build, wasted, low blood pressure, mild fever
Skin	Pigmentation, scanty hair, bruising, petechiae, blisters, clubbing, koilonychia, oedema
Mouth	Glossitis, aphthous ulcers
Abdomen	Thin, distension, visible peristalsis
Musculoskeletal	Proximal muscle weakness and wasting, waddling gait, rickets, tetany, tender bones
Neuropsychiatric	Peripheral neuropathy, cerebrospinal signs, anxiety/depressive features

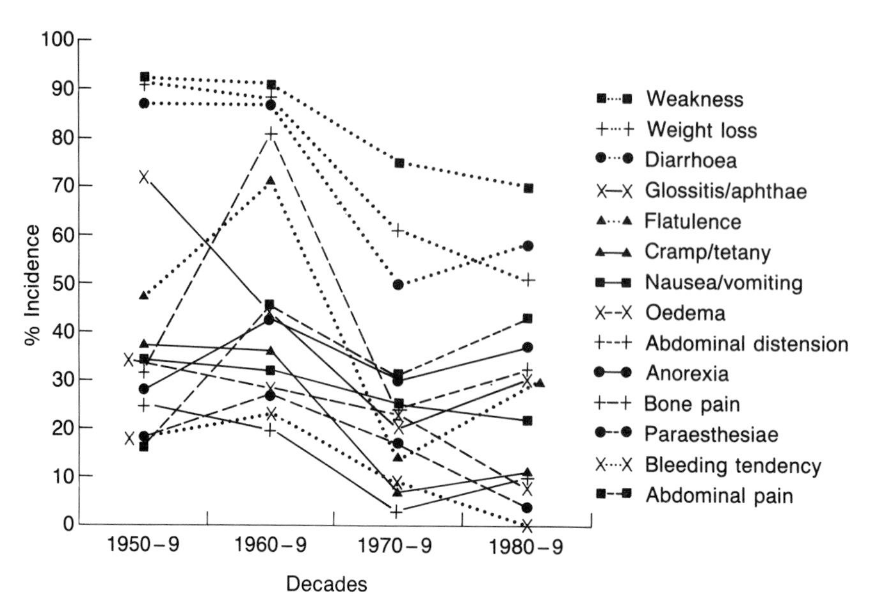

Fig. 3.5 The mean percentage incidence of symptoms and signs in coeliac patients at presentation over four decades. The major features of weakness, weight loss and diarrhoea, although still the most common, have decreased in incidence by 20–30%. Minor features of bone pain, bleeding tendency, paraesthesiae and oedema, which occur in severe disease, have decreased to less than 10% in incidence. (Data from [7,8,10,14,91].)

Diagnostic tests

Haematological investigations

Some haematological abnormality will almost invariably be present in an untreated coeliac patient [2], and in 50% will be responsible for symptoms of anaemia [3,29,90]. Since so many people have a blood test at some time during their lives, the diagnosis may be made, or suspicions raised, incidentally [7,8].

Iron deficiency is frequently seen (30–80%) [91] and may be the only abnormality demonstrable in an adult patient [2], although it may be subclinical [3,28]. Unresponsive iron deficiency should always raise the possibility of malabsorption and hence of a gluten-produced proximal mucosal abnormality at the site where iron is normally absorbed. Serum iron may be low due to impaired absorption and increased losses, especially from the high rate of enterocyte desquamation [92].

In 50% or more, a dimorphic picture is evident in the blood film, indicative of a combination of iron and folate deficiency. Folate deficiency is usual to some degree in all coeliac patients, and serum folate is markedly reduced in 60–80%, usually resulting in a megaloblastic bone marrow, and peripheral macrocytosis (mean corpuscular volume (MCV) >108 μm^3). Like iron, serum folate levels are low because absorption occurs predominantly in the upper jejunum [93]. Red cell folate, which is a measure of tissue folate stores, is also reduced in 80% of untreated patients. A low concentration of vitamin B_{12} is often present and may be <100 μg/ml in approximately 25% of patients. This is not due to mucosal disease affecting its absorptive site in the terminal ileum, but to some impairment of absorption [30], probably resulting from bacterial overgrowth [91]. It should be borne in mind, however, that severe folate deficiency causes a reduction in serum B_{12} concentration, the latter rising spontaneously on repletion of folate stores.

Splenic function may be variably impaired in approximately 20–80% of coeliac patients [94]. Typical changes on the blood film include Howell–Jolly bodies (nuclear remnants), acanthocytes, giant platelets and target cells, i.e. abnormal cellular remnants that physiologically would be rapidly cleared from the circulation in a normal person. Their persistence in coeliac patients, and presence in the blood film, indicate a severe degree of dysfunction, or atrophy of the spleen. In routine clinical practice, therefore, features of splenic atrophy are highly indicative of untreated gluten sensitivity. Their appearance on any 'casual' blood film should immediately alert the clinician to the underlying cause. Although iron deficiency, or folate deficiency, with or without the features of splenic atrophy, are the most important abnormalities suggested by a coeliac patient's blood film, other abnormalities may also be seen, such as thrombocytosis in about 50% [95], which is due partly to splenic dysfunction, and partly to the accompanying mucosal inflammatory reaction [96]. Some patients (approximately 10%) may have leucopaenia; lymphopaenia may also occur, although this is usually due to a redistribution of circulating T lymphocytes [97].

Tests of malabsorption

D-XYLOSE

This is an aldopentose not normally present in humans which has provided a means of testing small intestinal absorptive function by measuring urinary output after an oral dose (5 g or 25 g). Normally, at least 20% of the dose should appear in the urine within 6 hours of ingestion. In 80–100% of untreated coeliac patients, the 6-hour urinary excretion is likely to be markedly reduced [3,4,90,98]. The test is unreliable in the elderly because of reduced renal glomerular function [99].

The test enjoyed a popular vogue in screening children [100–102], but since the test lacks a high degree of sensitivity or specificity [103,104] its popularity has waned [105]. Nevertheless, it is an easy, non-invasive test that could be used sequentially in follow-up, or during a gluten challenge [106,107].

FAECAL FAT

Since approximately 70–100% [3,15] of patients have fat malabsorption, an increased mean faecal fat excretion (>6 g/day or 20 mmol/day) is useful in measuring the degree of intestinal dysfunction. It is an unpleasant test which is disliked by laboratories, so it is useless as a screening procedure although may be valuable for research purposes, or in monitoring the response to treatment.

Some indication, in the past, of vitamin stores was gained by estimating serum concentrations of vitamin A, carotene, vitamin D, vitamin E or prothrombin time (vitamin K) [91]. There is little indication for their measurement nowadays as a means of diagnosis.

SERUM ALBUMIN

A casual measurement of serum albumin concentration is a poor indicator of protein stores, or of protein synthesis. Note, however, that a persistently low albumin level (1) in an untreated coeliac may suggest a protein-losing enteropathy, and (2) in a well-treated patient may suggest the incipient development of intestinal lymphoma [3,16,108–110].

Immunological assays

ANTIGLIADIN ANTIBODIES

Apart from considerations of immunopathogenesis [111], there has been a continuing search for a simple serological test to help in the diagnosis and follow-up of coeliac patients. One of the major problems in the many studies published on circulating antigluten or antigliadin antibodies, both in adults and children [112–116] is the question of false negative and false positive results. However, in more recent studies in which the enzyme-linked immunoassay (ELISA) technique has been used [116–118], sensitivities and specificities just exceeding 90% have been achieved. Thus, testing for anti-α-gliadin (IgG) antibodies in the circulation seems to be, to date, the most stringent test available for screening and diagnosis. The highest antibody levels to α-gliadin are found in untreated subjects, and progressively fall during the early months of dietary gluten exclusion. This test is therefore helpful in following dietary compliance [117,119].

ANTICONNECTIVE TISSUE ANTIBODIES

Antibodies to reticulin were discovered in coeliac sera about 20 years ago [120,121] and initially were thought to be specific for gluten sensitivity until found in other conditions such as Crohn's disease [122,123]. Initial results comprised IgG antibody classes, but IgA type antibodies were subsequently found to be more specific [124,125]. 'Antireticulin' activity is ill-defined, but probably represents formation of antibodies to various connective tissue components of basal laminae and vascular basement membrane that are consequent upon severe mucosal damage [126].

Similarly, anti-endomysium antibodies (detected optimally on frozen monkey oesophagus) have been described, and probably bear some relationship to 'antireticulin' antibody [127]. That these antibodies are similarly dependent on tissue damage is shown by sensitivities or specificities approaching 100% in untreated coeliac and dermatitis herpetiformis patients with flat mucosae, decreasing with time during maintenance of a gluten-free diet [128].

It is unlikely that either antibody will play any major role in screening or diagnosis when compared with the specificity of anti-α-gliadin antibodies. This latter assay is now being increasingly performed in many major centres.

Tests of intestinal permeability

During the last few years, considerable interest has been shown in perturbations of intestinal permeability that occur in various enteropathies, including untreated CD. Such observations are based on the passage of various saccharides across the intestinal mucosa to appear in the urine. Paradoxically, untreated coeliac patients appear to show reduced permeation of small molecules (mannitol, rhamnose) and increased permeation of large molecules (lactulose, cellobiose). Tests based on urinary excretions of a pair of probes (mannitol : cellobiose), and expressed as a ratio, provide good discrimination between normal individuals, and those with mucosal disease including CD [129–131]. In this regard, the lactulose : mannitol test appears to have excellent screening value for suspected coeliac patients [132].

However, the success of these tests depends on severe mucosal damage, and they are much less useful in gluten-sensitive individuals with milder, or more subtle, mucosal lesions. Since, in the future, we will be more concerned with strategies to identify the undoubtedly large reservoir of 'latent' gluten-sensitive individuals, permeability tests with sugars, or ^{51}Cr-ethylenediamine tetra-acetic (EDTA) [133] are unlikely to fulfil this role. At the present time, therefore, there still appears to be no better substitute than to perform a jejunal biopsy.

Procedures for biopsy of the small intestine

As already suggested, it is necessary in the current state of knowledge to obtain a mucosal sample for diagnostic purposes. Since the disease is defined in morphological terms and in relation to whether the diet contains gluten or not, it is our view that tissue should be obtained on two occasions [134]. Mucosal appearances throughout the gluten-sensitive spectrum are detailed elsewhere in this volume (see Chapter 6).

Several capsules for obtaining peroral specimens of either distal duodenal or jejunal mucosa have been developed over the years [135–138] (Figs 3.6, 3.7). With the advent of modern, wide-channel fibreoptic endoscopes, however, it has become much easier to obtain biopsies from the proximal to mid-duodenum, and several studies suggest that CD can be reliably diagnosed in this way [139–142]. The problem of other disease states arises, particularly that of duodenitis, and whether such samples are always totally reliable. There is also a problem with the correct orientation of the mucosa with such small fragments [143] and this is another drawback to endoscopic biopsies. There can be no question that if the diagnosis is in doubt, a proper biopsy specimen of upper jejunum should be obtained with the correct instrument.

One further problem that creates confusion is related to sampling variations. Although in the majority of patients a diffuse abnormality of the upper jejunum is the norm, as originally described by Rubin *et al.* [144], there is convincing evidence that the severity of the mucosal lesions can vary, by one grade of abnormality, in about 10–20% of individuals sampled at the same time and in the same area

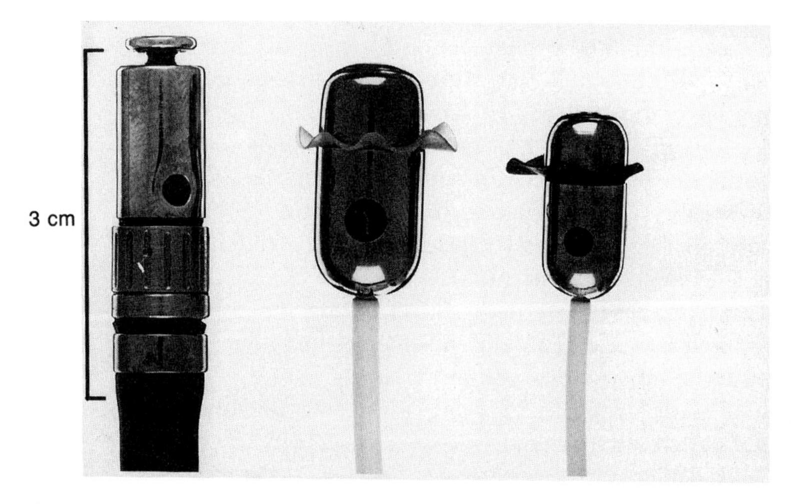

Fig. 3.6 Peroral intestinal biopsy capsules. Left to right: Quinton multiple hydraulic suction capsule, adult Crosby capsule and paediatric Crosby capsule.

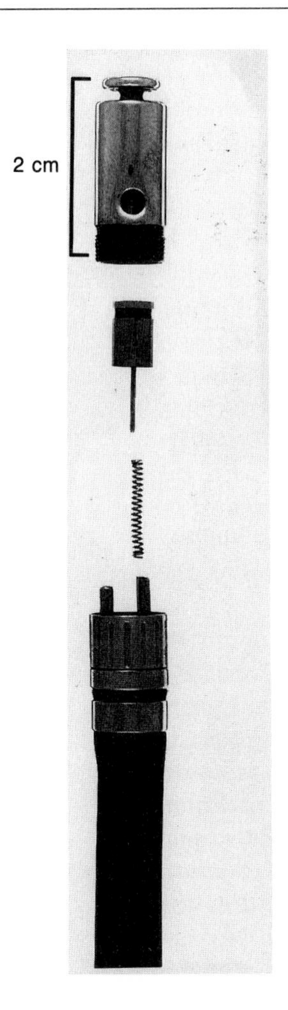

Fig. 3.7 An expanded view of the Quinton multiple hydraulic biopsy capsule, showing the circular blade and return spring. Biopsies are returned up the channel, the capsule remaining *in situ* in order to obtain further biopsies.

of the jejunum. These observations again suggest that if there is initial doubt, a further biopsy should be obtained [145,146]. It is also now becoming clear that in some patients taking a normal, gluten-containing diet, only a mild mucosal abnormality may be present [147].

If the mucosa fails to improve after gluten withdrawal then, by definition, CD cannot be diagnosed. Nevertheless, it has to be recognized that in many instances 'unresponsiveness', in terms of observed mucosal regeneration, is a secondary and often reversible phenomenon due either to: (1) the stage of the disease; (2) some other complication; or (3) the presence of some coexistent condition [148] such as chronic exocrine pancreatitis. Unresponsiveness of this kind (see p. 68) may occur in 20% patients [149] but, in our experience, is nearer 8% [150].

Another problem to confront the specialist is how to deal with patients who are taking a gluten-free diet and yet have never had an adequate pre-treatment biopsy. Thus, any subsequent biopsy will be uninterpretable and incapable of providing an incisive diagnosis. It is amazing that this state of affairs still exists, despite the voluminous literature regarding the proper diagnosis of CD! In these circumstances, a gluten challenge is mandatory.

Gluten challenge

Unfortunately, there is no universally applicable procedure for gluten challenge. The dose, and duration of challenge, have varied between different observers. Pollock *et al.* [151] added 30 g gluten each day to a gluten-free diet, or alternatively used a 'normal' gluten-containing diet. Schenk and Samloff [152] gave 10 g of gluten three times a day in addition to a gluten-containing diet; Bayless *et al.* [153] added the same amount of gluten to a gluten-free diet for 7 days. Weinstein [154] gave at least 20 g gluten per day for up to 30 weeks and induced morphological changes in patients with dermatitis herpetiformis and minimal jejunal lesions.

An average slice of bread contains approximately 1 g of gluten. The normal intake of gluten per day in the UK varies between 7 and 20 g [155,156]. In practice we ask patients to return to a normal gluten-containing diet, and ensure that they consume reasonable amounts of bread and other wheat-containing products. In some patients mucosal relapse occurs within days, but usually after a few weeks, and occasionally, only after many months [157]. In children it may take several years after commencement of a normal diet for a clinical relapse to occur [158,159]. In adults who have returned to a normal diet a biopsy should be obtained if they become symptomatic, otherwise biopsies should be repeated at 3, 6, 12 and 18 months. This implies that: (1) only a proportion of patients develop symptoms; (2) that mucosal changes occur in asymptomatic patients; and (3) that mucosal changes may be delayed for many months [157,160–162].

Many practitioners believe it is important that patients who have shown clinical and jejunal mucosal improvement on a gluten-free diet should be challenged with gluten to confirm the diagnosis, particularly with children [163,164] since coexisting and reversible causes of mucosal abnormality, such as cow's milk protein sensitivity and post-infectious enteropathy, are more likely to confuse the situation. Not all paediatricians adhere to such guidelines, which have recently been challenged [165]. With adults, there has been far less uniformity of approach, with some physicians believing that gluten challenge is necessary in order to correctly define the disorder [166], while others suggest that an initial flat jejunal mucosa without evidence of response may be diagnostically sufficient [167]. Scott and Losowsky [134] arrived at the compromise of requiring mucosal improvement following gluten exclusion, with gluten challenge only in difficult or borderline cases.

Recently, Loft *et al.* [168] have suggested a rectal challenge with gluten which will reveal mucosal changes diagnostic of CD. This approach clearly needs further confirmation.

Management of coeliac patients

The gluten-free diet

The cornerstone of the treatment of CD is life-long adherence to a gluten-free diet. Other treatment may be necessary in severely symptomatic patients (Fig. 3.8). For example, nutritional deficiencies (such as iron, folate and vitamin D) should be replaced and, if necessary, fluid and electrolytes repleted. In severely ill patients, parenteral nutrition may also be necessary. Patients should omit foods containing wheat, rye, barley or oats. There is some contention about oats, but their omission is recommended by the Coeliac Society of Great Britain [169].

Several immunological assays have recently been introduced to assess the gluten content of food as an aid to helping coeliac patients maintain their diet. None of these, however, is reliable for routine use [170].

The recommendation of a gluten-free diet for life has widespread implications, particularly for teenage patients who are often resentful of the limitations of the diet. This attitude is reinforced by the fact that teenagers and young adults often remain clinically well if they do stray from their diet, even though the small intestinal mucosa may show moderate abnormalities [13]. Every effort should be made to maintain contact with this age group, since some may have less than excellent health and may even not achieve their full physical and intellectual development [171–173]. In recent years some workers have suggested a much more liberal approach to teenage coeliac patients, perhaps based on pragmatism, since it is believed many youngsters do not maintain a strict gluten-free diet [174]. The majority of clinicians still recommend strict gluten withdrawal, not only in the belief that optimal health can be best maintained in this way, but also because evidence is now accumulating that malignancy in CD can be reduced by strict adherence to a gluten-free diet [175]. Such considerations raise the question of whether it is important to assess the strictness of the diet, which is difficult and requires the help of an experienced dietician. It has been demonstrated, however, that the degree of adherence assessed in such a way does relate to the degree of improvement in the small intestinal mucosa [18]. As already suggested, it is possible for some patients to consume gluten and remain clinically well; others, however, find they have to adhere strictly to their diet, even to the extent of avoiding communion wafers [176,177]. There is

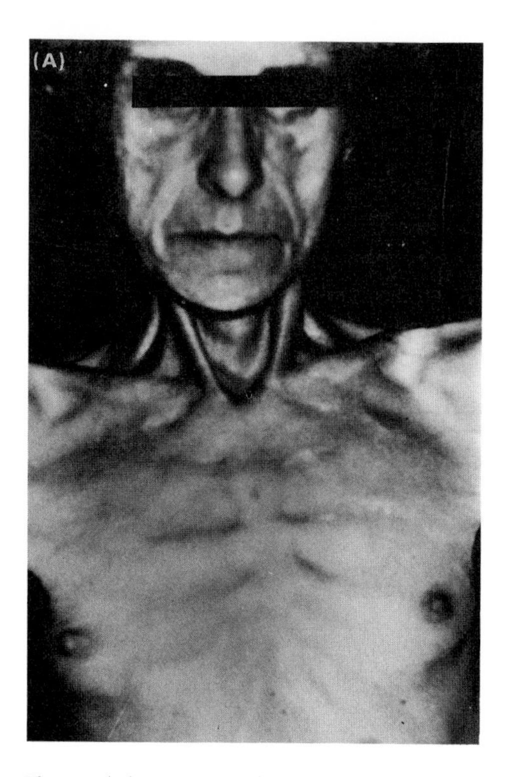

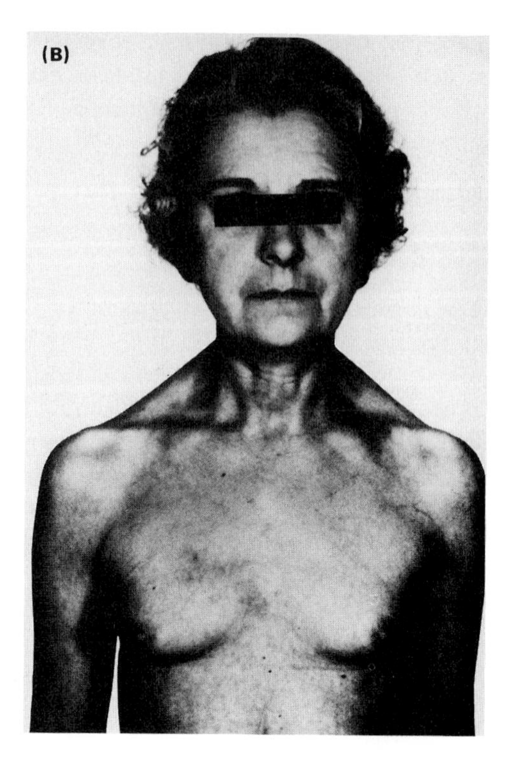

Fig. 3.8 (A) an untreated coeliac patient presenting with weakness, weight loss, diarrhoea and severe electrolyte disturbance. (B) the same patient after 6 months treatment with a gluten-free diet. (From Losowsky, *et al.* [11] with permission of Churchill Livingstone.)

no way of predicting how sensitive patients will be to small amounts of gluten.

If patients are to adhere to a gluten-free diet, they need help from a dietician and we advise them to join the Coeliac Society which publishes a handbook and up-to-date lists of gluten-free products. Some patients do have problems once dietary treatment has started. Initially, some put on weight, presumably as a result of their improved absorption. These patients need advice about weight reduction. It should be noted that in this situation diabetes may be unmasked, so the urine should be checked for sugar.

Constipation sometimes becomes a problem for other coeliac patients and reflects the fact that the bran from most cereals is omitted from the diet. Defatted rice bran or soya bran has been shown to help [178] and we also recommend bulking agents, such as ispaghula husk or methyl cellulose. It should also be noted that for some patients a gluten-free diet causes considerable confusion and fear of eating anything. These patients often, therefore, lose weight. It should be the task of the dietician to be satisfied that food intake is adequate and that only the right type of food is ingested. In order to help such patients, a positive approach should be employed to encourage them to build up a diet around fresh meat, vegetables, fish and fruit, and gradually to add other safe foods, using their Coeliac Society list. With care, this difficulty can gently be overcome.

Follow-up

We believe that coeliac patients should receive life-long follow-up and that it is important to observe the return to normal, or near normal, mucosal morphology during treatment. There is no evidence that subjective assessment of histology is any worse than the various methods of measurement [179]. Scanning electron microscopy may, however, show earlier improvement than gross villous changes [180], although access to such a machine may be limited.

In assessing morphological response, there are points for discussion. There is no agreement as to the time for a response to occur, nor to which features should be assessed. Epithelial cell improvement can occur very quickly, in 6–10 days [181], but other features such as an increase in villous height or decrease in crypt depth can take months or even years [182,183]. As to the degree of mucosal recovery, not all patients show a return to normal [18,148,181].

Some physicians place great reliance on a clinical response and while clinical and morphological responses can occur in parallel, there are well-documented cases where clinical improvement has occurred without morphological change [148,184,185]. Other means of assessing response include a decrease in intestinal permeability, maintenance of serum folate and iron levels, or reduction in α-gliadin antibody levels. None, however, reflects exactly morphological regeneration and we do not recommend any as the sole means of response to dietary exclusion.

The mucosa can also be assessed by criteria other than architectural features. Disaccharidase levels return to normal with treatment [18] and this occurs early [186] although lactase levels often remain low, even when morphological improvement has occurred [187].

There are many studies of immunological changes in the mucosa in CD both in the epithelium [188–191] and in the lamina propria [185,192]. Such changes almost always revert to normal, or near normal, on successful treatment and could, therefore, be used to assess mucosal response. Furthermore, intraepithelial lymphocyte numbers increase as an early and sensitive indicator of increasing gluten intake [193–195].

The final problem in follow-up is how often patients should be seen in the clinic. We believe that patients should be followed up for life. There are no guidelines as to whether or when further mucosal biopsies should be obtained. Some physicians do so only when there is a change in the patient's condition, perhaps a recurrence of diarrhoea or weight loss, or a nutritional deficiency. Others feel that regular biopsies, perhaps every few years, should be performed. The latter has been our practice. We believe this policy has demonstrated its value in detecting inadvertent non-compliance in individual patients and helps to motivate patients to maintain a strict diet.

Failure to respond to a gluten-free diet

Before accepting failure to respond, it should be realized that response may be delayed, even up to years, particularly if the diagnosis is made in adult life [183].

'Unresponsiveness' may manifest itself from the outset or later in the course of the disease. Particularly in the former situation, diagnostic questions are raised because, if the mucosa shows no response, the diagnosis by definition is not CD. Although in this situation one should always consider other, rarer, causes of a flat jejunal mucosa (Table 3.3) [196–216], many apparently unresponsive individuals do have a previous history of possible childhood disease, a positive family history, a typical HLA phenotype, or evidence on the blood film of hyposplenism, and it is difficult to deny these associations with CD [166].

There are several possibilities as to the cause of unresponsiveness, but by far the most common cause is inadequate dietary gluten exclusion. This may be conscious or inadvertent. The initial step is to assess dietary compliance. This requires the help of a well-informed dietician who carefully reviews the patient's diet. Even if patients intentionally ingest gluten, the act of reassessing the diet usually results in an improvement.

Other dietary factors may have to be considered. Cooke and Holmes [14] described a patient in whom a normal mucosa was achieved only after exclusion of milk and gluten. Secondary lactase deficiency has already been referred to and the omission of lactose in a milk-free diet provides symptomatic recovery in some patients, although clinical lactose intolerance is not common in CD [217].

Apart from milk, other food constituents have been reported to prevent mucosal recovery. Baker and Rosenberg [218] described a patient whose morphological improvement depended upon the exclusion of gluten, eggs, chicken and tuna. Mike and Asquith [219] described poorly responding coeliac patients who had a mucosal response on elimination of both gluten and soya.

Untreated coeliac patients are undoubtedly deficient in many nutritional factors [11]. There is very little evidence, however, that specific repletion of such deficiencies improves the response of the mucosa

Table 3.3 Causes of abnormal small intestinal mucosa, suggestive of CD

CD, including:
Non-responsive CD ('refractory' or 'collagenous sprue') [166,214–216]
Complications of CD (ulceration, malignancy) [196–201]
Cow's milk protein intolerance [202]
Soya protein intolerance [203]
Immunodeficiency syndromes [204]
Eosinophilic gastroenteropathy [205]
Immunoproliferative small intestinal disease (IPSID) [206]
Protein-energy malnutrition [207]
Intractable diarrhoea of infancy [208]
Gastroenteritis in children [209]
Infections:
Parasites, e.g. giardiasis [210]
Tuberculosis [211]
Human immunodeficiency virus [212]
Contaminated bowel syndrome [213]
Whipple's disease [214]
Tropical sprue [215]
Arterial disease of small intestine [216]
Drug and radiation damage [11]

beyond that produced by a gluten-free diet, even though many clinicians prescribe such supplements when initiating treatment. There is some evidence for the role of zinc in the treatment of non-responsive CD; Love *et al.* [220] reporting a dramatic clinical improvement in four of six patients, although jejunal mucosa was examined only in three of these. One patient also developed copper deficiency, suggesting that this and other trace elements may have some limited value in the treatment of CD, a suggestion supported by Goyens *et al.* [221].

Apart from attending to diet and nutritional supplementation, other manoeuvres must be considered in unresponsive patients. There is evidence that some untreated patients have bacterial overgrowth in the jejunum and that improvement occurs when the infection is treated with antibiotics [91,222]. In any unresponsive patient a trial of antibiotics would be reasonable, particularly if there was some evidence of bacterial overgrowth, or a possible additional reason for such contamination, such as jejunal diverticula or blind loops. Pancreatic insufficiency is another cause for treatment failure. Pink and Creamer [223] described a group of coeliac patients who failed to respond to gluten restriction and who showed evidence of pancreatic insufficiency. The pancreatic insufficiency seems to be secondary to the CD with impaired cholecystokinin–pancreozymin release from the abnormal mucosa leading to poor gall-bladder contraction and poor pancreatic secretion [224–226]. Pancreatic function usually improves on treatment of the CD [225,227] but if there is a poor response to gluten withdrawal, pancreatic supplements should be used in addition, particularly if tests of pancreatic function are abnormal [228,229].

More serious causes of unresponsiveness in CD are the ulceration–stricture sequence and malignancy. These specific complications are dealt with elsewhere in this volume (see Chapter 5).

The use of steroids

Steroids have been used in coeliac patients in whom response to a gluten-free diet is poor, or non-existent. Short-term mucosal and clinical improvement can be achieved with steroids, even without gluten restriction [230]; others have also confirmed this effect [14,231–233]. There are no long-term studies. Hamilton *et al.* [234] induced remission in a non-responsive coeliac patient with the use of steroids and azathioprine. Steroids may be used empirically in serious clinical situations where detailed assessment is not possible. Long-term steroids are, however, contraindicated if control can be achieved by other measures, in view of the risks of adrenal suppression and other complications such as osteoporosis and glucose intolerance.

Despite the known predisposing causes of unresponsiveness as outlined above, some cases fail to respond to all measures. Typical cases are described by Neale [235], Dowling and Henry [236] and van Tongeren *et al.* [237]. The symptomatology of these patients is very similar to that in CD, although abdominal pain, intestinal obstruction, finger clubbing and hypoalbuminaemia have been specifically noted. Booth [166] suggested these are coeliac patients in whom jejunal mucosal abnormalities have become irreversible. Before accepting this, however, it is necessary to work through all possible reasons for lack of response to a gluten-free diet and Fig. 3.9 shows a scheme for the follow-up of a patient with an abnormal intestinal mucosa and a presumptive diagnosis of CD.

Family counselling in CD

The tendency for CD to run in families has been recognized for many years. There are studies in which workers have investigated family members of coeliac patients by jejunal biopsy [238–243]. These show that the prevalence of severe mucosal abnormalities in first degree relatives is between 10.3 and 19.2%. In five of these six studies the range was 10.3–12.8%. Some of these individuals (approximately 50%) were asymptomatic. The mucosa in such subjects may respond to gluten withdrawal. With such studies there are, however, problems of interpretation since not all relatives undergo a small bowel biopsy and, in some, minor mucosal abnormalities are found which may or may not represent gluten sensitivity.

Coeliac patients or their relatives who seek advice should be informed of the risks of another member of the family being affected.

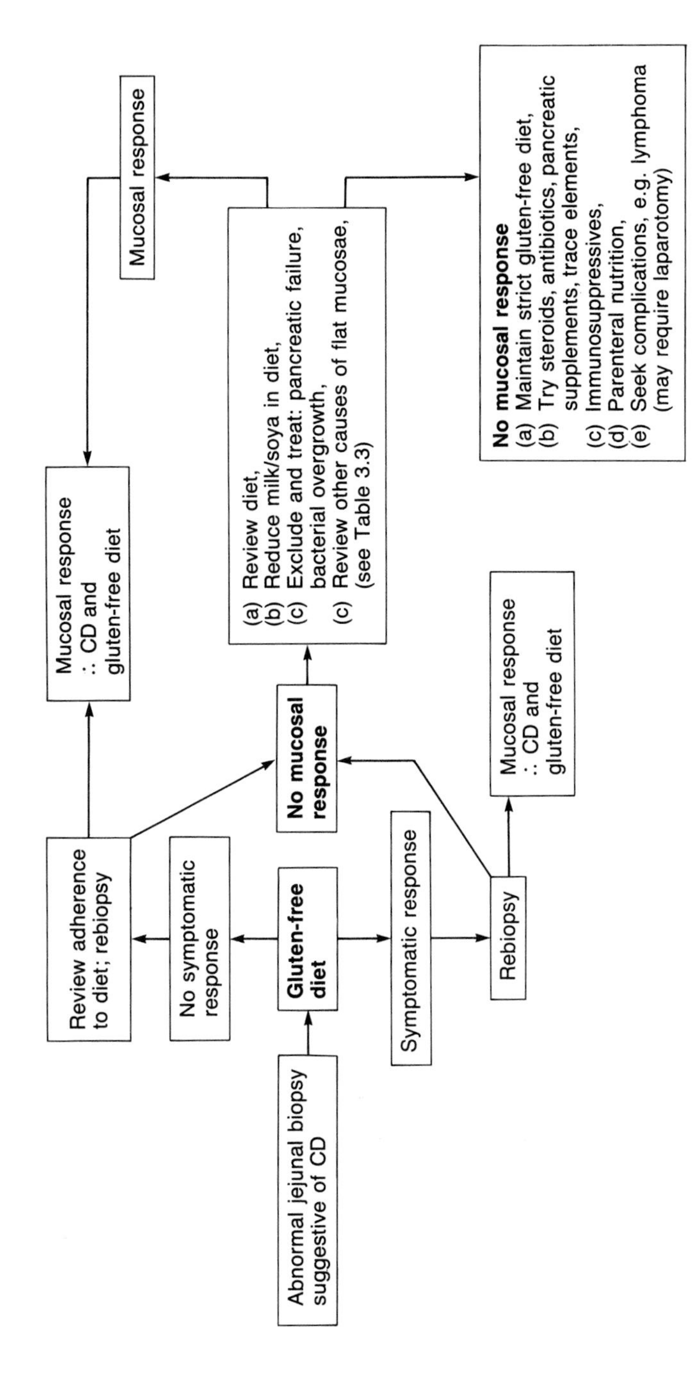

Fig. 3.9 A scheme for the management of a patient with an abnormal jejunal biopsy.

Symptomatic family members who present themselves for assessment should be investigated by small intestinal biopsy. In asymptomatic subjects, abnormalities in screening tests such as blood films, serum folate, antireticulin or antigliadin antibodies, or assessment of permeability may help to indicate the need for a biopsy. In view of the limitations of screening tests, however, there is a strong argument for small bowel biopsy being the primary investigation in family studies [240,241,244]. We recommend that the physician should perform a biopsy on all willing family members of coeliac patients. Indeed, such studies are more strongly indicated now that evidence is accumulating that treatment with a gluten-free diet does protect against malignancy [175]. Since so many relatives with presumptive CD are asymptomatic, a biopsy is vital in permitting assessment of jejunal morphology; if this is abnormal, a gluten-free diet should be recommended in the hope of preventing development of a malignancy in the longer term.

References

1 Losowsky MS. The protean clinical manifestations of coeliac disease. In: Ferguson A, ed. *Advanced Medicine 20*. London: Pitman, 1984:48–60.

2 Barry RE, Baker P, Read AE. The clinical presentation. *Clin Gastroenterol* 1974;3: 55–69.

3 Benson GD, Kowlessar OD, Sleisenger MH. Adult coeliac disease with emphasis upon response to the gluten free diet. *Medicine* 1964;43:1–40.

4 Brooks FP, Powell KC, Cerda JJ. Variable clinical course of adult coeliac disease. *Arch Intern Med* 1966;117:789–94.

5 Cooke WT, Peeney ALP, Hawkins CF. Symptoms, signs and diagnostic features of idiopathic steatorrhoea. *Q J Med* 1953;22: 59–77.

6 Gee S. On the coeliac affection. *St Bartholomew's Hosp Rep* 1888;24:17–20.

7 Swinson CM, Levi A. Is coeliac disease underdiagnosed? *Br Med J* 1980;281: 1258–60.

8 Logan RFA, Tucker G, Rifkind EA, Heading RC, Ferguson A. Changes in clinical features of coeliac disease in adults in Edinburgh and the Lothians 1960–79. *Br Med J* 1983; 1:95–7.

9 Corazza GR, Brocchi E, Caletti G, Gasbarrini G. Loss of duodenal folds allows diagnosis of unsuspected coeliac disease. *Gut* 1990;31:1080–1.

10 Dawson AM, Kumar PJ. Coeliac disease. In: Booth CC, Neale G, eds. *Disorders of the Small Intestine*. Oxford: Blackwell Scientific Publications, 1985:153–78.

11 Losowsky MS, Walker BE, Kelleher J. *Malabsorption in Clinical Practice*. Edinburgh: Churchill Livingstone, 1974.

12 Green PA, Wollaeger EE. The clinical behavior of sprue in the United States. *Gastroenterology* 1960;38:399–418.

13 Kumar PJ, Walker-Smith JA, Milla P, Harris G, Colyer J, Halliday R. The teenage coeliac: follow-up study of 102 patients. *Arch Dis Child* 1988;63:916–20.

14 Cooke WT, Holmes GKT. *Coeliac Disease*. Edinburgh: Churchill Livingstone, 1984.

15 Mann JG, Brown WR, Kern F. The subtle and variable clinical expressions of gluten-induced enteropathy (adult celiac disease, non-tropical sprue). *Am J Med* 1970;48: 357–66.

16 Cooper BT, Holmes GKT, Ferguson R, Cooke WT. Coeliac disease and malignancy. *Medicine (Baltimore)* 1980;59:249–61.

17 Salvesen HA. The blood pressure in idiopathic and symptomatic steatorrhoea. *Acta Med Scand* 1963;144:303–12.

18 Dissanayake AS, Truelove SC, Whitehead R. Jejunal mucosal recovery in coeliac disease in relation to the degree of adherence to a gluten-free diet. *Q J Med* 1974;43: 161–85.

19 Ross JR, Gibb SP, Hoffman DE, Stefanyk HN, Alvarez SZ. Systemic manifestations

of gluten enteropathy. *Med Clin North Am* 1966;50:515–27.

20 Thaysen TEH. *Non-Tropical Sprue*. London: Oxford University Press, 1932.

21 Finan PJ, Thompson MR. Surgical presentation of small bowel lymphoma in adult coeliac disease. *Postgrad Med J* 1980;56: 859–61.

22 Comfort MW. Non-tropical sprue: diagnosis and therapy. *Gastroenterology* 1958;34: 476–83.

23 Ferguson MM. Coeliac disease with recurrent aphthae. *Gut* 1980;21:223–6.

24 Ferguson R, Basu MK, Asquith P, Cooke WT. Jejunal mucosal abnormalities in patients with recurrent aphthous ulceration. *Br Med J* 1976;1:11–13.

25 Wright A, Ryan FP, Wilingham SE *et al.* Food allergy or intolerance in severe recurrent aphthous ulceration of the mouth. *Br Med J* 1986;292:1237–8

26 Challacombe SJ, Barkman P, Lehner T. Haematological features and differentiation of recurrent oral ulceration. *Br J Oral Surg* 1977;15:37–48.

27 Rose JDR, Smith DM, Allan FG, Sircus W. Recurrent aphthous ulceration and jejunal biopsy *Br Med J* 1978;1:1145.

28 Bonamico M, Vania A, Manti S *et al.* Iron deficiency in children with celiac disease. *J Pediatr Gastroenterol Nutr* 1987;6:702–6.

29 Hoffbrand AV. Anaemia in adult coeliac disease. *Clin Gastroenterol* 1974;3:71–89.

30 Stewart JS, Pollock DJ, Hoffbrand AV, Mollin DL, Booth CC. A study of proximal and distal intestinal structure and absorptive function in idiopathic steatorrhoea. *Q J Med* 1967;36:425–44.

31 Kowlessar OD, Phillips LD. Coeliac disease. *Med Clin North Am* 1970;54:647–56.

32 Badenoch J. Steatorrhoea in the adult. *Br Med J* 1960;2:879–87.

33 Bennett TI, Hunter D, Vaughan JM. Idiopathic steatorrhoea (Gee's disease). A nutritional disturbance associated with tetany, osteomalacia and anaemia. *Q J Med* 1932;1: 603–77.

34 McNicholl B. Childhood coeliac disease. *J Irish Med Assoc* 1970;63:1–7.

35 Visakorpi JK, Kuitunen P, Pelkonen P. Intestinal malabsorption: a clinical study of 22 children over 2 years of age. *Acta Paediatr Scand* 1970;59:273–80.

36 Hamilton JR, Lynch MJ, Reilly BJ. Active coeliac disease in childhood. Clinical and laboratory findings in 42 cases. *Q J Med* 1969;38:135–58.

37 Molteni N, Caraceni MP, Barbella MT, Ortolani S, Gandolini GG, Bianchi P. Bone mineral density in adult celiac patients and the effect of gluten-free diet from childhood. *Am J Gastroenterol* 1990;85:51–3.

38 Cooke WT, Smith WT. Neurological disorders associated with adult coeliac disease. *Brain* 1966;89:683–722.

39 Morris JS, Ajdukiewicz AB, Read AE. Neurological disorders and adult coeliac disease. *Gut* 1970;11:549–54.

40 Hallert C, Derefelt T. Psychic disturbances in adult coeliac disease. I. Clinical observations. *Scand J Gastroenterol* 1982;17: 17–19.

41 Hallert C, Astrom J. Psychic disturbances in adult coeliac disease. II. Psychological findings. *Scand J Gastroenterol* 1982;17: 21–4.

42 Dohan FC. Coeliac disease and schizophrenia. *Lancet* 1970;i:897–8.

43 Stevens FM, Lloyd RS, Geraghty SMH *et al.* Schizophrenia and coeliac disease — the nature of the relationship. *Psychol Med* 1977;7:259–63.

44 Wollaeger EE, Scribner BH. Delayed excretion of water with regular nocturnal diuresis in patients with non-tropical sprue (idiopathic steatorrhoea). *Gastroenterology* 1951;19:224–40.

45 Taylor WH. Water diuresis in idiopathic steatorrhoea. *Clin Sci* 1954;13:239–45.

46 Taylor WH. Water diuresis in idiopathic steatorrhoea. *Clin Sci* 1955;14:725–30.

47 Morris JS, Ajdukiewicz AB, Read AE. Coeliac infertility: an indication for dietary gluten restriction. *Lancet* 1970;i:213–14.

48 Green JRB, Goble HL, Edwards CRW, Dawson AM. Reversible insensitivity to androgens in men with untreated gluten enteropathy. *Lancet* 1977;i:280–2.

49 Baker PG, Read AE. Reversible infertility in male coeliac patients. *Br Med J* 1975;2: 316–17.

50 Cummiskey J, Keelan P, Weir DG. Coeliac disease and diffuse pulmonary disease. *Br Med J* 1976;1:1401.

51 Robinson TJ, Nelson SD, Haire M, Middleton D, McMillan SA, Evans JP. Jejunal villous changes associated with farmer's lung. *Postgrad Med J* 1981;57: 697–701.

52 Berrill WT, Eade OE, Fitzpatrick PF, Hyde I, Macleod WM, Wright R. Bird fancier's lung and jejunal villous atrophy. *Lancet* 1975;ii:

1006–8.
53 Faux JA, Hendrick DJ, Anand BS. Precipitins to different avian serum antigens in bird fancier's lung and coeliac disease. *Clin Allergy* 1978;8:101–8.
54 Karlish AJ. Coeliac disease and diffuse lung disease. *Lancet* 1971;i:1077.
55 Smith BDO. Sarcoidosis with recurrent thrombophlebitis and idiopathic steatorrhoea. *Proc R Soc Med* 1966;59:569–70.
56 Edwards C, Williams A, Asquith P. Bronchopulmonary disease in coeliac patients. *J Clin Pathol* 1985;38:361–7.
57 Hendrick DJ, Faux JA, Anand B, Piris J, Marshall R. Is bird fancier's lung associated with coeliac disease? *Thorax* 1978;33: 425–8.
58 Anon. Coeliac lung disease. *Lancet* 1978; i:917–18.
59 Walsh CH, Cooper BT, Wright AD, Malins JM, Cooke WT. Diabetes mellitus and coeliac disease: a clinical study. *Q J Med* 1978;47:89–100.
60 Cacciari E, Salardi S, Volta U *et al.* Prevalence and characteristics of coeliac disease in type 1 diabetes mellitus. *Acta Paediatr Scand* 1987;76:671–2.
61 Mäki M, Hällström O, Huupponen T, Vesikari Y, Visakorpi JK. Increased prevalence of coeliac disease in diabetes. *Arch Dis Child* 1984;59:739–42.
62 Stokes PL, Ferguson R, Holmes GKT, Cooke WT. Familial aspects of coeliac disease. *Q J Med* 1976;45:567–82.
63 Carter C, Sheldon W, Walker C. The inheritance of coeliac disease. *Ann Hum Genet* 1959;23:266–78.
64 Craxi A, Pinzello G, Oliva L, Pagliaro L. Primary biliary cirrhosis and coeliac disease. *Lancet* 1978;i:713–14.
65 Hagander B, Berg NO, Brandt L, Norden A, Sjolund D, Stenstam M. Hepatic injury in adult coeliac disease. *Lancet* 1977;i:270–2.
66 Lee FI, Murray SM, Norfolk D, Vasudev KS. Primary biliary cirrhosis and coeliac disease. *Lancet* 1978;i:713.
67 Logan RFA, Ferguson A, Finlayson NDC, Weir DG. Primary biliary cirrhosis and coeliac disease. An association? *Lancet* 1978;i:230–3.
68 Pollock DJ. The liver in coeliac disease. *Histopathology* 1977;1:421–30.
69 Swarbrick ET, Fairclough PD, Campbell PJ, Levison DA, Greenwood RH, Baker LRI. Coeliac disease, chronic active hepatitis and mesangiocapillary glomerulonephritis in the same patient. *Lancet* 1980;ii:1084–5.
70 Naschitz JE, Yeshurun D, Zuckerman E, Arad E, Boss JH. Massive hepatic steatosis complicating adult celiac disease: report of a case and review of the literature. *Am J Gastroenterol* 1987;82:1186–9.
71 Maggiore G, De Giacomo C, Scotta MS, Sessa F. Celiac disease presenting as chronic hepatitis in a girl. *J Pediatr Gastroenterol Nutr* 1986;5:501–3.
72 Behr W, Barnert J. Adult celiac disease and primary biliary cirrhosis. *Am J Gastroenterol* 1986;81:796–9.
73 Miller DG. Coeliac disease with autoimmune haemolytic anaemia. *Postgrad Med J* 1984;60:629–30.
74 Toivonen S, Pitkanen E, Siurala M. Collagen disease associated with intestinal malabsorption and sprue-like changes in the intestinal mucosa. *Acta Med Scand* 1964; 175:91–5.
75 Siurala M, Julkunen H, Toivonen S, Pelkonen R, Saxen E, Pitkanen E. Digestive tract in collagen diseases. *Acta Med Scand* 1965;178:13–25.
76 Henriksson KG, Hallert C, Walan A. Gluten-sensitive polymyositis and enteropathy. *Lancet* 1976;ii:317.
77 Pittman FE, Holub DA. Sjögren's syndrome and adult coeliac disease. *Gastroenterology* 1965;48:869–76.
78 MacLaurin BP, Matthews N, Kilpatrick JA. Coeliac disease associated with autoimmune thyroiditis, Sjögren's syndrome and a lympho-cytotoxic serum factor. *Aust NZ J Med* 1972;2:405–11.
79 Mayberry JF, Smart HL, Toghill PJ. Familial association between coeliac disease and ulcerative colitis: preliminary communication. *J R Soc Med* 1986;79:204–5.
80 Nugent FW, Gonyea RJ. Development of gluten enteropathy after ileostomy for ulcerative colitis. *Am J Digest Dis* 1968;13: 186–9.
81 Falchuk KR, Falchuk ZM. Selective immunoglobulin A deficiency, ulcerative colitis and gluten-sensitive enteropathy — a unique association. *Gastroenterology* 1975;69:503–6.
82 Kumar PJ, O'Donoghue DP, Gibson J, Stansfield A, Dawson AM. The existence of inflammatory bowel lesions in gluten-sensitive enteropathy. *Postgrad Med J* 1979;55:753–6.
83 Kitis G, Holmes GKT, Cooper BT, Thompson H, Allan RN. Association of

coeliac disease and inflammatory bowel disease. *Gut* 1980;2:636–41.
84 Shuster S, Watson AJ, Marks J. Coeliac syndrome in dermatitis herpetiformis. *Lancet* 1968;i:1101–6.
85 Marks J, Shuster S. Intestinal malabsorption and the skin. *Gut* 1971;12:938–47.
86 McCrae WM, Sandor G, Sangani AP, Stalker R. Finger print changes in coeliac disease. *Br Med J* 1971;3:109–10.
87 Mylotte MJ, Egan-Mitchell B, Fottrell PF, McNicholl B, McCarthy CF. Fingerprints in patients with coeliac disease and their relatives. *Br Med J* 1972;4:144–6.
88 David TJ, Ajdukiewicz AB, Read AE. Finger print changes in coeliac disease. *Br Med J* 1970;2:594–6.
89 David TJ, Ajdukiewicz AB, Read AE. Dermal and epidermal ridge atrophy in coeliac sprue. *Gastroenterology* 1973;64: 539–44.
90 Cooke WT, Fone DJ, Cox EV, Meynell MJ, Gaddie R. Adult coeliac disease. *Gut* 1963; 4:279–91.
91 Cluysenaer OJJ, van Tongeren JHM. *Malabsorption in Coeliac Sprue.* The Hague: Martinus Nijhoff, 1977.
92 Sutton DR, McLean Baird I, Stewart JS, Coghill NF. 'Free' iron loss in atrophic gastritis, post-gastrectomy states and adult coeliac disease. *Lancet* 1970;ii:387–91.
93 Hepner GW, Booth CC, Cowan J, Hoffbrand AV, Mollin DL. Absorption of crystalline folic acid in man. *Lancet* 1968;ii:302–6.
94 Corazza GR, Gasbarrini G. Defective splenic function and its relation to bowel disease. *Clin Gastroenterol* 1983;12:651–69.
95 Nelson EW, Ertan A, Brooks FP, Cerda JJ. Thrombocytosis in patients with coeliac sprue. *Gastroenterology* 1976;70:1042–4.
96 Bullen AW, Losowsky MS. Consequences of impaired splenic function. *Clin Sci* 1979; 57:129–37.
97 Bullen AW, Losowsky MS. Lymphocyte subpopulations in adult coeliac disease. *Gut* 1978;19:892–7.
98 Mortimer PE, Stewart JS, Norman AP, Booth CC. Follow-up study of coeliac disease. *Br Med J* 1968;3:7–9.
99 Kendall MJ. The influence of age on the xylose absorption test. *Gut* 1970;11: 498–501.
100 Rolles CJ, Kendall MJ, Nutter S, Anderson CM. One-hour blood xylose screening test for coeliac disease in infants and young children. *Lancet* 1973;ii:1043–5.
101 Buts JP, Morin CL, Roy CC, Weber A, Bonin A. One-hour blood xylose test: a reliable index of small bowel function. *J Pediatr* 1978;92:729–33.
102 Hawkins KI. Paediatric xylose absorption test: measurements in blood preferable to measurements in urine. *Clin Chem* 1970; 16:749–52.
103 Krawitt EL, Beeken WL. Limitations of usefulness of D-xylose absorption test. *Am J Clin Pathol* 1975;63:261–3.
104 Sladen GE, Kumar PJ. Is the xylose test still a worthwhile investigation? *Br Med J* 1973; 3:223–6.
105 Badé S, Gudman-Hoyer E. The diagnostic value of the D-xylose absorption test in adult coeliac disease. *Scand J Gastroenterol* 1987;22:1217–22.
106 Kendall MJ, Nutter S, Hawkins CF. Testing gluten sensitivity by the xylose test. *Lancet* 1972;i:667–8.
107 Kendall MJ, Cox PS, Schneider R, Hawkins CF. Gluten subfractions in coeliac disease. *Lancet* 1972;ii:1065–7.
108 Jarnum S, Jensen KB, Soltoft J, Westergaard H. Protein loss and turnover of albumin IgG and IgM in adult coeliac disease. In: Booth CC, Dowling RH, eds. *Coeliac Disease.* Edinburgh: Churchill Livingstone, 1970:163–72.
109 Parkins RA. Protein-losing enteropathy in the sprue syndrome. *Lancet* 1960;ii:1366–9.
110 Waldman TA, Wochner RD, Strober W. The role of the gastrointestinal tract in plasma protein metabolism. *Am J Med* 1969;46:275–85.
111 Howdle PD, Losowsky MS. The immunology of coeliac disease. *Ballieres Clin Gastroenterol* 1987;1:507–29.
112 Taylor KB, Thompson DL, Truelove SC, Wright R. An immunological study of coeliac disease and idiopathic steatorrhoea. Serological reactions to gluten and milk proteins. *Br Med J* 1961;2:1727–31.
113 Katz J, Kantor FS, Herskovic T. Intestinal antibodies to wheat fractions in celiac disease. *Ann Int Med* 1968;69:1149–53.
114 Ferguson A, Carswell F. Precipitins to dietary proteins in serum and upper intestinal secretions of coeliac children. *Br Med J* 1972;1:75–7.
115 Volta V, Lazzari R, Bianchi FB *et al.* Antibodies to dietary antigens in coeliac disease. *Scand J Gastroenterol* 1986;21:935–40.
116 Friis SU, Gudmand-Hoyer E. Screening for coeliac disease in adults by simultaneous

determination of IgA and IgG gliadin antibodies. *Scand J Gastroenterol* 1986;21: 1058–62.
117 Kelly J, O'Farrelly C, Rees JPR, Feighery C, Weir DGW. Humoral response to α-gliadin as serological screening test for coeliac disease. *Arch Dis Child* 1987;62:469–73.
118 Husby S, Foged N, Oxelius V-A, Svehag SE. Serum IgG subclass antibodies to gliadin and other dietary antigens in children with coeliac disease. *Clin Exp Immunol* 1986; 64:526–35.
119 O'Farrelly C, Kelly J, Hekkens W *et al.* α-gliadin antibody levels: a serological test for coeliac disease. *Br Med J* 1983;i: 2007–10.
120 Alp MH, Wright R. Autoantibodies to reticulin in patients with idiopathic steatorrhoea, coeliac disease and Crohn's disease, and their relation to immunoglobulins and dietary antibodies. *Lancet* 1971;ii:682–5.
121 Seah PP, Fry L, Hoffbrand AV, Holborrow EJ. Tissue antibodies in dermatitis herpetiformis and adult coeliac disease. *Lancet* 1971;i:834–6.
122 Seah PP, Fry L, Holborrow EJ *et al.* Antireticulin antibody: incidence and diagnostic significance. *Gut* 1973;14:311–15.
123 Magalhaes AFN, Peters TJ, Doe WF. Studies on the nature and significance of connective tissue antibodies in adult coeliac disease and Crohn's disease. *Gut* 1974;15:284–8.
124 Eade OE, Lloyd RS, Lang C, Wright R. IgA and IgG reticulin antibodies in coeliac disease and non-coeliac patients. *Gut* 1977; 18:991–3.
125 Mallas EG, Williamson N, Cooper BT, Cooke WT. IgA-class reticulin antibodies in relatives of patients with coeliac disease. *Gut* 1977;18:647–50.
126 Williamson N, Asquith P, Stokes PL, Jowett AW, Cooke WT. Anticonnective tissue and other antitissue 'antibodies' in the sera of patients with coeliac disease compared with the findings in a mixed hospital population. *J Clin Pathol* 1976;29:484–94.
127 Chorzelski TP, Sulej J, Tchorzewska H. IgA class endomysium antibodies in dermatitis herpetiformis and coeliac disease. *Ann NY Acad Sci* 1983;420:325–34.
128 Hällström O. Comparison of IgA-class reticulin and endomysium antibodies in coeliac disease and dermatitis herpetiformis. *Gut* 1989;30:1225–32.
129 Menzies IS, Laker MF, Pounder RE. Abnormal intestinal permeability to sugars in villous atrophy. *Lancet* 1979;ii:1107–9.
130 Cobden I, Dickinson RJ, Rothwell J, Axon ATR. Intestinal permeability assessed by excretion ratios of two molecules: results in coeliac disease. *Br Med J* 1978;2:1060–1.
131 Hamilton I, Cobden I, Rothwell AJ, Axon ATR. Intestinal permeability in coeliac disease: the response to gluten withdrawal and single dose gluten challenge. *Gut* 1982; 23:202–10.
132 Juby L, Rothwell AJ, Axon ATR. Lactulose/Mannitol test: an ideal screening rest for coeliac disease. *Gastroenterology* 1989;96: 79–85.
133 Bjarnason I, Marsh MN, Price A, Levi AJ, Peters TJ. Intestinal permeability in patients with coeliac disease and dermatitis herpetiformis. *Gut* 1985;26:1214–19.
134 Scott BB, Losowsky MS. The definition and diagnosis of coeliac disease. *J R Coll Phys Lond* 1977;11:405–11.
135 Shiner M. Jejunal biopsy tube. *Lancet* 1956; i:85.
136 Crosby WH, Kugler HW. Intraluminal biopsy of the small intestine: the intestinal biopsy capsule. *Am J Dig Dis* 1957;2:236–41.
137 Brandborg LL, Rubin CE, Quinton WE. A multipurpose instrument for suction biopsy of the oesophagus, stomach, small bowel and colon. *Gastroenterology* 1959;37:1–16.
138 Flick AL, Quinton WE, Rubin CE. A peroral hydraulic biopsy tube for multiple sampling at any level of the gastrointestinal tract. *Gastroenterology* 1961;40:120–6.
139 Gillberg R, Ahren C. Coeliac disease diagnosed by means of duodenoscopy and endoscopic duodenal biopsy. *Scand J Gastroenterol* 1977;12:911–16.
140 Holdstock G, Eade OE, Isaacson PG, Smith CL. Endoscopic duodenal biopsies in coeliac disease and duodenitis. *Scand J Gastroenterol* 1979;14:717–20.
141 Scott BB, Jenkins D. Endoscopic small intestinal biopsy. *Gastrointest Endos* 1981; 27:162–7.
142 Mee AS, Burke M, Vallon AG, Newman J, Cotton PB. Small bowel biopsy for malabsorption: comparison of the diagnostic adequacy of endoscopic forceps and capsule biopsy specimens. *Br Med J* 1985;291: 769–72.
143 Perera DR, Weinstein WM, Rubin CE. Small intestinal biopsy. *Hum Pathol* 1975;6: 157–217.
144 Rubin CE, Brandborg LL, Phelps PC, Taylor HC. Studies of coeliac disease. I. The

apparent identical and specific nature of the duodenal and proximal jejunal lesion in coeliac disease and idiopathic sprue. *Gastroenterology* 1960;38:28–49.
145 Roy-Choudhury DC, Cooke WT, Banwell JG, Smits BJ. Multiple jejunal biopsies in adult coeliac disease. *Am J Dig Dis* 1967; 12:657–63.
146 Scott BB, Losowsky MS. Patchiness and duodenal–jejunal variation of the mucosal abnormality in coeliac disease and dermatitis herpetiformis. *Gut* 1976;17:984–92.
147 Scott BB, Losowsky MS. Coeliac disease with mild mucosal abnormalities: a report of four patients. *Postgrad Med J* 1977;53: 134–8.
148 Collins BJ, Bell PM, Thomson JM, Free DB, Wilson EA, Love AHG. Dietary history and nutrition state in treated coeliac patients. *J R Soc Med* 1986;79:206–9.
149 Douglas AP. Long term prognosis and relation to diets. In: Hekkens WTJM, Pena AS, eds. *Coeliac Disease*. Leiden: Stenfert-Kroese, 1974:399–405.
150 Howdle PD. Coeliac disease: therapeutic choices in non-responders to conventional therapy. In: Dobrilla G, Bardhan KD, Steele A, eds. *Non-Responders in Gastroenterology*. Verona: Cortina International, 1991:129–39.
151 Pollock DJ, Nagle RE, Jeejeebhoy KN, Coghill NF. The effect on jejunal mucosa of withdrawing and adding dietary gluten in cases of idiopathic steatorrhoea. *Gut* 1970; 11:567–75.
152 Schenk EA, Samloff IM. Clinical and morphological changes following gluten administration to patients with treated celiac disease. *Am J Pathol* 1968;52: 579–93.
153 Bayless TM, Rubin SE, Topping TM, Yardley JH, Hendrix TR. Morphologic and functional effects of gluten feeding on jejunal mucosa in coeliac disease. In: Booth CC, Dowling RH, eds. *Coeliac Disease*. Edinburgh: Churchill Livingstone, 1970; 76–89.
154 Weinstein WM. Latent celiac sprue. *Gastroenterology* 1974;66:489–93.
155 Baker PG, Barry RE, Read AE. Detection of continuing gluten ingestion in treated coeliac patients. *Br Med J* 1975;1:486–8.
156 Weinstein WM, Piercey JRA, Dossetor JB. Dermatitis herpetiformis and coeliac sprue. In: Hekkens WTJM, Pena AS, eds. *Coeliac Disease*. Leiden: Stenfert Kroese, 1974: 361–73.
157 Kumar PJ, O'Donaghue DP, Stenson K, Dawson AM. Reintroduction of gluten in adults and children with treated coeliac disease. *Gut* 1979;20:743–9.
158 McNicholl B, Egan-Mitchell B, Fottrell PF. Variability of gluten intolerance in treated childhood coeliac disease. *Gut* 1979;20: 126–32.
159 Kuitunen P, Savilahti E, Verkasalo M. Late mucosal relapse in a boy with coeliac disease and cow's milk allergy. *Acta Paediatr Scand* 1986;75:340–2.
160 Hamilton JR, McNeill LK. Childhood coeliac disease: Response of treated patients to a small uniform daily dose of wheat gluten. *J Paediatr* 1972;81:885–93.
161 Rolles CJ, McNeish AS. Standardised approach to gluten challenge in diagnosing childhood coeliac disease. *Br Med J* 1976;1: 1309–11.
162 Shmerling DH, Franckx J. Childhood celiac disease: a long-term analysis of relapses in 91 patients. *J Pediatr Gastroenterol Nutr* 1986;5:565–9.
163 Meeuwisse GW. Diagnostic criteria in coeliac disease. *Acta Paediatr Scand* 1970; 59:461–3.
164 McNeish AS, Harms HK, Roy J, Shmerling DH, Visakorpi JK, Walker-Smith JA. The diagnosis of coeliac disease. A commentary on the current practices of members of the European Society for Paediatric Gastroenterology and Nutrition (ESPGAN). *Arch Dis Child* 1979;54:783–6.
165 Guandalini S, Ventura A, Ansaldi N *et al*, Diagnosis of coeliac disease: time for a change? *Arch Dis Child* 1989;64:1320–5.
166 Booth CC. Definition of adult coeliac disease. In: Hekkens WTJM, Pena AS, eds. *Coeliac Disease*. Leiden: Stenfert Kroese, 1974:17–24.
167 Cooke WT. Adult coeliac disease. In: Jerzy Glass GB, ed. *Progress in Gastroenterology*. Vol. 1. New York: Grune & Stratton, 1968: 299–338.
168 Loft DE, Marsh MN, Sandle GI *et al*. Studies of intestinal lymphoid tissue. XII. Epithelial lymphocyte and mucosal responses to rectal gluten challenge in celiac sprue. *Gastroenterology* 1989;97:29–37.
169 Segal E. Oats and coeliac disease. *Br Med J* 1974;4:589.
170 Howdle PD, Losowsky MS. A review of methods for measuring gliadins in food. *Gut* 1990;31:712–13.

171 McCrae WM, Eastwood MA, Martin MR, Sircus W. Neglected coeliac disease. *Lancet* 1975;i:187–90.
172 McNeish AS. Coeliac disease: duration of gluten free diet. *Arch Dis Child* 1980;55: 110–11.
173 Colaco J, Egan-Mitchell B, Stevens FM, Fottrell PF, McCarthy CF, McNicholl B. Compliance with a gluten-free diet in coeliac disease. *Arch Dis Child* 1987;62: 706–8.
174 Kumar PJ, Clark M, Dawson A. Adult coeliac disease and low gluten diets. In: Kumar PJ, Walker-Smith JA, eds. *Coeliac Disease: 100 Years*. Leeds: Leeds University Printing Service, 1990:289–93.
175 Holmes GKT, Prior P, Lane MR, Allan RN. Malignancy in coeliac disease — effect of a gluten-free diet. *Gut* 1989;30:333–8.
176 Price H, Zownir J, Prokipchuk E. Coeliac disease. *Lancet* 1975;ii:920–1.
177 Guiraldes E, Gutierrez C. Coeliac disease and Holy Communion. *Lancet* 1988;i:57.
178 Barry RE, Henry C, Read AE. The patient's view of a gluten free diet. In: McNicholl B, McCarthy CF, Fottrell PF, eds. *Perspectives in Coeliac Disease*. Lancaster: MTP Press, 1978:487–93.
179 Corazza GR, Frazzoni M, Dixon MF, Gasbarrini G. Quantitative assessment of the mucosal architecture of jejunal biopsy specimens: a comparison between linear measurement, stereology and computer-aided microscopy. *J Clin Pathol* 1985;38: 765–70.
180 Carpino F, Ceccamea A, Magliocca FM, Familiari G, Lombardi ME, Bonamico M. Scanning electron microscopy of jejunal biopsies in patients with untreated and treated coeliac disease. *Acta Paediatr Scand* 1985;74:775–81.
181 Yardley JH, Bayless TM, Norton JH, Hendrix TR. Coeliac disease: a study of the jejunal epithelium before and after a gluten free diet. *New Engl J Med* 1962;267:1173–9.
182 Stewart JS. Clinical and morphologic response to gluten withdrawal. *Clin Gastroenterol* 1974;3:109–26.
183 Grefte JMM, Bouman JG, Grond J, Jansen W, Kleibeuker JH. Slow and incomplete histological and functional recovery in adult gluten sensitive enteropathy. *J Clin Pathol* 1988;41:886–91.
184 MacDonald WC, Brandborg LL, Flick AL, Trier JS, Rubin CE. Studies in coeliac sprue. IV. The response of the whole length of the small bowel to a gluten free diet. *Gastroenterology* 1964;47:573–89.
185 Holmes GKT, Asquith P, Stokes PL, Cooke WT. Cellular infiltrate of jejunal biopsies in adult coeliac disease in relation to gluten withdrawal. *Gut* 1974;15:278–83.
186 Riecken EO, Stewart JS, Booth CC, Pearse AGE. A histochemical study on the role of lysosomal enzymes in idiopathic steatorrhoea before and during a gluten-free diet. *Gut* 1966;7:317–32.
187 Pena AS, Truelove SC, Whitehead R. Disaccharidase activity and jejunal morphology in coeliac disease. *Q J Med* 1972;41:457–76.
188 Ferguson A. Intraepithelial lymphocytes of the small intestine. *Gut* 1977;18:921–37.
189 Dobbins WO. Human intestinal intraepithelial lymphocytes. *Gut* 1986;27: 972–85.
190 Malizia G, Trejdosiewicz LK, Wood GM, Howdle PD, Janossy G, Losowsky MS. The microenvironment of coeliac disease: T cell phenotypes and expression of the T2 'T-blast' antigen by small bowel lymphocytes. *Clin Exp Immunol* 1985;60:437–46.
191 Marsh MN. Studies of intestinal lymphoid tissue. III. Quantitative analyses of epithelial lymphocytes in the small intestine of human control subjects and patients with celiac sprue. *Gastroenterology* 1980;79:481–92.
192 Brandtzaeg P, Baklien K. Immunoglobulin-producing cells in the intestine in health and disease. *Clin Gastroenterol* 1976;5: 251–69.
193 Freedman AR, Macartney JC, Nelufer JM, Ciclitira PJ. Timing of infiltration of T lymphocytes induced by gluten into the small intestine in coeliac disease. *J Clin Pathol* 1987;40:741–5.
194 Ferguson A. Lymphocytes in coeliac disease. In: Hekkens WTJH, Pena AS, eds. *Coeliac Disease*. Leiden: Stenfert Kroese, 1974: 265–76.
195 Lancaster-Smith M, Kumar PJ, Dawson AM. The cellular infiltrate of the jejunum in adult coeliac disease and dermatitis herpetiformis following the reintroduction of dietary gluten. *Gut* 1975;16:683–8.
196 Mills PR, Brown IL, Watkinson G. Idiopathic chronic ulcerative enteritis. *Q J Med* 1980; 194:133–49.
197 Bayless TM, Kapelowitz RF, Shelley WM, Ballinger WR, Hendrix TR. Intestinal ulceration, a complication of coeliac disease. *New Engl J Med* 1967;276:996–1002.
198 Bayless TM, Baer A, Yardley JH, Hendrix

TR. Intestinal ulceration, flat mucosa and malabsorption: report of registry of 33 patients. In: McNicoll B, McCarthy CF, Fottrell PF, eds. *Perspectives in Coeliac Disease*. Lancaster: MTP Press, 1987: 311–12.

199 Cooper BT, Read AE. Coeliac disease and lymphoma. *Q J Med* 1987;63:269–74.

200 Swinson CM, Coles CC, Slavin G, Booth CC. Coeliac disease and malignancy. *Lancet* 1983;i:111–5.

201 Isaacson PG, O'Connor NTJ, Spencer J *et al.* Malignant histiocytosis of the intestine: a T cell lymphoma. *Lancet* 1985;ii:688–91.

202 Iyngkaran N, Robinson MJ, Sumithran E, Lam SK, Puthucheary SD, Yadav M. Cows' milk protein-sensitive enteropathy: combined clinical and histological criteria for diagnosis. *Arch Dis Child* 1978;53:20–6.

203 Ament ME, Rubin CE. Soy protein, another cause of the flat intestinal lesion. *Gastroenterology* 1972;62:227–34.

204 Ross IN. Primary immunodeficiency and the small intestine. In: Marsh MN, ed. *Immunopathology of the Small Intestine.* Chichester: John Wiley & Sons, 1987: 283–332.

205 Leinbach GE, Rubin CE. Eosinophilic gastroenteritis: a simple reaction to food allergens? *Gastroenterology* 1970;59: 874–89.

206 Khojasteh A. Immunoproliferative small intestinal disease. *New Engl J Med* 1983; 309:1127.

207 Freeman HJ, Kim YS, Sleisenger MH. Protein digestion and absorption in man. Normal mechanisms and protein-energy malnutrition. *Am J Med* 1979;67:1030–6.

208 Rossi TM, Lebenthal E, Nord KS, Fazili RR. Extent and duration of small intestinal mucosal injury in intractable diarrhoea of infancy. *Pediatrics* 1980;66:730–5.

209 Walker-Smith JA. Postenteritis diarrhoea. In: Lebenthal E, ed. *Textbook of Gastroenterology and Nutrition in Infancy*. New York: Raven Press, 1989:1171–86.

210 Yardley JH, Takano J, Hendrix TR. Epithelial and other mucosal lesions in the jejunum in giardiasis. Jejunal biopsy studies. *Bull Johns Hopkins Hosp* 1964;115:389–406.

211 Fung WP, Tan KK, Yu SF, Kho KM. Malabsorption and subtotal villous atrophy secondary to pulmonary and intestinal tuberculosis. *Gut* 1970;11:212–16.

212 Miller ARO, Griffin GE, Batman P *et al.* Jejunal mucosal architecture and fat absorption in male homosexuals infected with human immunodeficiency virus. *Q J Med* 1988;69:1009–19.

213 Isaacs PET, Kim YS. Blind loop syndrome and small bowel bacterial contamination. *Clin Gastroenterol* 1983;12:395–414.

214 Maizel H, Ruffin JM, Dobbins WO. Whipple's disease: a review of 19 patients from one hospital and a review of the literature since 1950. *Medicine (Baltimore)* 1970;49:175–205.

215 Klipstein FA. Tropical sprue in travellers. *Gastroenterology* 1981;80:590–600.

216 McDonald GSA, Hourihane DO. Ischaemic lesions of the alimentary tract. *J Clin Pathol* 1972;25:99–105.

217 Kerlin P, Wong L. Lactose tolerance despite hypolactasia in adult coeliac disease. *J Gastroenterol Hepatol* 1987;2:233–7.

218 Baker AL, Rosenberg IH. Refractory sprue: Recovery after removal of non-gluten dietary proteins. *Ann Int Med* 1978;8:505–8.

219 Mike N, Asquith P. Soya protein sensitivity in non-responsive coeliac disease. *Gut* 1984;25:A1190.

220 Love AHG, Elmes M, Golden MK, McMaster D. Zinc deficiency and coeliac disease. In: McNicholl B, McCarthy CF, Fottrell PP, eds. *Perspectives in Coeliac Disease*. Lancaster: MTP Press, 1978: 335–42.

221 Goyens P, Brasseur D, Cadranel S. Copper deficiency in infants with active coeliac disease. *J Pediatr Gastroenterol Nutr* 1985; 4:677–80.

222 Roufail WM, Ruffin JM. Effect of antibiotic therapy on gluten sensitive enteropathy. *Am J Dig Dis* 1966;11:587–93.

223 Pink IJ, Creamer B. Response to a gluten free diet of patients with the coeliac syndrome. *Lancet* 1967;i:300–4.

224 DiMagno EP, Go VLW, Summerskill WHJ. Impaired cholecystokinin-pancreozymin secretion, intraluminal dilution and malabsorption of fat in sprue. *Gastroenterology* 1972;63:25–32.

225 Maton PN, Seblen AC, Fitzpatrick ML, Chadwick VS. Reversible defect of gallbladder emptying and plasma cholecystokinin (CCK) release in coeliac disease. *Gastroenterology* 1985;88:391–6.

226 Regan PT, DiMagno EP. Exocrine pancreatic insufficiency in celiac sprue: a cause of treatment failure. *Gastroenterology* 1980; 78:484–7.

227 Kilander AF, Hanssen LE, Gillberg RE.

Secretin release in coeliac disease. *Scand J Gastroenterol* 1983;18:765–9.
228 Collins BJ, Bell PM, Boyd S, Kerr J, Buchanan KD, Love AHG. Endocrine and exocrine pancreatic function in treated coeliac disease. *Pancreas* 1986;1:143–7.
229 Weizman Z, Hamilton JR, Kopelman HR, Cleghorn G, Durie PR. Treatment failure in celiac disease due to coexistent exocrine pancreatic insufficiency. *Pediatrics* 1987; 80:924–6.
230 Wall AJ, Douglas AP, Booth CC, Pearse AGE. The response of the jejunal mucosa in adult coeliac disease to oral prednisolone. *Gut* 1970;11:7–14.
231 Kumar PJ, Silk DBA, Marks R, Clarke ML, Dawson AM. Treatment of dermatitis herpetiformis with corticosteroids and a gluten-free diet: a study of jejunal morphology and function. *Gut* 1973;14:280–3.
232 Peters TJ, Jones PE, Jenkins WJ, Wells G. Analytical subcellular fractionation of jejunal biopsy specimens: enzyme activities, organelle pathology and response to corticosteroids in patients with non-responsive coeliac disease. *Clin Sci Mol Med* 1978;55: 293–300.
233 Zaitoun A, Record CO. Morphometric studies in duodenal biopsies from patients with coeliac disease: the effect of the steroid fluticasone propionate. *Aliment Pharmacol Therap* 1991;5:151–60.
234 Hamilton JD, Chambers RA, Wynn-Williams A. Role of gluten, prednisolone and azathioprine in non-responsive coeliac disease. *Lancet* 1976;i:1213–16.
235 Neale G. A case of coeliac disease resistant to treatment. *Br Med J* 1968;1:678–84.
236 Dowling RH, Henry K. Non-responsive coeliac disease. *Br Med J* 1972;3:624–31.
237 van Tongeren JAM, Cluysenaer OJJ, Schillings PAM. Refractory Sprue. In: McNicholl B, McCarthy CF, Fottrell PF, eds. *Perspectives in Coeliac Disease.* Lancaster: MTP Press, 1978:323–9.
238 MacDonald WC, Dobbins WO, Rubin CE. Studies of the familial nature of coeliac sprue using biopsy of the small intestine. *New Engl J Med* 1965;272:448–56.
239 Robinson DC, Watson AJ, Wyatt EH, Marks JM, Roberts DF. Incidence of small intestinal mucosal abnormalities and of clinical coeliac disease in the relatives of children with coeliac disease. *Gut* 1971;12: 789–93.
240 Shipman RT, Williams AL, Kay R, Townley RRW. A family study of coeliac disease. *Aust NZ J Med* 1975;5:250–5.
241 Mylotte M, Egan-Mitchell B, Fottrell PF, McNicholl B, McCarthy CF. Familial studies in coeliac disease. *Q J Med* 1974;43: 359–69.
242 Stokes PL, Ferguson R, Holmes GKT, Cooke WT. Familial aspects of coeliac disease. *Q J Med* 1976;45:567–82.
243 Ellis A, Evans DAP, McConnell RB, Woodrow JC. Liverpool coeliac family study. In: McConnell RB, ed. *The Genetics of Coeliac Disease.* Lancaster: MTP Press 1981:265–90.
244 Rolles CJ, Kyaw-Myint TB, Wai-Kee Sin, Anderson CM. The familial incidence of asymptomatic coeliac disease. In: McConnell RB, ed. *The Genetics of Coeliac Disease.* Lancaster: MTP Press, 1981: 235–50.

Chapter 4/Dermatitis herpetiformis

LIONEL FRY

The American dermatologist Dühring first used the term dermatitis herpetiformis (DH) in Philadelphia in 1884. Although recognized as a specific entity from that time onwards, DH was included within a group of conditions known collectively for over 100 years as the bullous disorders, which also included pemphigus and pemphigoid. Pemphigus was shown to be a specific condition by Civatte (1943) because its blister is intraepidermal, rather than subepidermal as in DH and pemphigoid [1]. The distinction between the two latter conditions and between DH and linear IgA dermatosis was effected with the later advent of immunofluorescence techniques.

A further significant milestone was passed in 1940 with Costello's observation that the rash of DH clears after a few days with sulphapyridine treatment [2]. The use of this drug was originally based on the premise that DH is an allergic reaction to a bacterium, a view quickly dispelled by the failure to eradicate the condition following antibiotic therapy. In 1950, Esteves and Brandao showed that dapsone was also effective, and probably more so than sulphapyridine, in suppressing the rash of DH [3].

The next landmark in the history of DH was in 1966 with the demonstration of an enteropathy in nine of 12 patients by Marks and her colleagues [4]. In the following year [5] attention was drawn to the similarities between DH and coeliac enteropathy, such as iron and folate deficiency, a low serum IgM concentration and evidence of splenic atrophy on blood film (Howell–Jolly bodies, thrombocytosis). Subsequent studies by the same authors [6,7] confirmed that both the enteropathy and rash are gluten dependent, thereby indicating that DH is uniquely distinction pathogenesis from the other bullous dermatoses.

Finally, in 1969, Van der Meer [8] reported that immunoglobulin IgA deposits are present in uninvolved skin. Two patterns of IgA deposition were subsequently observed, the more common granular IgA deposition in dermal papillae and the rare linear deposition along the line of the basement membrane. In reviewing the features of DH, Fry and Seah [9] stated: 'IgA deposition in the uninvolved skin is the most reliable diagnostic criterion of DH, and [that] the diagnosis should not be made without the presence of IgA'. This has now become accepted practice.

During the last decade it has become universally accepted that IgA deposition in DH exists in two forms, both of which show 'granular' deposits of IgA either in the dermal papillae or along the line of the dermoepidermal junction. A third pattern of IgA deposition, in which the deposits form a 'homogeneous' linear band along the dermo-epidermal junction, is now termed linear IgA disease (LAD), and is a separate disorder. Further, the distribution of the rash [10], lack of response to gluten withdrawal [11], and human leucocyte antigen (HLA) studies [12] provide further support for this view.

Thus, within almost a century of its original description by Dühring, the pathogenesis and specific diagnostic features, together with the drug and dietary treatment of DH have been established. In addition, skin biopsy has been shown to permit separation of true DH from LAD and from other bullous skin disorders both in adults and also, importantly, in children.

Presentation

DH apparently can occur at any age, the youngest patient being 10 months old [13] and the oldest >90 years-of-age [14]. In less than one-fifth of patients (18%) the rash begins later than 50, and in only 5% beyond the 80th birthday. In the majority, DH occurs in young adults within the age range of 15–40 years (median, 30). This figure seems consistent in studies from Finland [15], three UK centres (Edinburgh [16], Cardiff [17] and our own unit at St Mary's Hospital, London) and two of three Swedish groups [18,19]; the other from southern Sweden [14] reported a higher mean age. The condition is much rarer in children, and in only two of our patients did the rash commence before the 10th year. Childhood DH may be more common in Italy [13] and Hungary; generally, the eruption usually begins around the 7th year of life [13,20]. The enteropathy is more severe in children compared with adult DH patients.

On average, the male : female ratio is 3 : 2 (adults) compared with 1 : 2 in children [13]. This preponderance of female children is consistent with the higher prevalence of DH in women less than 40 years-of-age. The reason why DH presents earlier in females is unknown.

In the few studies published, the prevalence of DH in Edinburgh [16] and Finland [15] was approximately 12 : 100 000, being much lower than that reported in various Swedish centres per 100 000 population, such as 20 Malmo [14], 27 Kristianstad [14], 40 central Sweden [14] and 23 western Sweden [18], respectively. In order to be accurate, strict diagnostic criteria must be employed in population studies if the figures are to have any real meaning. For this reason, the reported incidence

(1 : 500–1700) in Northern Ireland [21] is impossible to interpret. Diagnostic stringency and accuracy also impinge on the utility of comparisons between DH and coeliac disease (CD), particularly as it is generally regarded that CD is underdiagnosed on account of the high number of asymptomatic, subclinical cases.

Thus, while the incidence between DH and CD in Sweden is apparently 1 : 2, there is a five-fold difference compared with Edinburgh (1 : 10 000 and 1 : 2000), respectively.

There are sparse data concerning geographical distribution although like CD, DH appears to be more common in Europe and other countries to which Europeans have emigrated. It is also seen, like CD, in the Middle and Far East although with a considerably lower rate than in the West. At St Mary's Hospital, London, which serves a large and predominantly Black/Asian community, no DH patient out of a total of 170 cases was seen in these ethnic groups, with the possible exception of one with Indian/Portuguese parentage. Among our patients, however, is a very high proportion of individuals of Irish descent and one would expect that the incidence of both diseases would be largely congruent, and in similar ratios, throughout the world where wheat is a dietary staple. Ireland, particularly in its western parts, is reported to have the highest incidence of CD in the world [22], and it is likely that the incidence of both DH and CD, and the ratio of CD : DH, would be similar among the Irish domiciled in England.

Cutaneous distribution of the rash

The rash of DH is extremely symmetrical. The most common site of involvement is the extensor surfaces of the elbow and proximal forearms (Fig. 4.1), with over 90% of patients having lesions at this site [23]. The next is the buttocks (Fig. 4.2) occurring in some two-thirds of patients, while the third most common site is the extensor surfaces of the knees (Fig. 4.3). Other sites frequently affected are the back, particularly over the scapulae, and the face. Involvement of all areas, apart from the soles of the feet, has been described. In some patients the rash may be confined to one or two areas, e.g. elbows and buttocks, whilst in others, the eruption is widespread. Lesions also appear, apparently from trauma, e.g. from belts, braces and bras. If there is a 'breakthrough' in patients whose eruption is treated by drugs, the face will be commonly affected in addition to the elbows and buttocks. Where breakthrough occurs in any individual, due to inadequate drug control, the rash will involve the same sites on each occasion.

In our experience, mucous membrane involvement is rare and occurs in less than 5% of patients. IgA deposition does occur in the oral mucosa [24] but as with uninvolved skin, does not necessarily lead to clinical lesions. In one study [25] a high incidence of oral lesions (12 of

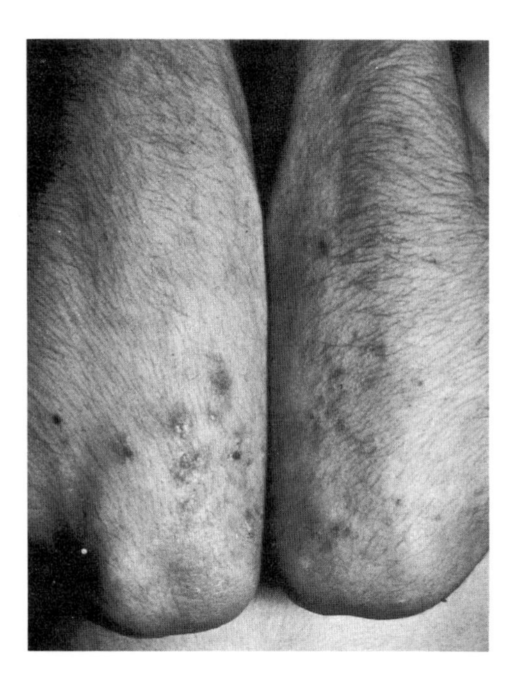

Fig. 4.1 Blisters and excoriated papules on the elbows and extensor forearms which are the most common sites for DH.

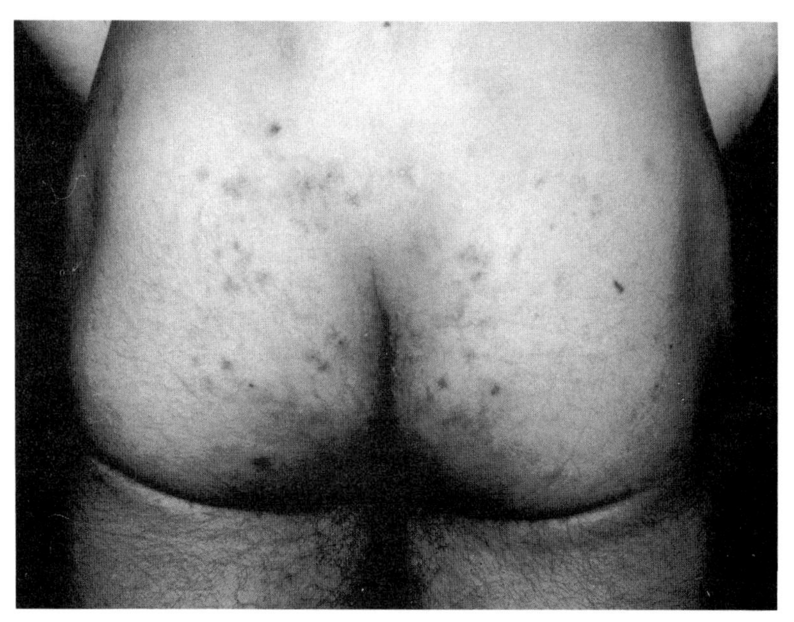

Fig. 4.2 Grouped lesions on the buttocks.

15 patients) was noted but in only two patients were they symptomatic. It is possible that in some earlier reports of oral involvement, the patients may not have had DH, but LAD, in which over 25% of patients develop symptomatic oral lesions (Table 4.1).

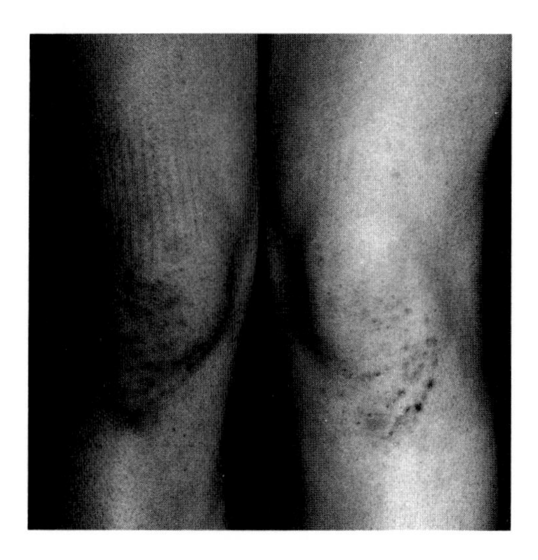

Fig. 4.3 Symmetrical lesions on the knees.

Morphology of lesions

The classical lesion of DH is a small blister situated on an erythematous urticarial plaque. It has to be stressed that DH is an intensely irritating disorder so that patients can hardly resist scratching their lesions. Thus, in practice, it is often rare to find intact blisters; instead the lesions most frequently appear as excoriated and scabbed papules. Moreover, if the rash is chronic and well-established there are often lichenified patches at the sites of involvement. The absence of blisters (because of scratching) cannot be too strongly emphasized for the practising clinician. The distribution of the rash is far more likely to suggest the diagnosis than lesional morphology. Indeed, the rash of DH is of variable morphology. Occasionally, blisters and excoriations are the only lesions, and no urticarial plaques are present. Alternatively, urticarial patches may be the predominant lesion with no clinical blister formation. Rarely, large blisters (>1 cm diameter) are seen. Scarring is not a feature of DH despite the fact that the primary site of the skin lesion is dermal.

It has already been mentioned that in some patients the eruption may be widespread, whilst in others only a few lesions are present. In some patients with mild disease, the rash may be intermittent with intervening periods of remission, a presentation that occurs in <10% of patients.

There is no doubt that in some female patients an exacerbation of the rash occurs premenstrually. However, the effect of pregnancy is variable; in some patients the rash improves, in others it worsens, while in others it seems to precipitate the eruption. DH may also occur for the first time in pregnancy which subsequently clears after

Table 4.1 Comparison of bullous disorders

	DH	LAD	Pemphigus	Pemphigoid	Eczema
Most common age of presentation	15–40	Any age	40–60	60+	Any age
Sex ratio male : female	3 : 2	2 : 3	1 : 1	1 : 1	1 : 1
Irritation	+++	+	Nil	+	++
Distribution of rash	Elbows, knees and buttocks	Anywhere	Anywhere	Mainly trunk and limbs	Anywhere
Morphology of lesions	Small blisters or urticarial plaques	Small and/or large blisters. Urticarial base lesions; may be annular	Erosions and flaccid blisters	Small and/or large blisters on urticarial base	Blisters and excoriated papules
Oral lesions	Rare	25%	60%	Rare	Nil
Main site of pathology	Dermis	Dermoepidermal junction	Intraepidermal	Dermoepidermal junction	Epidermal and dermal
Immunofluorescence skin	IgA in upper dermis	Linear IgA along dermoepidermal junction	IgG on surface of epidermal cells	IgG along dermoepidermal junction	Negative
Circulating autoantibodies	Antireticulin antigliadin	Rarely IgA (to dermoepidermal junction)	IgG (to surface antigen of epithelial cells)	IgG (dermoepidermal junction)	Nil

MHC associations	B8/DR3/DQW2	B8/DR3/DQW1/DR2/DRW6	A10/A26/BW38/DRW4	Nil	Nil
Organ specific antibodies	ANA ++, GPC ++, Thyroid ++, ARA ++	ANA +, GPC +, Thyroid +	Nil	Nil	Nil
Aetiology	Gluten sensitivity	? Autoimmune	Autoimmune	Autoimmune	Unknown
Treatment	Gluten-free diet, dapsone, sulphapyridine, sulphamethoxy-pyridazine	Dapsone, sulphapyridine, sulphamethoxy-pyridazine, systemic steroids?	Systemic steroids, azathioprine, cyclosporine	Systemic steroids, azathioprine, dapsone	Topical steroids, systemic steroids, photochemotherapy
Course	Persistent 10% remission	Persistent; 20% remission	Variable; possible remission	Variable; possible remission	Persistent; possible remission
Prognosis	Good; increased incidence of lymphoma	Good; increased incidence of malignancy	Mortality ~ 10%; morbidity ++ from high-dose steroids	Good	Good

ANA, antinuclear antibodies; ARA, antireticulin antibodies; DH, dermatitis herpetiformis; GPC, gastric parietal cell antibodies; LAD, linear IgA disease; MHC, major histocompatibility complex.

delivery. Thus, while female sex hormones appear to have a modifying effect on the disease process, there is no indication for their use clinically.

Differential diagnosis

The differential diagnosis depends on the duration and nature of the eruption. There are a number of other conditions apart from DH which respond to sulphones, and the beneficial response may thus lead to an incorrect diagnosis of DH. The conditions which respond to sulphones include LAD, chronic bullous dermatosis of childhood, subcorneal pustular dermatosis, erythema elevatum diutinium, some forms of vasculitis and in some patients, eczema, pemphigus and pemphigoid (see Table 4.1). In one study the most common diagnosis in patients who were incorrectly thought to have DH was eczema [26].

In adults, the two most common diseases that have to be distinguished from DH are LAD and eczema. In LAD, the rash does not show a predilection for the elbows, knees and buttocks but tends to be more generalized and commonly affects the groins and axillae. In both conditions the blisters are often situated on an urticarial base so that it is not often possible to distinguish between either, on clinical grounds. If eczema involves the extensor forearms and has blisters, a trial of dapsone may be given. There is no doubt that dapsone does often decrease the pruritus associated with eczema; this symptomatic relief produces both subjective and objective improvement.

Pemphigoid tends to occur predominantly in the elderly and does not show a predilection for the extensor surfaces of the limbs. However, the morphology of the lesions may be similar although the blisters tend to be larger and more widespread. These are generalizations, and at times, it is not possible to make the diagnosis on clinical features alone. In these circumstances, diagnosis requires a biopsy from uninvolved skin for immunofluorescent studies.

Pemphigus tends to produce superficial erosions and flaccid bullae rather than urticarial plaques, but as mentioned above, a few patients with pemphigus may respond dramatically to sulphones.

Erythema multiforme may produce similar lesions to DH. However, erythema multiforme is usually self-limiting, shows no response to dapsone and frequently affects the hands.

Scabies has in the past been misdiagnosed as DH because, in both disorders, there is involvement of the buttocks and intense irritation. The presence of burrows on the hands, and papules on the male genitalia, may help to distinguish the two disorders. A trial of a scabicide such as γ-benzene hexachloride is advisable if there is any doubt.

Chronic papular urticaria (insect bites) has certainly been misdiagnosed as DH in the past. Blisters are a feature in some patients with papular urticaria and the lesions are intensely irritating. The distribution of the eruption follows no particular pattern, unlike DH.

Some forms of cutaneous vasculitis present as urticarial plaques and may respond to dapsone. The distribution is usually not that of DH and blisters are not usually a feature.

Subcorneal pustular dermatosis is a rare disorder with numerous small blisters and pustules. There is a good response to dapsone, but the distribution and presence of pustules argue against DH.

In children, chronic bullous dermatosis of childhood (now sometimes referred to as LAD of childhood), should be distinguished from DH because of the therapeutic implications. The characteristic rash in this dermatosis comprises small blisters often arising on annular urticarial lesions. The most common sites are the pubic area and thighs. The rash responds well to dapsone. The diagnosis is established and distinguished from DH by a biopsy from uninvolved skin which shows a linear homogeneous IgA band at the dermoepidermal junction by immunofluorescence.

Investigations

From among the conditions listed above that might be confused with DH either because of their resemblance to the rash, or because of a response to dapsone, it is important that gluten-responsive DH is recognized and a correct diagnosis made. The investigation of choice, as emphasized by Fry and Seah [9], is to demonstrate IgA deposits in uninvolved skin. The diagnosis of DH cannot be entertained if, after careful sectioning of the biopsy and examination of a second skin biopsy (if the first proves negative for IgA), no granular IgA deposits are found in the papillary dermis or along the line of the basement membrane [27]. It is also important to understand that these criteria cannot be met if biopsies from active lesions are examined. IgA is present in all uninvolved skin although to a variable degree as assessed by immunofluorescence [28]. For diagnostic purposes, skin from the upper outer buttock is preferred.

In practice, a punch biopsy (4 mm diameter) of uninvolved skin should be immediately frozen in liquid Nitrogen, embedded in Tissue Tek II OCT compound (Lamb, London, UK) and stored at −80°C.

Patterns of IgA deposition in DH

Papillary

This term is used because the IgA deposits are found in the dermal papillae (Fig. 4.4). This is the common pattern in DH, the IgA deposits appearing as small 'granules' or sometimes as a 'fibrillar' network,

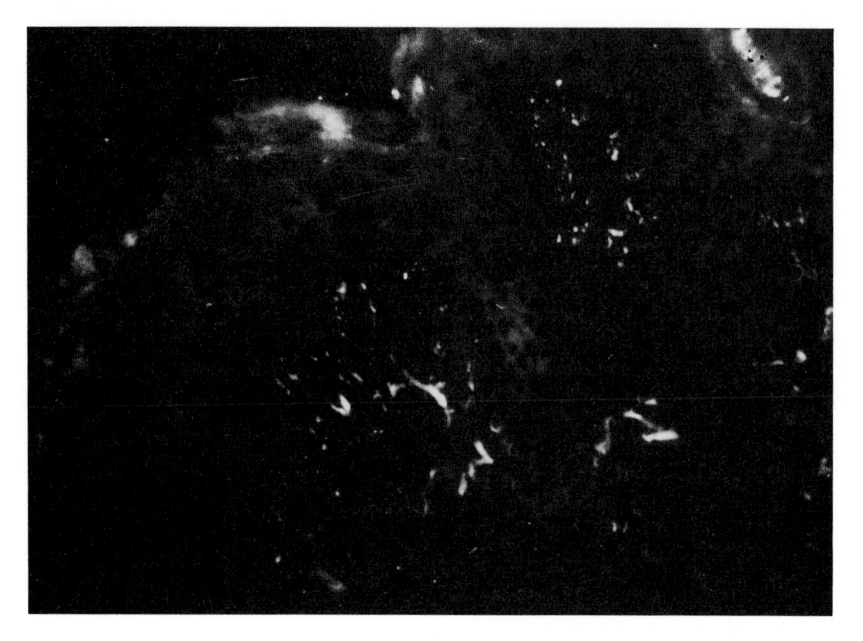

Fig. 4.4 Granular deposits of IgA in the dermal papillae.

depending on the plane of section of the reticulin fibres (where the IgA is deposited). Granular deposits, however, are not always confined to the dermal papillae but may also be seen in the upper dermis below the rete pegs.

Linear granular

It is most important to be able to distinguish between a linear granular pattern of IgA deposition (Fig. 4.5) and a linear homogeneous pattern (Fig. 4.6). It has now been shown that the linear granular pattern relates to DH, whereas the linear homogeneous pattern implies LAD [10]. Follow-up studies in our department have shown that over a period of time the linear granular pattern may revert to a papillary pattern, but the homogeneous pattern does not, and thus always implies a different condition.

Treatment of the rash with sulphones or sulphonamides does not alter the IgA deposits in the skin, and therefore, biopsies can be taken for diagnostic purposes once drug therapy has begun. A gluten-free diet has no immediate effect on IgA deposition although after many years, the quantity of IgA decreases and may eventually disappear [29,30]. It is difficult to quantitate IgA by immunofluorescence and thus, the gradual decrease is difficult to monitor. Total disappearance of IgA in our patients takes at least 7 years after the start of a gluten-free diet.

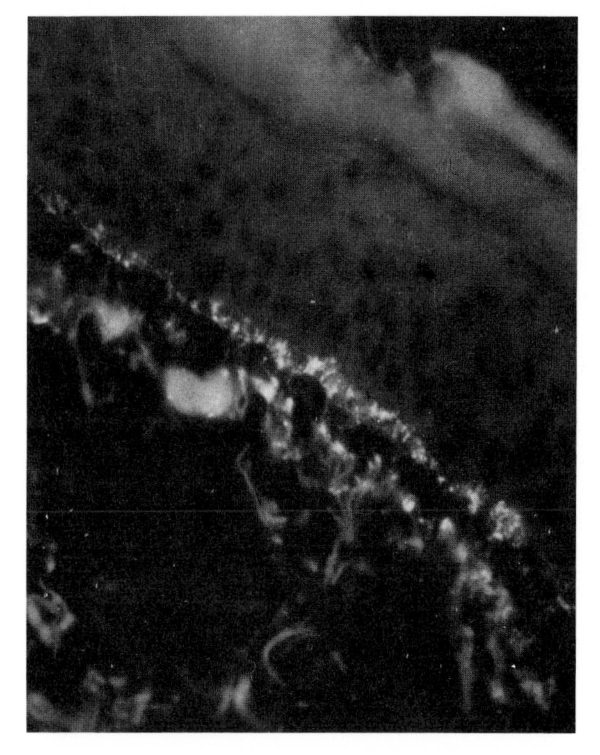

Fig. 4.5 Linear *granular* IgA deposits along the line of the basement membrane in DH.

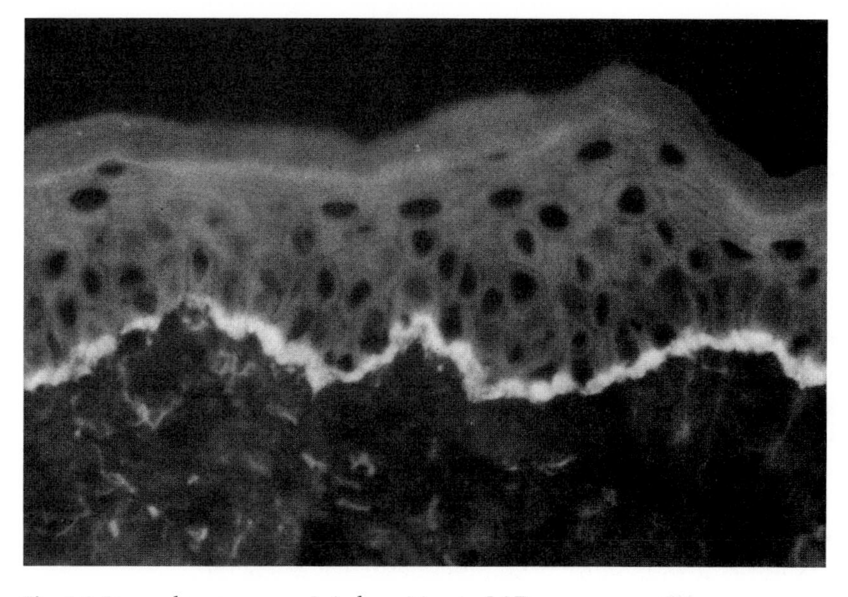

Fig. 4.6 Linear *homogeneous* IgA deposition in LAD.

The C3 component of complement is also found in approximately two-thirds of patients taking a normal diet [29,31] and codistributes with IgA. IgG and IgM may also be present, in addition to IgA, in uninvolved skin. IgM is seen in about one-third, and IgG in 10% of biopsies; their distribution tends to follow that of IgA [27].

If the clinical features of the rash and its response to sulphones suggest DH but no IgA is detected, serial sections of the biopsy should be taken. Of 50 patients, only two required a second biopsy to detect IgA [27].

Histological features of lesional skin

Biopsy of lesional skin for diagnostic purposes has now been superseded by biopsies from uninvolved skin. However, knowledge of the histological features of the DH skin lesion is helpful in understanding likely pathogenetic mechanisms. The characteristic features of DH are a subepidermal blister (bulla) and microabscesses in the surrounding dermal papillae. Neutrophils are the predominant cell in the bullae and microabscesses, and leukocytoclasis and fibrin deposition are commonly seen. Eosinophils are present in approximately 25% of bullae [32]. In the dermis there is also a perivascular infiltrate of lymphocytes and histiocytes which has been claimed to be the initial feature of the developing skin lesion.

Both pemphigoid and LAD have similar histological features. Thus, detection of the pattern and class of immunoglobulin deposition in uninvolved skin by immunofluorescence is a more reliable way of excluding these other possibilities, and of establishing the diagnosis of DH with certainty.

Small intestinal biopsy

Ideally, this should be performed in all patients once DH has been unequivocally diagnosed. Approximately two-thirds of patients will have an abnormal mucosa as judged on dissecting microscopy and routine histology. If multiple biopsies are taken the frequency of abnormalities will rise since the enteropathy is often patchy, rather than confluent, in the upper small intestine in DH [33]. The histological features are those characteristic of a gluten-sensitive enteropathy.

Approximately 60% of subjects have a moderate-to-severe mucosal abnormality. The remainder have an essentially normal appearing mucosal architecture in which villous epithelium is infiltrated by an increased number of intraepithelial lymphocytes. In 10% of DH patients no abnormality of the intestinal mucosa can be demonstrated [34], although there is latent gluten sensitivity, since gluten loading can induce features of an enteropathy [35].

Gluten-induced malabsorption

Given that the biopsy of uninvolved skin reveals the presence of granular IgA deposits, further investigations of the patient are advisable in (1) evaluating the degree of associated malabsorption, in addition to jejunal biopsy and (2) excluding other associated conditions.

One key to determining the type of malabsorption is a full haematological work-up. Anaemia may be present which is due to iron deficiency (~30%), or folate deficiency which may be inferred from the presence of macrocytosis and hypersegmented polymorphs. Howell–Jolly bodies identify splenic dysfunction and thus strengthen the gluten-sensitive basis of the dermatitis. In addition to iron and folate levels, the serum B_{12} level should also be measured to exclude the rarer association with pernicious anaemia.

Despite the enteropathy, few DH patients have corresponding symptoms of diarrhoea and steatorrhoea. Any functional upset can be quantitated by a 5-day faecal fat determination or a D-xylose absorption test. In practice these are rarely abnormal in adults [5] but are more likely to show abnormalities in children [13]. Weight and height, likewise, are invariably within reference range for adults although in a study of 75 children, 11 (15%) had reduced weights and 10 (13%) reduced heights. Nevertheless, many (38%) of the children had abdominal pain [13]. The spectrum of jejunal mucosal changes is described elsewhere (see Chapter 6).

Associated conditions

There is a significant increase in thyroid disease and pernicious anaemia (PA) in patients with DH. In addition, other conditions such as systemic lupus erythematosus, myasthenia gravis and chronic active hepatitis are also prevalent.

Thyroid disease is the most common 'autoimmune' disease associated with DH. The prevalence of thyroid antibodies was found in our series to be 48% of 115 patients [36], while overt thyroid disease occurred in only six patients (5%). In addition, a further six patients were found to have raised thyroid-stimulating hormone levels implying some degree of thyroid failure; a similar degree of overt thyroid disease was found in two other studies [16,17]. Their incidence of thyroid disease and antibodies were considerably lower compared with the study in Salt Lake City [37] where 34% (of 50 DH patients) were reported to have thyroid disease and 38% had thyroid antibodies. It is possible that there are local factors in Salt Lake City which predispose to thyroid disease resulting in such very high rates, compared with the UK.

Other autoimmune phenomena involve the stomach. In 170 patients from St Mary's Hospital, ~30% revealed gastric parietal cell antibodies

(GPC), while five patients (3%) actually developed PA. In a study from Edinburgh Royal Infirmary [16] ~15% had GPC, although 3% (2/76) also developed PA.

A good correlation between the presence of GPC and achlorhydria has been demonstrated [38] with rates >68% for achlorhydria and <10% for those with normal acid secretion [38]. Of 116 DH patients, 30 (26%) were found to have achlorhydria, and >90% of those were shown to have biopsy appearances consistent with atrophic gastritis (see p. 178).

A few patients develop insulin-dependent diabetes. Annual urine tests are advised to check on this occurrence.

Our work (unpublished) in London has shown that a gluten-free diet does not influence the subsequent development of, nor the course of, established autoimmune disorders; neither does it have any effect on autoantibody production.

Lymphoma

Following a series of case reports [39–45] associating DH with lymphoma, it was subsequently shown that there is a true increase in lymphoma in this condition [46]. Of 109 patients, three developed lymphoma, giving a relative risk of 100. It was also found that those patients who were not taking a strict gluten-free diet had microscopic evidence of enteropathy on biopsy. However, another four cases of lymphoma were described in DH patients taking a gluten-free diet [47]. Although the majority of lymphomas, like CD, arise within the gastrointestinal tract, they may also occur elsewhere. The immunohistological classification of lymphomas is described in detail elsewhere in this volume (see Chapter 5).

Treatment

Virtually all patients with DH require treatment to control the rash and severe irritation. Patients with very mild disease are the exception and may not even find their way to a dermatological clinic. There are two ways of treating DH, one with drugs and the other with a gluten-free diet. It is imperative to realize that immediate relief of irritation and suppression of the rash can be obtained with drugs, but that control of the rash by diet takes several months. Therefore, initial treatment is with drugs, whether combined with a gluten-free diet or not.

Three drugs, sulphapyridine, dapsone and sulphamethoxypyridazine, effectively control the rash but have no effect on the enteropathy. Their mechanism of action in suppressing the skin lesions is unknown, but probably results from blocking the production or action of the chemical mediators involved in the inflammatory process. Adequate dosage relieves the irritation within 48 hours and clears the rash soon after; conversely, rash and irritation return rapidly after cessation of therapy.

The initial dose of *dapsone* for an adult should be 100 mg daily and reviewed when the patient is seen 2 weeks later (Table 4.2). If the rash is completely controlled, the dose should be reduced to 50 mg daily, and if control is still achieved with this dose subsequent reductions should be advised, increasing the interval between successive doses to every second or third day, and so on, until 'breakthrough' of the rash occurs. In our experience, the minimum dose necessary to control the rash in adults is 50 mg twice weekly. If, after 2 weeks, the eruption is not controlled with 100 mg daily the dose should be increased to 200 mg daily for a further 2-week period. If no control is achieved on this dosage the diagnosis should be reviewed, and another skin biopsy performed for the detection of IgA. Of 160 patients with DH seen at St Mary's over the last 18 years, only two required a dose >300 mg daily to suppress the rash. One required 400 mg daily and another 700 mg daily, but even then there was not complete control in this latter patient. Eventual control was achieved with the addition of sulphapyridine 2.0 g daily, but because of severe haematological side-effects this patient was persuaded to take a gluten-free diet; finally, success was achieved with a gluten-free diet and dapsone 100 mg daily.

It is important that the minimum dose necessary to suppress the rash is found, and that patients do not take excess dapsone because the frequency and severity of side-effects is generally related to the dosage. It is also important to be aware that, in the longer term, patients' dose requirements may fall; thus, they should always be advised to reduce the dose. In a follow-up study of 36 patients over a mean period of 7.4

Table 4.2 Drug usage in DH

Dosage	Dapsone/day	Sulphapyridine/ day	Sulphamethoxy-pyridazine/day
Initial dose	100 mg	2 g	0.5 g
If good control of rash, reduce dose to	50 mg	1 g	0.5 g alternate days
If control is maintained, reduce dose further every second and third day, etc., until breakthrough occurs. Maintenance at a dose to stop breakthrough			
If rash not controlled increase dose to	200 mg	3 g	1.0 g
Maximum dose	300 mg	4 g	1.5 g
If no control repeat skin biopsy? Diagnosis. Alternatively, use drugs in combination			

years [30], the dose of dapsone remained constant in 13 and decreased in 15, among whom five no longer required treatment. In eight patients drug dosage increased, which probably represents an alteration in disease 'activity'.

In general, dapsone is a very safe drug, although the majority of patients have a haemolytic anaemia which is dose related (Table 4.3). In patients destined to develop severe haemolysis, its characteristic features will be present in the blood count from the outset (i.e. 2–4 weeks after commencement of treatment). If haemolysis has not developed, then subsequent blood tests are performed at 3 monthly intervals during the first year, and at 6 monthly intervals thereafter. Any degree of haemolysis is best monitored by the reticulocyte count.

Methaemoglobinaemia, although not dose related, presents as cyanosis; the importance of this side-effect lies in its reduction of the oxygen-carrying capacity of the blood. Therefore, people with known ischaemic disease (cerebral, cardiac, arterial) or those beyond 50 years-of-age, should receive alternative treatment. Agranulocytosis is a very rare complication.

One of the most common and more troublesome side-effects is headache which may warrant other therapy. Occasionally, lethargy, insomnia or depression may be encountered and rarely, mononeuropathy. Teratogenicity has not been reported with dapsone and at St Mary's Hospital there have been four patients who have had normal pregnancies whilst taking dapsone. Infertility (male) has never been encountered. Gastrointestinal symptoms do not usually accompany treatment, although severe hypoalbuminaemia has been reported.

With *sulphapyridine*, the initial daily dose should be 2 g and should never exceed 4 g daily; in many patients the rash will be controlled within this dose range. As with dapsone, the initial dose (2 g) should be reviewed within 2 weeks and the dose increased, or decreased; the aim being to determine the least dosage necessary to prevent 'break-

Table 4.3 Side-effects of drugs

Dapsone	Sulphapyridine	Sulphamethoxy-pyridazine
Haemolysis (dose related)	Haemolysis	Skin rash
Methaemoglobinaemia	Agranulocytosis	Gastrointestinal upset
Lethargy, insomnia, depression, headache	Marrow aplasia	Agranulocytosis
Mononeuropathy		
Agranulocytosis		
Hypoalbuminaemia	Skin rash	Pneumonitis

through' (Table 4.2). Again, in the longer term, dose requirements may fall and this must be borne in mind during each patient's follow-up.

The important side-effects are marrow depression (agranulocytosis or complete marrow depression) and skin rashes. Other features may be nausea, lethargy and depression (Table 4.3).

A third agent is *sulphamethoxypyridazine* which is commenced at a dosage of 0.5 g daily (Table 4.2). At review 2 weeks later, the dose is either decreased or increased to a maximum not exceeding 1.5 g daily. In our experience with these dose levels, side-effects are infrequent, although may include skin rashes, nausea or lethargy (Table 4.3).

The combination of either two, or three drugs can be employed when the dose of individual drugs exceeds their safe maximum (dapsone 300 mg, sulphapyridine 4 g and sulphamethoxypyridazine 1.5 g, daily). From our experience, it is an unproven view that dapsone is superior to sulphas in controlling the DH rash, and therefore is the drug of choice. However, sulphonamide-induced side-effects are less than with dapsone. Because of haemolysis and methaemoglobinaemia with dapsone, our practice is now not to use dapsone routinely in patients over 50 years-of-age because of the risk of inducing, or exacerbating, existing ischaemic symptoms. Thus, sulphamethoxypyridazine is preferable in such patients.

Gluten-free diet

It has been established by several centres that a gluten-free diet is effective in controlling the rash of DH. However, it is imperative to remember that for the diet to be effective, it must be strict and that its ultimate impact on the rash can only finally be assessed on average, after 2 years [48]. However, some effect on drug dosage may be seen within 3 months after the commencement of the diet, although the average is about 8 months. Lesser benefits will be achieved by those who are not strict with their diet. In a study of 42 patients taking a gluten-free diet, 23 maintained a strict gluten-free diet and 22, (96%) were able to cease taking drugs within 0.5–2.5 years (mean 2 years) while those who knowingly took gluten-containing foods (even if only once per week), were not able to discontinue their drugs [30]. In 17 patients with occasional (and presumably unintentional) lapses, eight (45%) were able to stop taking drugs within a period of 0.5–9 years (mean 3.5 years). As with coeliac patients, DH sufferers need to join their local branch of the National Coeliac Society and to have their diet supervised closely by a trained dietician.

Apart from reducing, or even removing, the need for drug treatment, a gluten-free diet often brings a subjective improvement in well-being and energy. Furthermore, strict adherence to the diet lessens the occurrence or severity of drug-induced side-effects and permits restoration of intestinal mucosal architecture. It is also likely that the diet will protect against the risk of developing lymphoma, as shown in CD [49].

It must be stressed that, in addition to the enteropathy, the rash is also *gluten driven* [30] irrespective of the intestinal abnormality (a point sometimes unappreciated not only by gastroenterologists but also by some dermatologists). Thus, benefit can be expected from the diet, including reduction of drug dosage and side effects.

Criteria for the suitability of a gluten-free diet probably vary between physicians, some of whom may feel it proper to attempt starting all patients on this course of treatment. Our view is that the diet may be inappropriate in the elderly whose rash can be adequately controlled by tablets. In addition, social and professional reasons may not allow strict adherence to the diet, and in these circumstances, drug treatment may be more suitable, provided that adequate control of the rash can be achieved without troublesome side-effects. However, because of the benefits of a gluten-free diet, all patients with DH should be offered and advised to take the diet although age, (i.e. the elderly) and social circumstances are understandable reasons for refusal.

Pathogenesis

There are two important clues regarding the nature of the skin rash in DH. Firstly, it has been shown to be gluten dependent [5,6,7,50] and secondly, that immunoglobulin A is deposited within uninvolved skin and produces a granular pattern on immunofluorescence [8].

Despite the fact that gluten withdrawal lessens the severity of the rash with time, and that gluten challenge causes an abrupt return of skin irritation and blistering, it is not known whether the presence of gluten in skin is a necessary prerequisite for the eruption to occur. Attempts to demonstrate gluten peptides within DH skin have been unsuccessful. Gluten may be surrounded by IgA antibodies thus rendering its detection by exogenous antibody impracticable. Furthermore, attempts to elute gluten from involved skin have not proved successful [51–53]. The chemicals needed to extract IgA suggest that if gluten is present, the association is not by the usual forces of attachment for immune complexes; furthermore, their use might render any gluten present antigenically 'inert' to the antigluten antibody employed for detection.

Thus, much greater interest has centred on the dermal deposits of IgA because of the associated gluten-induced enteropathy and because IgA is predominantly an antibody derived for gastrointestinal secretions. It was thus important to establish whether the IgA deposits in DH could arise from the intestine (as opposed to bone marrow). The dimeric nature of skin IgA was established [54] although in a later study [55] it was proposed that only IgA1 was demonstrable in that site, thus questioning its origin. However, more recently IgA1 and IgA2 immunoglobulins were successfully eluted from skin [51].

It has been suggested [56] that IgA is bound to reticulin fibres in the papillary dermis. Immunoelectron microscopy has indicated that IgA is associated with microfibrillar bundles and the microfibrillar component of elastic tissue [57,58]; the latter work also suggested that there may be an abnormal component in DH skin that acts as a receptor for IgA.

It is unclear whether IgA is deposited because of an affinity for some connective tissue component in DH patients, or whether it binds to gluten that has already become lodged there (for which there is no evidence) or represents IgA/gluten complexes. Unfortunately, studies of elastin have not identified any antigen to which the IgA could bind. It is conceivable that only small amounts of IgA actually bind to the skin and that larger aggregates are built up by further deposition of IgA. Given that it takes so many years of gluten withdrawal before IgA deposits finally clear from the skin (or at least are no longer detectable by immunofluorescence) [29] and reappear rapidly after gluten challenge [50] it is possible (1) that the immunoglobulin is very tightly bound to skin, and (2) that the antibody is likely to have a direct relationship to antigenic epitopes in gluten.

Since antireticulin antibodies (ARA) [59] were discovered in DH and coeliac patients, the IgA isotype antibodies correlate best with the gluten-driven nature of DH and CD. Since gluten binds to reticulin [60,61], it was thought that ARA might result from reticulin rendered immunogenic by damage caused by circulating gluten/IgA antibody complexes [56]. However, neither prevalence of circulating complexes, nor of ARA (~20%) are sufficient to suggest that IgA ARA bind to skin and lead to the rash, unless of course, antibody and complex in the circulation represent excess, and do not correlate with their presence in skin.

Another IgA class antibody reactive to endomysial smooth muscle fibres (AEMA) was described in 1983 [62]. It occurs in ~70% of all cases of DH and CD. It is seen in those with the more severe forms of enteropathy [63,64]. Like ARA, the reason for the presence of AEMA in gluten-sensitive subjects is unknown. While it may possibly reflect damage to skin components, it could also be an antibody to a dietary component that is cross reactive with certain (undefined) macromolecules of connective tissue and thus, unrelated to the pathogenesis of the skin lesions. Similar sentiments could also be attributed to availability of antigluten IgA antibodies [65,66] in DH.

Although Ig deposits other than IgA are found in DH skin, the latter (IgA) is consistently present. Some points that argue against IgA having a direct role in blister formation are its continued presence (1) in patients with spontaneous remission, and (2) in patients adhering strictly to a gluten-free diet. However, it may be necessary for additional triggers to be operative in order to place the IgA into the appropriate pathogenetic mechanism(s). Because of their localization, skin movement or friction may be necessary to initiate the inflammation related to blister formation.

In addition to IgA, the C3 component of complement has also been demonstrated by immunofluorescence in uninvolved skin [30,32] and in blisters [67]; C3 also disappears with time if a gluten-free diet is strictly followed [29]. As C3 is found in the uninvolved skin in two-thirds of patients (not receiving a gluten-free diet), it is possible it is in an inactive form such as C3d. It has been assumed that the IgA in uninvolved skin is responsible for activating complement and hence lesion formation, but that view is unlikely to be correct.

It has recently been demonstrated in our laboratory that dendritic cells collect beneath the dermoepidermal junction, at the site of IgA deposition. IgA may bind to their F_c receptors so that these cells are activated and elaborate cytokines which then initiate the inflammatory process.

Iodine and iodides

It is an interesting yet unexplained observation that potassium iodide, whether taken orally or applied to the skin, will induce lesions of DH in the previously uninvolved skin. In fact, the potassium iodide patch was often used to diagnose DH before the introduction of more specific tests. The clinical response to iodides is not seen in patients whose rash is controlled by dapsone or a gluten-free diet, even though IgA is still present in the skin [68]. The response is also negative in patients in spontaneous remission despite the presence of IgA deposits in the skin.

The skin lesions produced by iodides in DH patients are identical to the spontaneous eruption. It would appear that in some way, iodides lower the threshold for activation of the final inflammatory pathways responsible for the production of a DH lesion. This could possibly involve complement activation or the production of chemical mediators. Dapsone appears to have the opposite effect to iodides. It does not seem to influence complement deposition or activation, but more likely inhibits the synthesis, or activity of, chemical mediators involved in production of the lesion.

Prognosis

The ultimate prognosis in DH is related to the gluten sensitivity and risk of developing lymphoma. What order of 'risk' this might be has not been adequately documented in any major follow-up study.

With regard to the rash, it usually pursues a chronic course with a low rate of spontaneous remission. Based on three series of approximately 200 patients followed for a mean of 17 years (11–25), 24 remissions were observed, or 12% [16,30,69]. Nevertheless, the remission is rarely complete and may be interrupted by periods of irritation accompanied by a few skin lesions; remission on average takes about 5 years from onset of the rash. There is also a tendency for the rash to be less severe over the age of 60 irrespective of the length of previous history [14]. Detailed studies of DH from Sweden suggest a somewhat different natural history of the rash, compared with UK experiences [18,19].

Summary of pathogenesis

It is an accepted fact that both the rash and enteropathy of DH are gluten dependent. Genetic factors appear to be important in determining these abnormalities (see Chapter 8). While it is likely that the intestinal lesion is produced by a delayed hypersensitivity response against gluten [70] the mechanism(s) by which the skin lesions are produced is still poorly understood. It was originally argued that the skin lesions were produced by gluten : antigluten IgA immune complexes arising in the intestine and transported to the skin. However, contradicting this hypothesis is that in only 30% of DH patients are IgA containing complexes detectable. In addition, the IgA in the skin does not appear to be deposited in the form of an immune complex and gluten has not yet been detected, either in the skin or within circulating immune complexes. Finally, it takes on average 2 years for the rash of DH to be completely controlled with a gluten-free diet. It is unlikely that the immune complexes would persist for this length of time in the skin, once gluten was withdrawn from the diet. Possibly, a new mechanism, distinct from circulating immune complexes, should be invoked to explain the development of the skin lesions.

It has been known for many years that there is an infiltration of lymphocytes and histiocytes (macrophages) around the dermal blood vessels in DH, and these cells could play an important pathogenetic role. Gluten could be transported to the skin by macrophages to which IgA would bind. Antigen specific T cells might then be attracted by these macrophages. Two possible pathways could now be involved to recruit neutrophils into the skin to cause the eruption. First, macrophage-bound IgA can activate complement which then produces chemoattractant breakdown products for neutrophils. Second, cytokines produced by the T helper cells could also permit emigration of neutrophils from the local microvasculature, and hence into regions of gluten deposition. At least these possible mechanisms for the occurrence of skin lesions in DH are testable and hopefully might yield some new interesting clues about this condition in the near future.

However, whatever mechanism is involved in the production of skin lesions, it has to be argued why gluten sensitivity in one group of patients (CD) produces only the enteropathy, and in the other (DH), both enteropathy and skin lesions. This would seem to imply a difference in genetic factors, still to be demonstrated, or possibly an additional environmental factor, still to be identified.

References

1 Civatte A. Diagnostic histopathologique de la dermatite polymorphe douloureuse ou Maladie de Dühring-Brocq. *Ann Dermatol Syph (Paris)* 1943;3:1–30.
2 Costello M. Dermatitis herpetiformis treated with sulphapyridine. *Arch Dermatol Syph* 1940;41:134.
3 Esteves J, Brandao FN. Au sujet de l'action des sulfamides et des sulphones dans la maladie de Dühring. *Trab Soc Port Dermatol* 1950;8:209.
4 Marks J, Shuster S, Watson AJ. Small bowel changes in dermatitis herpetiformis. *Lancet* 1966;ii:1280–2.
5 Fry L, Keir P, McMinn RMH, Cowan JD, Hoffbrand AV. Small intestinal structure and function, and haematological changes in dermatitis herpetiformis. *Lancet* 1967;ii: 729–34.
6 Fry L, McMinn RMH, Cowan JD, Hoffbrand AV. Effect of gluten-free diet on dermatological, intestinal and haematological manifestations of dermatitis herpetiformis. *Lancet* 1968;i:557–61.
7 Fry L, McMinn RMH, Cowan JD, Hoffbrand AV. Gluten-free diet and re-introduction of gluten in dermatitis herpetiformis. *Arch Dermatol* 1969;100:129–35.
8 Van der Meer JB. Granular deposits of immunoglobulins in the skin of patients with dermatitis herpetiformis. An immunofluorescent study. *Br J Dermatol* 1969;81: 493–503.
9 Fry L, Seah PP. Dermatitis herpetiformis: an evaluation of diagnostic criteria. *Br J Dermatol* 1974;90:137–46.
10 Leonard JN, Haffenden GP, Ring NP *et al.* Linear IgA disease in adults. *Br J Dermatol* 1982;107:301–6.
11 Leonard JN, Griffiths CEM, Powles AV, Haffenden GP, Fry L. Experience with a gluten-free diet in the treatment of linear IgA disease. *Acta Derm Venereol* 1987;67: 145–8.
12 Sachs JA, Leonard JN, Awad J *et al.* A comparative serological and molecular study of linear IgA disease and dermatitis herpetiformis. *Br J Dermatol* 1987;118:759–64.
13 Ermacora E, Prampolini L, Tribbja G *et al.* Long term follow up of dermatitis herpetiformis in children. *J Am Acad Dermatol* 1986;15:24–30.
14 Christensen OB, Hindsen M, Svensson A. Natural history of dermatitis herpetiformis in southern Sweden. *Dermatologica* 1986; 1973:271–7.
15 Reunala T, Lokki J. Dermatitis herpetiformis in Finland. *Acta Derm Venereol* 1978;58: 505–10.
16 Gawkrodger DJ, Blackwell JN, Gilmore HM, Rifkind EA, Heading RC, Barneston RSt C. Dermatitis herpetiformis: diagnosis, diet and demography. *Gut* 1984;25:151–7.
17 Davies MG, Marks G. Dermatitis herpetiformis: a skin manifestation of a generalised disturbance in immunity. *Q J Med* 1978;186: 221–48.
18 Mobracken H, Kastrup W, Nilsson LA. Incidence and prevalence of dermatitis herpetiformis in western Sweden. *Acta Derm Venereol* 1984;64:400–4.
19 Moi H. Incidence and prevalence of dermatitis herpetiformis in a county in central Sweden, with comments on the course of the disease and IgA deposits as diagnostic criterion. *Acta Derm Venereol* 1984;64: 144–50.
20 Marsden RA, McKee PH, Bhogal B, Black MM, Kennedy LA. A study of benign chronic bullous dermatosis of childhood and comparison with dermatitis herpetiformis and bullous pemphigoid. *Clin Exp Dermatol* 1980;5:159–76.
21 Love AHG. Epidemiological and genetic aspects of the coeliac syndrome in relation to dermatitis herpetiformis. In: McConnell RB, ed. *The Genetics of Coeliac Disease.* Lancaster: MTP Press, 1981:95–9.
22 Mylotte M, Egan-Mitchell B, McCarthy CF, McNicholl B. Incidence of coeliac disease in the west of Ireland. *Br J Med* 1973;1:703–5.
23 Leonard JN. *Dermatitis herpetiformis — a*

comparison between adult patients with papillary and linear deposits of IgA. MD Thesis: University of London, 1982.
24 Nisengard RJ, Chorzelski T, Mariejowska E, Kryst L. Dermatitis herpetiformis: IgA deposits in gingiva, buccal mucosa and skin. *Oral Surgery* 1982;54:22–5.
25 Fraser NG, Kerr NW, Donald D. Oral lesions in dermatitis herpetiformis. *Br J Dermatol* 1973;89:439–50.
26 Fry L, Walkden V, Wojnarowska F, Haffenden GP, McMinn RMH. A comparison of IgA positive and IgA negative dapsone responsive dermatoses. *Br J Dermatol* 1980;103:371–82.
27 Seah PP, Fry L. Immunoglobulins in the skin in dermatitis herpetiformis and their relevance in diagnosis. *Br J Dermatol* 1975;92: 157–66.
28 Haffenden GP, Wojnarowska F, Fry L. Comparison of immunoglobulin and complement deposition in multiple biopsies from the uninvolved skin in dermatitis herpetiformis. *Br J Dermatol* 1979;101:39–45.
29 Reunala T. Gluten-free diet in dermatitis herpetiformis. *Br J Dermatol* 1978;98:69–78.
30 Fry L, Leonard JN, Swain AF, Tucker WFG, Haffenden GP, Ring NP, McMinn RMH. Long term follow up of dermatitis herpetiformis with and without dietary gluten withdrawal. *Br J Dermatol* 1982;107:631–40.
31 Fry L, Haffenden GP, Wojnarowska F, Thompson BR, Seah PP. IgA and C3 complement in the uninvolved skin in dermatitis herpetiformis after gluten withdrawal. *Br J Dermatol* 1978;99:31–7.
32 Blenkinsop WK, Fry L, Haffenden GP, Leonard JN. Histology of linear IgA disease, dermatitis herpetiformis and bullous pemphigoid. *Am J Dermatopathol* 1983;5: 547–54.
33 Brow J, Parker F, Weinstein W, Rubin CE. The small intestinal mucosa in dermatitis herpetiformis: severity and distribution of the small intestinal lesion and associated malabsorption. *Gastroenterology* 1971;60:355–61.
34 Fry L, Seah PP, Harper PG, Hoffbrand AV, McMinn RMH. The small intestine in dermatitis herpetiformis. *J Clin Pathol* 1974; 27:817–24.
35 Weinstein WM. Latent coeliac sprue. *Gastroenterology* 1973;64:489–93.
36 Weetman AP, Burrin JM, Mackay D, Leonard JN, Griffiths CEM, Fry L. The prevalence of thyroid auto-antibodies in dermatitis herpetiformis. *Br J Dermatol* 1988;118: 377–83.
37 Cunningham MJ, Zone JJ. Thyroid antibodies in dermatitis herpetiformis: prevalence of clinical thyroid disease and thyroid antibodies. *Ann Intern Med* 1985;102:194–6.
38 Gillberg R, Kastrup W, Mobacken H, Stockbrugger R, Ahren C. Gastric morphology and function in dermatitis herpetiformis and in coeliac disease. *Scand J Gastroenterol* 1985; 20:133–40.
39 Andersson H, Dotevall G, Mobacken H. Malignant mesenteric lymphoma in a patient with dermatitis herpetiformis, hypochlorhydria and small bowel abnormalities. *Scand J Gastroenterol* 1971;6:397–9.
40 Mansson T. Malignant disease in dermatitis herpetiformis. *Acta Derm Venereol* 1971;51: 379–82.
41 Goodwin P, Fry L. Reticulum cell sarcoma complicating dermatitis herpetiformis. *Proc R Soc Med* 1973;66:625–6.
42 Tonder M, Sorlie D, Keaney M. Adult coeliac disease. A case with ulceration, dermatitis herpetiformis and reticulosarcoma. *Scand J Gastroenterol* 1976;11:107–11.
43 Silk DBA, Mowat NAG, Riddell RH, Kirby JD. Intestinal lymphoma complicating dermatitis herpetiformis. *Br J Dermatol* 1977; 96:555–60.
44 Gould DJ, Howell R. Dermatitis herpetiformis and reticulum cell sarcoma, a rare complication. *Br J Dermatol* 1977;96:561–2.
45 Freeman HJ, Weinstein WM, Shritka TK, Piercy JRA, Wensel RH. Primary abdominal lymphoma. Presenting manifestation of coeliac sprue or complicating dermatitis herpetiformis. *Am J Med* 1977;63:385–94.
46 Leonard JN, Tucker WFG, Fry JS *et al.* Increased incidence of malignancy in dermatitis herpetiformis. *Br Med J* 1983;i:16–8.
47 Reunala T, Heling J, Kuokkaned K, Hakala R. Lymphoma in dermatitis herpetiformis: report of four cases. *Acta Derm Venereol* 1982;62:343–5.
48 Fry L, Seah PP, Riches DJ, Hoffbrand AV. Clearance of skin lesions in dermatitis herpetiformis after gluten withdrawal. *Lancet* 1973;i:288–91.
49 Holmes GKT, Prior P, Lane MR, Pope W, Allan RN. Malignancy in coeliac disease — effect of a gluten-free diet. *Gut* 1989;30: 333–8.
50 Leonard JN, Haffenden GP, Tucker W *et al.* Gluten challenge in dermatitis herpetiformis. *N Engl J Med* 1983;308:816–19.
51 Jones P, Kumar V, Beutner EH, Chorzelski TP. A simple method for elution of IgA

deposits from the skin of patients with dermatitis herpetiformis. *Arch Dermatol Res* 1989;281:406–10.
52 Egelrud T, Back O. Dermatitis herpetiformis: biochemical properties of the granular deposits of IgA in papillary dermis. Characterisation of SDS soluble IgA-like material and potentially antigen-binding IgA fragments released by pepsin. *J Invest Dermatol* 1985;84:239–45.
53 Meyer LJ, Carioto L, Zone JJ. Dermatitis herpetiformis: Extraction of intact IgA from granular deposits in dermal papillae. *J Invest Dermatol* 1987;88:559–63.
54 Unsworth DJ, Payne AW, Leonard JN, Fry L, Holborow EJ. IgA in dermatitis herpetiformis skin is dimeric. *Lancet* 1982;i:478–80.
55 Olbricht SM, Flotte TJ, Collins AB, Chapman CM, Harrist TJ. Dermatitis herpetiformis: cutaneous deposition of polyclonal IgA1. *Arch Dermatol* 1986;122:418–21.
56 Seah PP, Fry L, Stewart JS, Chapman BL, Hoffbrand AV, Holborow EJ. Immunoglobulins in the skin in dermatitis herpetiformis and coeliac disease. *Lancet* 1972;i: 611–14.
57 Stingl G, Honigsmann H, Holubar K, Wolff K. Ultrastructural localisation of immunoglobulins in skin of patients with dermatitis herpetiformis. *J Invest Dermatol* 1976;67: 507–12.
58 Yaoito H. Indentification of IgA binding structures in skin of patients with dermatitis herpetiformis. *J Invest Dermatol* 1978;71: 213–16.
59 Seah PP, Fry L, Hoffbrand AV, Holborow EJ. Tissue antibodies in dermatitis herpetiformis and coeliac disease. *Lancet* 1971;ii:834–6.
60 Unsworth DJ, Johnson GD, Haffenden GP, Fry L, Holborow EJ. Binding of wheat gliadin *in vitro* to reticulin in normal and dermatitis herpetiformis skin. *J Invest Dermatol* 1981; 76:88–93.
61 Unsworth DJ, Leonard JN, Hobday DM *et al.* Gliadins bind to reticulin in a lectin-like manner. *Arch Dermatol Res* 1987;279: 232–5.
62 Chorzelski TP, Sulej J, Tchorzewska H, Jablonska S, Beutner EH, Kumar V. IgA class endomysium antibodies in dermatitis herpetiformis and coeliac disease. *Ann NY Acad Sci* 1983;420:325–34.
63 Sulej J, Leonard JN. Anti-endomysial antibodies in dermatitis herpetiformis and coeliac disease In: Chorzelski TP, Kumar VJ, eds. *Immunopathology of the Skin.* New York: Wiley, 1987:477–82.
64 Leonard JN, Chorzelski TP, Beutner EH *et al.* IgA anti-endomysial antibody detection in the serum of patients with dermatitis herpetiformis following gluten challenge. *Arch Dermatol Res* 1985;277:349–51.
65 Unsworth DJ, Leonard JN, McMinn RMH, Swain AF, Holborow EJ, Fry L. Anti-gliadin antibodies and small intestinal mucosal damage in dermatitis herpetiformis. *Br J Dermatol* 1981;105:653–8.
66 Kilander AF, Gillberg RE, Kastrup W, Mobacken H, Nilsson LA. Serum antibodies to gliadin and intestinal morphology in dermatitis herpetiformis. *Scand J Gastroenterol* 1985;20:951–8.
67 Seah PP, Fry L, Mazaheri MR, Mowbray JF, Hoffbrand AV, Holborow EJ. Alternate pathway complement fixation by IgA in the skin in dermatitis herpetiformis. *Lancet* 1973;ii:175–7.
68 Haffenden GP, Blenkinsop WK, Ring NP, Wojnarowska F, Fry L. The potassium iodide patch tests in dermatitis herpetiformis in relation to treatment with a gluten-free diet and dapsone. *Br J Dermatol* 1980;102:313–17.
69 Alexander JO'D. *Dermatitis Herpetiformis.* London: WB Saunders, 1975:28–9.
70 Marsh MN. Studies of intestinal lymphoid tissue. XI. The immunopathology of cell-mediated reactions in gluten-sensitivity and other enteropathies. *Scanning Microsc* 1988; 2:1663–84.

Chapter 5/Malignancy as a complication of coeliac disease

GEOFFREY K.T. HOLMES AND
HENRY THOMPSON

Historical background

The early literature on malabsorption records that patients often died of malignancy, particularly lymphoma [1]. Lehmkuhl in 1927 [2] and Golden in 1936 [3] reported patients with lymphosarcoma of the small intestine and malabsorption, and speculated that this was due to infiltration of the gut with tumour. On the other hand Fairley and Mackie in 1937 [4] and Salvesen and Kobro in 1939 [5] considered that enlarged mesenteric glands, by obstructing the lymphatics, were the main cause of malabsorption. Subsequently, many patients with lymphoma in association with steatorrhoea were reported [6–12].

In papers up to 1961 the steatorrhoea, in every case, was considered secondary to lymphoma. In 1962 however, Gough *et al.* [13] suggested that lymphoma is a complication of coeliac disease (CD) and that the mucosal lesion is a pre-malignant condition. Further work from this group strengthened their hypothesis [14] which was also supported by additional evidence from Birmingham [15].

It then became evident that other malignant tumours occur in CD; Harris *et al.* [15] called attention to the increased frequency of gastrointestinal cancer in general, and carcinoma of the oesophagus, in particular. Carcinoma of the upper small bowel in association with CD was first reported from the Massachusetts General Hospital in 1958 [16] and is now known to be the second most common invasive malignancy after lymphoma [17].

Lymphoma as a complication of CD

Much that is known about malignancy in CD is reviewed in this chapter, but there is still much to unravel and many contentious issues which are also addressed. Lymphoma at presentation is usually widespread and the prognosis is very poor, although occasionally a tumour obstructing the small intestine can be resected successfully. In view of this poor outlook, can the diagnosis of lymphoma be made earlier to allow more effective treatment and so improve the prognosis? A gluten-free diet has a dramatic beneficial effect on the health of patients with CD and so a more fundamental question is whether strict adherence to the diet offers protection against the development of malignant complications. What type of lymphoma occurs and is it specific to CD? What is the relationship between chronic ulceration of the small bowel and lymphoma or a flat small intestinal mucosa and lymphoma? All these questions are considered in this section.

Prevalence

Many reports where CD is complicated by lymphoma have appeared since 1961 [1]. Larger series have allowed an assessment of prevalence, but the precise frequency of malignancy is unknown for several reasons: (1) the incidence of CD in the general population is uncertain since many patients without symptoms or only mild upset may never present or have the diagnosis established; (2) if post-mortem examinations are not performed, the presence of malignancy, and particularly of lymphoma, will be underestimated; and (3) seven patients with primary abdominal lymphoma were subsequently found to have CD [18]. Such patients with overt lymphoma are not usually subjected to small intestinal biopsy, so that CD may not be detected and thus its association with malignancy underestimated.

Nevertheless, despite these reservations, information is available for the prevalence of malignancy among groups of patients followed up for many years. Harris *et al.* [15] defined a series of 202 patients with CD or idiopathic steatorrhoea diagnosed between 1941 and 1965 in Birmingham and found that 27 of 77 deaths were attributable to cancer, 14 being due to lymphoma; altogether, 32 malignancies occurred. This same series was reviewed at the end of 1975 when four more lymphomas had arisen, making 18 (9%) for the whole group out of a total of 43 cancers [19]. A series of 210 patients with biopsy proven CD who had attended the General Hospital, Birmingham, was analysed with regard to malignant complications [20]. Of 21 deaths, 13 were due to lymphoma when the expected was 0.1 (Table 5.1). A cancer morbidity study of these same 210 patients showed the relative risk of developing lymphoma compared with the general population was about 40 (Table 5.2) [20]. Of 74 coeliac patients diagnosed in Sweden between 1965 and 1977, five developed lymphoma (7%) [21]. In Galway, an area with a high prevalence of CD, 16 patients with malignant complications were seen between 1969 and 1981 of whom 10 had lymphoma [22]. During these years 198 coeliac patients over the age of 12 years were diagnosed so the proportion who developed malignancy was 8%. Selby and Gallagher [23] recognized malignancy in 10 of 93 patients (11%) seen between 1958 and 1978. Five of these had oesophageal cancer and four lymphoma. In a further series of 100 patients followed for 18 years, malignancy was confirmed in eight and suspected in another three [24]. In a

Table 5.1 Deaths due to malignancy among 210 patients with CD [19]

Group	Observed	Expected	Probability
Total group (*n* = 210)			
All malignancies	21	5.048	<0.001
Lymphoma	13	0.114	<0.001
Cancer of the oesophagus	2	0.098	<0.01
Cancer of the pharynx	2	0.027	<0.001
Men (*n* = 94)			
All malignancies	12	2.878	<0.001
Lymphoma	6	0.062	<0.001
Cancer of the oesophagus	2	0.053	<0.01
Cancer of the pharynx	2	0.013	<0.001
Women (*n* = 116)			
All malignancies	9	2.170	<0.001
Lymphoma	7	0.052	<0.001
Cancer of the oesophagus	0	0.045	NS
Cancer of the pharynx	0	0.014	NS

Table 5.2 Cancer morbidity in 210 patients with CD [20]

Site of cancer	ICD* 8	Observed number	Expected number	Observed : expected number of tumours	Probability
All sites	140–208	31	15.48	2.0	<0.001
Mouth and pharynx	140–147	3	0.31	9.7	<0.01
Oesophagus	150	3	0.24	12.3	<0.01
Non-Hodgkin's lymphoma	200, 202	9	0.21	42.7	<0.001
Gastrointestinal tract	151–154	3	3.07	1.0	NS
Remainder		13	11.65	1.1	NS

* International Classification of Disease (8th edn).

cohort of 653 patients with CD in Edinburgh and the Lothian region of Scotland of whom 115 were dead, 20 were certified as having lymphoma and in 17 this was listed as the cause of death [25]. Of 77 deaths among members of the Coeliac Society, 31 were due to malignancy of which 10 resulted from lymphoma [26].

Age and sex incidence

The diagnosis of lymphoma is made almost exclusively in adult life. Although a report of this occurrence in a child with CD has appeared [27], further studies revealed the tumour was a B cell lymphoma and

Table 5.3 Diagnosis of lymphoma in relation to diagnosis of CD

Age at diagnosis of CD (years)		Age at diagnosis of lymphoma (years)		Length of coeliac history preceding diagnosis of lymphoma (years)		Interval between the diagnosis of CD and diagnosis of lymphoma (years)		
Mean	Range	Mean	Range	Mean	Range	Mean	Range	Reference
51	32–71	55	35–82	15	0.5–60	5	0–20	[28]
58	54–63	61	56–65	9	3–21	3	0.5–6	[21]
43	29–64	47	29–64	11	2–26	4	2–7	[23]

Table 5.4 Sex incidence of malignancy in CD

	Total patients	Male	Female	Reference
Lymphoma	27	15	12	[28]
Carcinoma	25	16	9	
Lymphoma	4	1	3	[23]
Carcinoma (oesophagus)	5	1	4	
Lymphoma	5	3	2	[21]
Lymphoma	17	8	9	[25]
Carcinoma (oesophagus)	4	1	3	
Carcinoma (small bowel)	29	21	8	See p. 122

hence to be unassociated with CD (see p. 36). While the diagnosis can be made under the age of 30 [23,29] or 40 years [28,30] in three other series the mean age was 61 [21], 47 [23] and 55 years [28] (Table 5.3). Although CD is more common in women [31], the numbers of men and women affected with lymphoma are similar, which is unlike adenocarcinoma of the small bowel which has, for unknown reasons, a marked male preponderance (Table 5.4).

Symptoms and signs

The diagnosis of lymphoma arising on a background of CD is difficult and may be delayed because the presenting features are often non-specific and indistinguishable from uncomplicated CD itself, either at presentation or in relapse. In most patients the tumour is widely disseminated at diagnosis and the prognosis is correspondingly poor. The diagnosis was only made at autopsy in one-third of cases in one series, and at laparotomy in a further one-third [28].

The most common presenting symptoms are weight loss, lethargy, diarrhoea and abdominal pain (Fig. 5.1). A striking symptom which afflicts about one-half of patients is profound weakness which affects voluntary muscles and gradually becomes more marked as the illness progresses, thus severely impairing walking and other motor functions. Apart from lymphoma, marked muscle weakness is usually only seen in coeliac patients with osteomalacia [32] or neuropathy [33]. In the majority of patients the illness is insidious although some present acutely, for example, with intestinal perforation or obstruction [34], haemorrhage from a bowel tumour, or with an opportunistic infection [29]. The early signs are also often vague and non-specific (Fig. 5.2), although the presence of unexplained fever should always arouse suspicion. Lymphadenopathy and hepatomegaly occur late and indicate widespread malignancy. Thus, muscle weakness, pyrexia and lymphadenopathy are useful and important pointers to the presence of lymphoma, for these features are unusual or otherwise only rarely encountered in CD [35–37].

Some unusual manifestations of coeliac lymphoma may be encountered. Mycosis fungoides d'emblee corresponds to skin lymphomatous deposits appearing rapidly in association with coeliac lymphoma, but without the characteristic preceding history of skin rash which occurs in true mycosis fungoides. Pautrier microabscesses

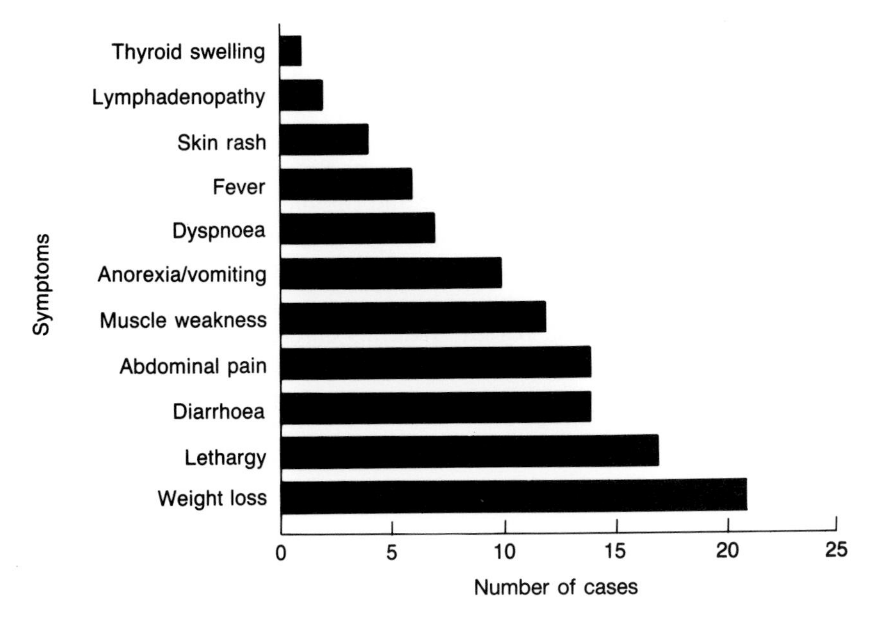

Fig. 5.1 Coeliac lymphoma. Presenting symptoms in 27 patients.

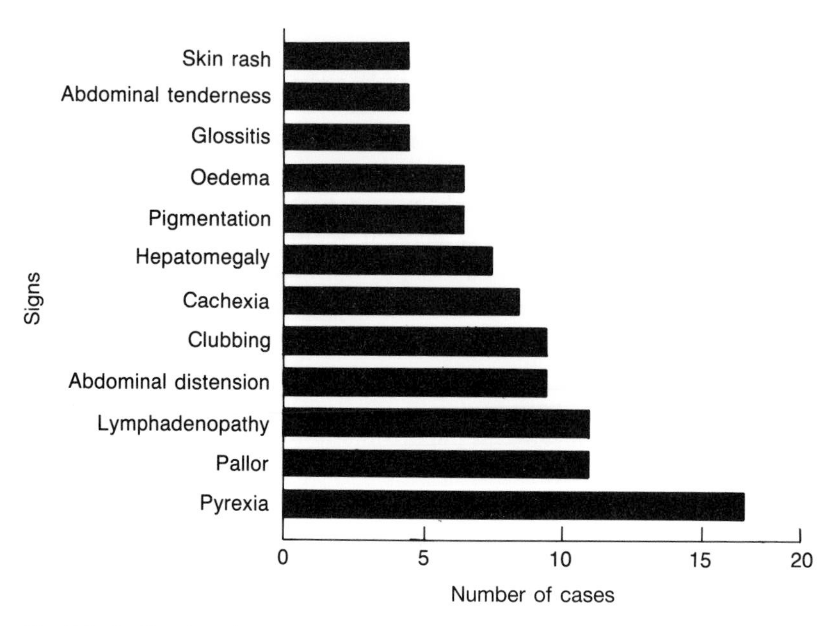

Fig. 5.2 Coeliac lymphoma. Presenting signs in 27 patients.

can occur presumably because this is a T cell lymphoma, although it is gut- rather than skin-orientated [38]; one such patient at The General Hospital, Birmingham, died rapidly. Raynaud's phenomenon and digital gangrene, haemolytic anaemia and disseminated intravascular coagulation are other rare manifestations of malignant lymphomas which we have encountered.

Coeliac patients with malignancy may present in one of two ways. There are patients with well-established CD who have responded to a gluten-free diet but then deteriorate because of the development of lymphoma. In others, who may or may not have a history compatible with CD, the demonstration of a flat jejunal biopsy and the diagnosis of lymphoma occur more or less at the same time [19,25]. There is considerable evidence to indicate that the latter group are gluten sensitized and do have CD, as discussed below.

Finally, the newly diagnosed coeliac patient requires careful observation for in one study [39] one in 20 patients developed lymphoma within 4 years of the diagnosis; over the age of 50 years, the risk was increased to one in 10 [39].

Diagnosis

Laboratory data

Many haematological and biochemical abnormalities occur in patients with lymphoma, but no pattern emerges which permits early diagnosis [29]. A progressive rise in serum IgA levels is sometimes seen but this is of little value as raised levels may also be found in uncomplicated coeliac patients [40]. Increased levels of lysozyme were observed in malignant histiocytosis but this is not a reliable indicator of coeliac lymphoma [41–43]. Reduced responses of lymphocytes from coeliac patients with lymphoma to phytohaemagglutinin were found in one small study [44] but poor responses also occur in uncomplicated patients, particularly those taking a normal diet [45].

Small intestinal mucosal biopsy

Changes in the inflammatory cell infiltrate of the small intestinal mucosa have been described in those patients who eventually develop malignancy, and which differ quantitatively from those who do not [46,47]. These consist of lower plasma cell counts and higher lymphocyte counts in the lamina propria and lower lymphocyte counts in the epithelium compared with biopsies from untreated coeliac patients. Comment has also been made on the presence of hypoplastic crypts [48] and histiocytic aggregates [49]. Prospective studies, however, have never been mounted and these observations, even if true, are unlikely to be helpful in the individual case.

Radiology

A radiological examination of the intestinal tract may be carried out if lymphoma is suspected but will not always reveal the diagnosis. Of examinations in 15 patients at presentation, 10 showed an uncomplicated malabsorption pattern, although five were subsequently found to have small gut involvement. Lymphoma of the stomach producing stenotic lesions may prevent adequate visualization of the more distal bowel so that lesions there may remain undetected. Multiple, irregular, narrowed segments are characteristic of small bowel lymphoma (Fig. 5.3) but this pattern is not commonly seen [29].

Endoscopy

CD may be diagnosed reliably by endoscopic small bowel biopsy and is now the preferred method [50,51]. The technique allows inspection of the upper gastrointestinal tract and the opportunity to diagnose other abnormalities, particularly tumours. Lymphoma of the stomach has been diagnosed in this way [52] and an early malignant lesion of the duodenum, probably a primitive lymphoma, was also detected and successfully treated [53].

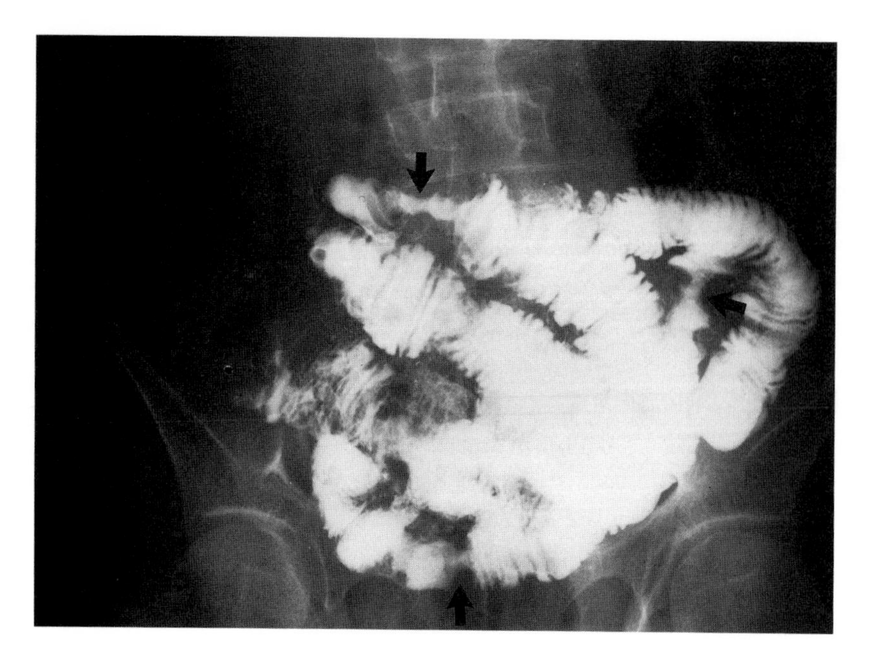

Fig. 5.3 Strictures in the small bowel due to lymphoma (arrows); two in the mid-abdomen and one in the left iliac fossa. The mucosa is destroyed and the lumen is irregular. (With permission of Churchill Livingstone.)

Ultrasound and computed tomographic scanning

These techniques have the potential to detect abnormalities of bowel and abdominal lymph nodes [54,55] but how useful they will be in the diagnosis of coeliac lymphoma is still to be determined. Scanning, however, may reveal mesenteric lymph node enlargement or cavitation in a patient with abdominal masses thought clinically to be due to malignancy [56].

Laparotomy

It may be necessary to resort to laparotomy when suspicion of malignant lymphoma is high and other approaches have failed to make a firm diagnosis [29]. This can be a difficult decision to make in an ill patient and must not be left so late that the patient is unable to withstand surgery. When cancer is found it is usually widespread, although occasionally it is possible to perform a curative operation especially when a localized bowel lymphoma is present (Fig. 5.4).

Pathology

The lymphomas in the Bristol and Birmingham series were originally classified in terms of intestinal reticulosis, reticulum cell sarcoma or

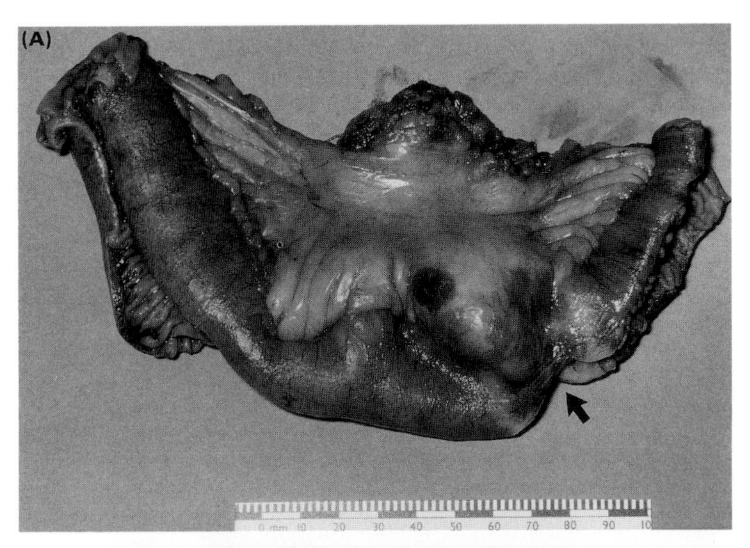

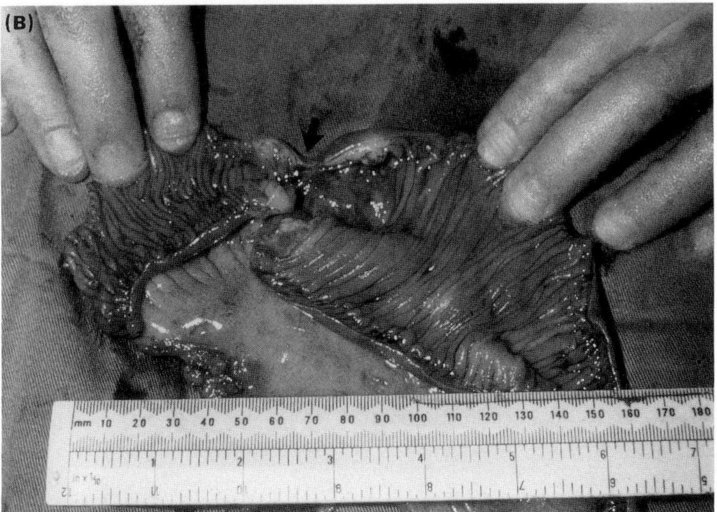

Fig. 5.4 Lymphoma confined to the jejunum in CD. This single lesion was resected and the patient remains healthy 5 years later. (A) external and (B) internal appearances.

Hodgkin's disease, in line with the classification system then in use. Taylor [57] suggested that the lymphoma originated from B lymphocytes since the tumour cells displayed surface immunoglobulins. Henry and Farrer Brown [58] also believed that the tumours were of B cell origin because of their plasmacytoid appearance and ultrastructural morphology. Isaacson and Wright [59] and Isaacson *et al.* [60,61] classified the lymphoma as malignant histiocytosis of the intestine based on morphological, immunological and histochemical considerations. The tumour cells did not appear to be of T cell origin but reacted with the histiocytic marker α_1-antitrypsin.

However, with the development of a wide range of monoclonal antibodies which allowed more accurate typing of malignant lymphoma and the use of DNA hybridization techniques, it became clear that the tumours were of T cell origin [62], a contention supported by others [63,64]. This makes more sense than derivation from histiocytes, because T cells are abundant in the small intestinal mucosa and may be involved in the development of the various mucosal lesions seen in CD [65,66], while malignant transformation of such cells would result in lymphoma. In this context, the observations of Isaacson *et al.* [67], Spencer *et al.* [68] and Stein *et al.* [69] are of interest. They demonstrated that a monoclonal antibody, HML-1, developed against intraepithelial lymphocytes (IEL) [70] also stains the cells of the T cell lymphoma which complicates CD. Alfsen *et al.* [71] reported a patient with low-grade intestinal lymphoma of IEL with concomitant enteropathy associated T cell lymphoma (EATL). The intraepithelial tumour cells represented small cell lymphoma which stained with HML-1 monoclonal antibody. The presence of two tumours suggests the possibility that EATL derives from IEL and that the small cell lymphoma arising from IEL represents an intermediate stage in the development of the large cell tumour. An epitheliotropic lymphoma has been reported in one patient with intractable malabsorption [72].

These cases, therefore, broaden the clinical and morphological spectrum of intestinal T cell disorders. However, according to Pallesen and Hamilton-Dutoit [73] HML-1 is not an absolutely specific or sensitive marker since it occasionally reacts with other peripheral T cell lymphomas while some enteropathy lymphomas have nil, or poor, expression. It is still uncertain whether these lymphomas derive either from IEL or lamina propria lymphocytes, although the fact that tumour cells react with HML-1 favours the former.

Site and gross appearance

In the Birmingham series the majority of lymphomas were located in the jejunum, but they also occurred in the ileum, lymph nodes and less commonly, in the stomach and colon. Occasionally, patients present with the primary tumour apparently involving the thyroid, liver, peripheral lymph nodes or some other extragastrointestinal site. The tumours occur as solitary or multiple circumferential ulcerating lesions (Figs 5.5, 5.6) or as mucosal plaques or nodules (Figs 5.7, 5.8). Very rarely they present as solid lesions forming a discrete tumour mass extending outside the wall of the gastrointestinal tract. Perforation is a well-recognized complication that is associated with generalized or localized peritonitis, with abscess formation (Figs 5.6, 5.9). Metastatic

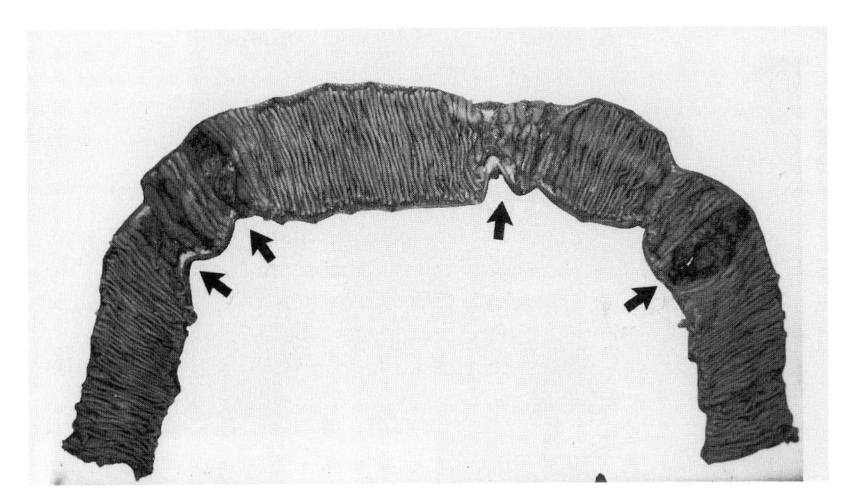

Fig. 5.5 Segment of small intestine showing circumferential ulcerated lesions (arrows) due to lymphoma complicating CD.

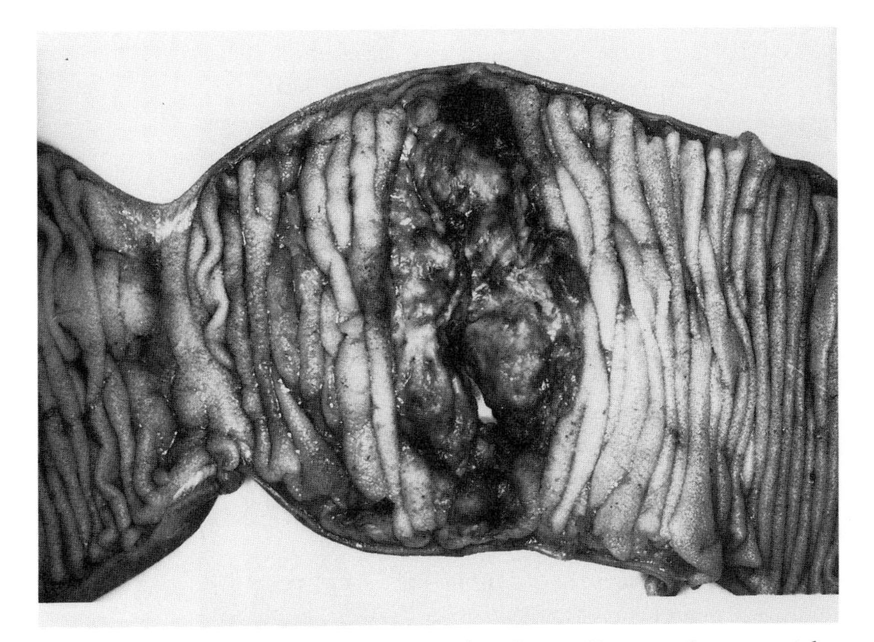

Fig. 5.6 Perforated ulcerated tumour due to lymphoma. Close up of extreme right-hand lesion seen in Fig. 5.5.

tumour may be present in mesenteric, abdominal and occasionally other lymph nodes including those in the neck and axilla. Deposits may be present in the liver, spleen and bone marrow, and particularly of the vertebrae and long bones. Other organs such as the thyroid or adrenals may occasionally and unexpectedly be involved.

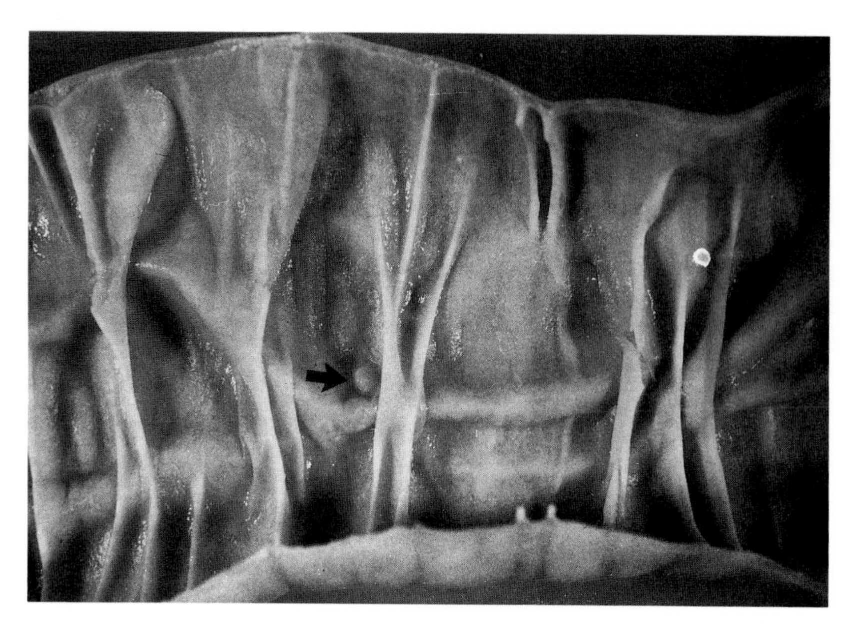

Fig. 5.7 Intact nodule of malignant lymphoma in CD.

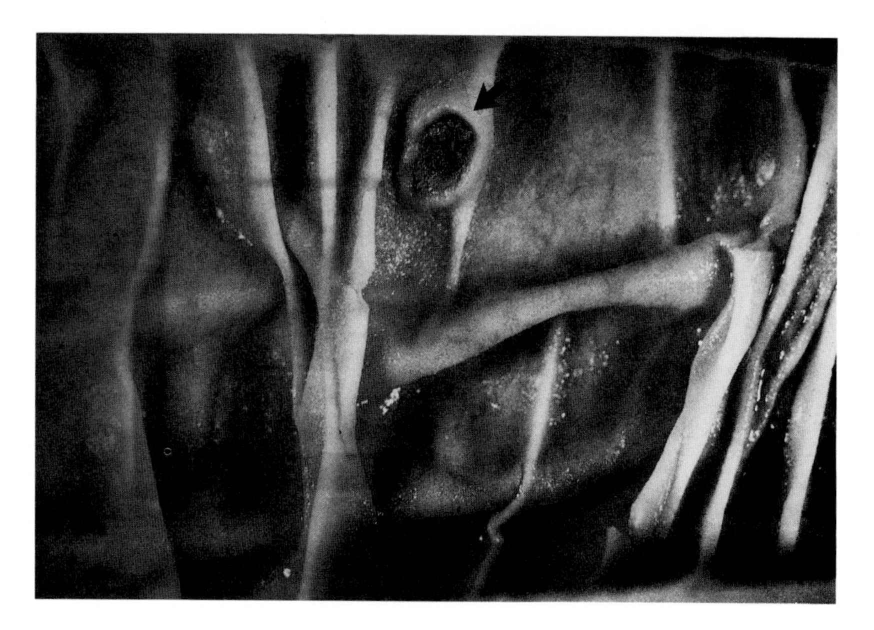

Fig. 5.8 Ulcerated nodule of lymphoma in CD.

Histology

The histological appearance of these lymphoid tumours is variable. Pleomorphic neoplastic lymphoid cells of a high grade and large cell

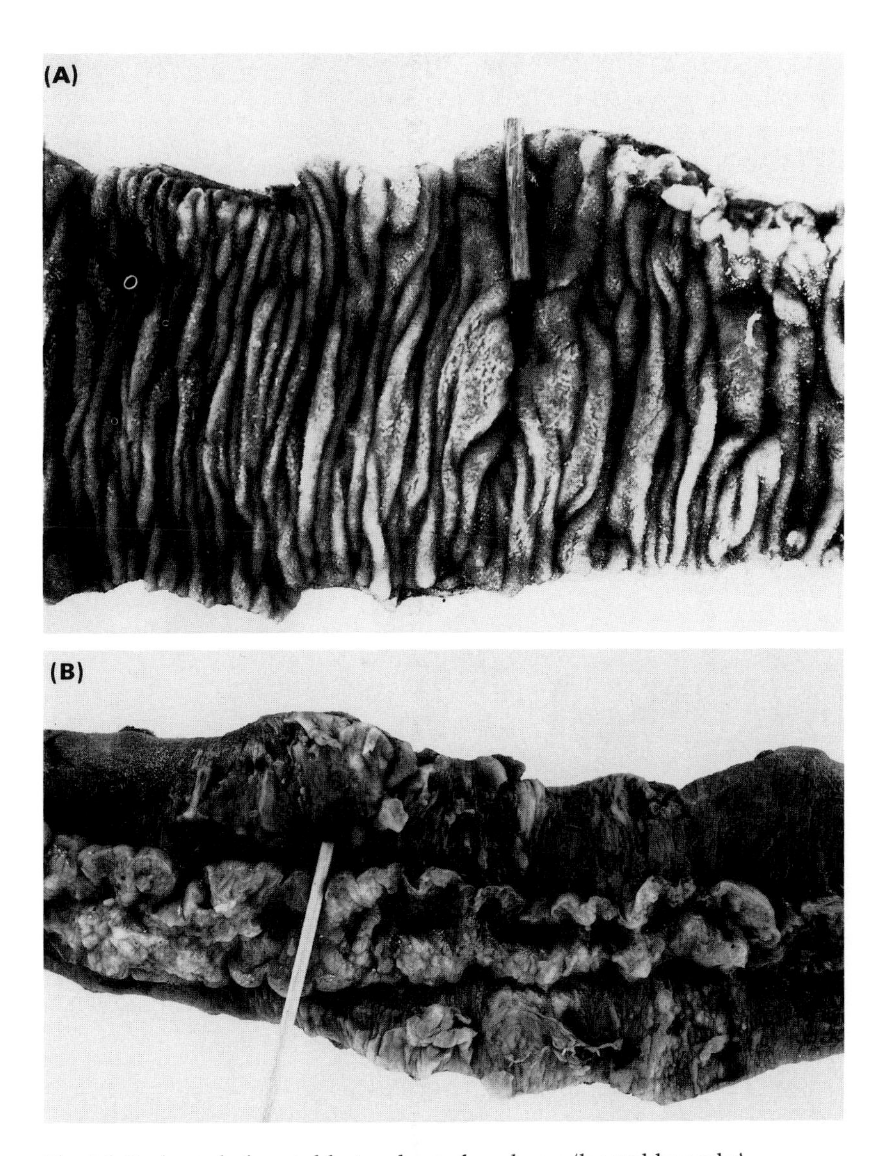

Fig. 5.9 Perforated ulcerated lesion due to lymphoma (located by probe). (A) mucosal surface and (B) serosal aspect.

type predominate (Fig. 5.10) while multinucleated cells resembling Reed–Sternberg cells are present in many cases, such that the histological features are not unlike Hodgkin's disease (Fig. 5.11). The lymphoma cells may have a plasmacytoid appearance (Fig. 5.12). Mitoses and disintegration of nuclei are prominent. Necrosis and inflammatory cell infiltration are frequently observed with reactive neutrophils, plasma cells, B lymphocytes, eosinophils, macrophages and histiocytes. Lymphoma extends diffusely through all layers of the bowel. Fibrosis

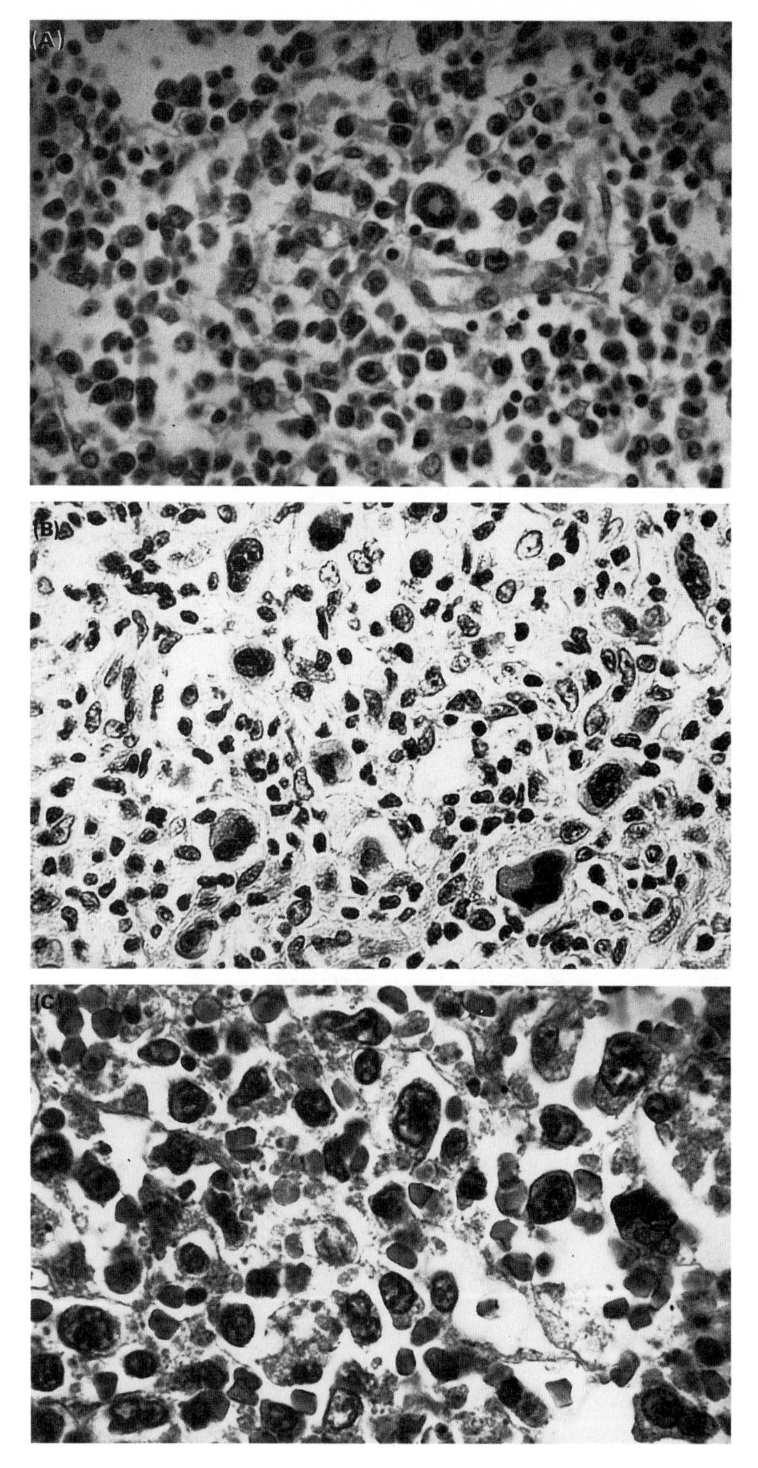

Fig. 5.10 (A) pleomorphic T cell lymphoma complicating CD (low power magnification); (B) with several multinucleated and polylobed nuclei (high power magnification); (C) with immature cell nuclei (high power magnification).

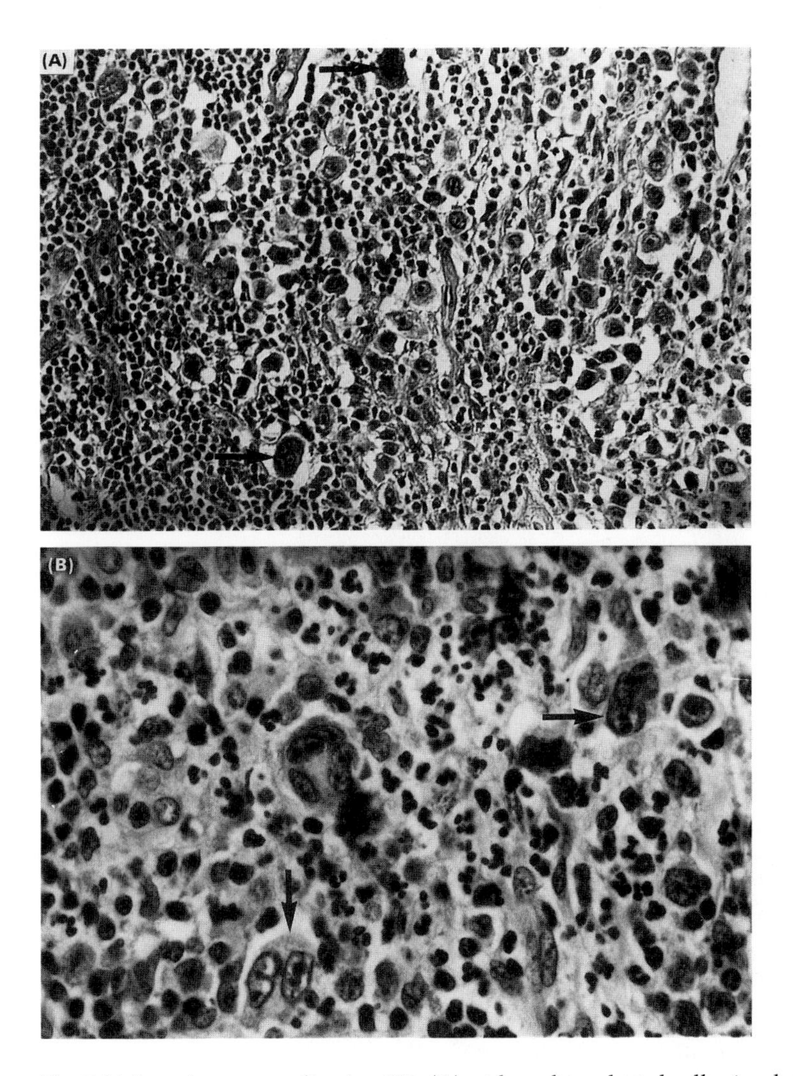

Fig. 5.11 Lymphoma complicating CD: (A) with multinucleated cells simulating Hodgkin's disease in a cervical lymph node; (B) Reed–Sternberg cells in same node (high power magnification).

is found but is not a prominent feature. Vascular invasion with necrosis of vessels may occur. Erythrophagocytosis may be encountered but it probably involves reactive macrophages and histiocytes rather than neoplastic cells. Malignant nodes show sinusoidal infiltration and loss of architecture with cells extending outside the capsule. In some cases the histological diagnosis of malignant lymphoma can be exceedingly difficult.

Occasionally, at autopsy, there is no gross evidence of tumour tissue but malignancy may be present as microscopic foci which can only be identified by painstaking histological examination. Tumour

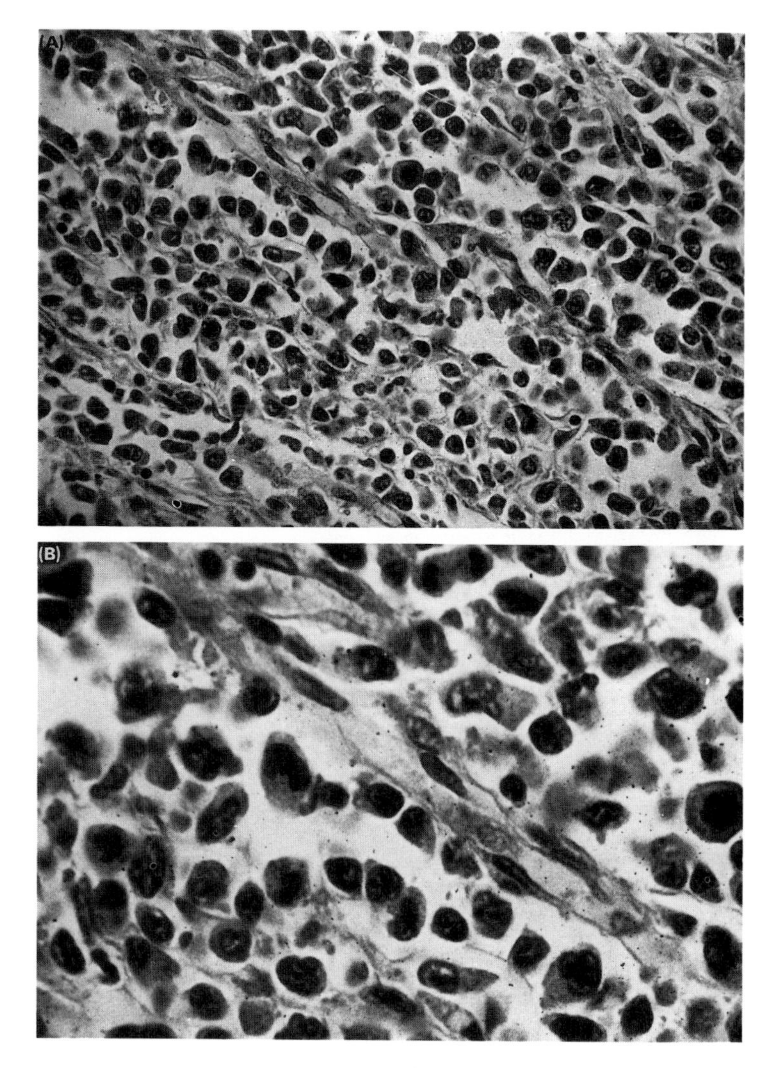

Fig. 5.12 Lymphoma with plasmacytoid features complicating CD: (A) low power magnification and (B) high power magnification.

deposits may be present, for example, in the liver, spleen and bone marrow but only detected microscopically. In two of our cases no gross evidence of tumour or ulceration was found in the bowel yet two foci of lymphoma were identified histologically in the lamina propria of the jejunal mucosa.

Lymphadenopathy

Whitehead [74] claimed that lymphomas arise from cellular elements in the lamina propria of the bowel wall and regional lymph nodes, through a stage of progressive hyperplasia of reticuloendothelial lymphoid tissue. Mesenteric lymphadenopathy does occur in CD [75–77] and it is conceivable that malignant lymphoma cells emerge from this hyperplastic state. Horowitz and Shiner [78] studied five fatal cases of presumed CD and three with terminal lymphoma. They identified occasional abnormal cells with features suspicious of malignancy by electron microscopic examination. We have noted mesenteric lymphadenopathy in a number of our patients but this has not caused problems in differential diagnosis. It is possible that the diagnosis of early lymphoma may be overlooked in patients with mesenteric lymphadenopathy by histopathologists with relatively little experience in lymphoma pathology. The diagnosis can be made, however, by lymphoma experts with the use of sensitive immunocytochemical techniques.

Treatment and prognosis

Surgery, radiotherapy and chemotherapy may be used in suitable cases depending on the pathological staging. If the disease is confined to the intestine the affected segment (or segments) will usually be resected with good prognosis, many patients surviving for more than 5 years [17]. Unfortunately, in the majority of cases, lymphoma is widespread at diagnosis and the outlook is very poor so that few patients survive for longer than 1 year [17,29,30].

Carcinoma as a complication of CD

Carcinoma occurs in patients with CD much as in the general population and the clinical features and prognosis are often very similar [29]. However, certain gastrointestinal carcinomas, notably those of the mouth, pharynx and oesophagus [15,19,20,23,25] and of the small intestine [17] occur more commonly than expected. The site and type of tumour largely determine the presentation and outlook, but in addition, the development of cancer may exacerbate, or provoke symptoms of CD itself. Thus, patients who relapse unexpectedly after a period of good health on a gluten-free diet, or who do not respond to gluten withdrawal from the outset, will require careful assessment from this point of view.

Carcinoma of the small intestine

Until recently carcinoma of the small intestine was thought to be a rare phenomenon. In a review in 1980 [79], only 14 cases could be found in the literature and it was commented that: 'it is perhaps surprising that there are so few reports of carcinoma occurring in coeliac disease, as this part of the bowel is characteristically abnormal in untreated patients and may show features of malignancy'. In a later British collaborative study [17], 19 patients with small intestinal carcinoma were discovered, thus making this the second most common invasive malignancy after lymphoma. This observation illustrates the value of pooling results from many centres. At present there are 23 patients reported in some detail in the literature [16,80–99] and the authors of this chapter have personal experience of a further six, bringing the total series to 29 patients for consideration, as outlined below.

Age and sex incidence

Although this type of tumour may arise in relatively young adults the mean age at presentation is 59 years which is similar to that of lymphoma. Unlike lymphoma, however, there is a marked male preponderance with 21 or the 29 patients being men, although why this should be is not clear (Table 5.4).

Symptoms and signs

An analysis of presentation in the 29 cases is shown in Fig. 5.13. Anaemia is common and often associated with gastrointestinal blood loss either overt or occult. Weight loss, abdominal pain and intestinal obstruction are also prominent features. The presence of an abdominal mass suggests carcinoma rather than lymphoma [29] and intestinal

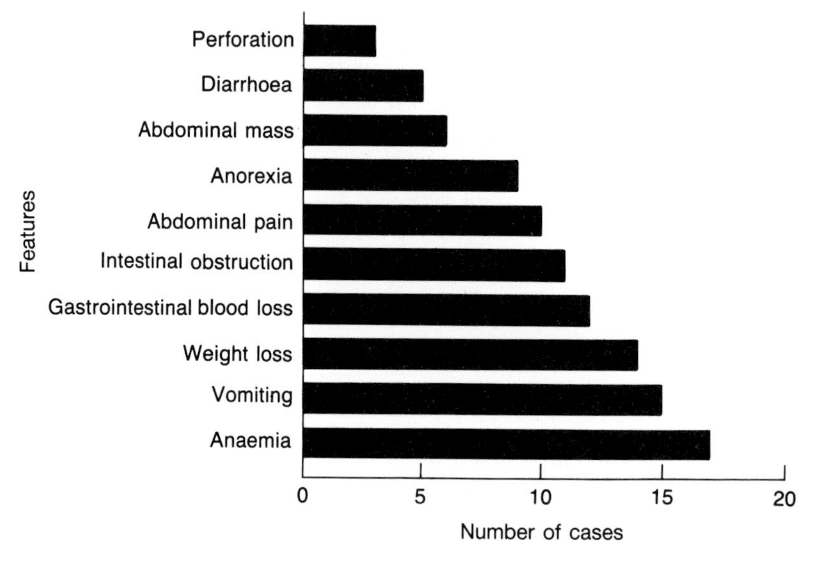

Fig. 5.13 Presenting features of 29 patients with carcinoma of the upper small intestine as a complication of CD.

perforation may occur. The profound muscle weakness which accompanies lymphoma is not seen.

Diagnosis

Laboratory data

There is little in routine blood tests of particular significance although anaemia which is sometimes severe is commonly found. The major contributing factor appears to be blood loss into the bowel. It is essential to test for the presence of blood in the stools of all patients suspected to have this diagnosis.

Radiology

In contrast to lymphomatous involvement of the bowel where radiology may be unhelpful, barium studies are most reliable for detecting small intestinal cancer, for the lesion can usually be seen (Fig. 5.14) or its presence inferred from features suggesting intestinal obstruction.

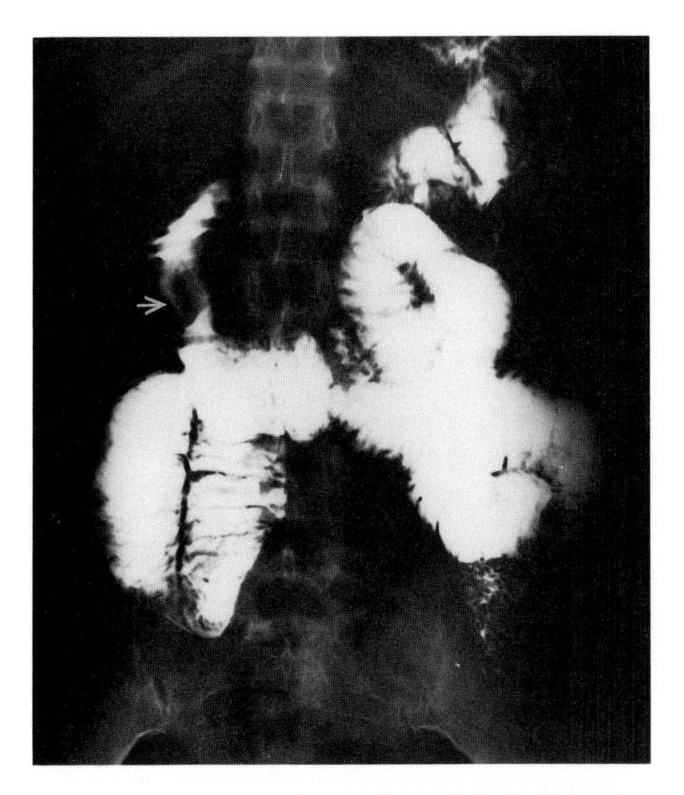

Fig. 5.14 A carcinoma in the second part of the duodenum in a patient with CD. This lesion was seen and biopsied with a fibreoptic endoscope. (With permission of Churchill Livingstone and R. Cockel.)

Endoscopy

This technique, performed with standard instruments, is being used increasingly in the diagnosis of CD and also allows inspection of the upper gastrointestinal tract for other abnormalities including malignancy (Fig. 5.14). Unfortunately, only very proximal lesions can be seen but inspection of the duodenum to the limit of the instrument should always be attempted. Whether the technique of fibreoptic enteroscopy [100] will facilitate the diagnosis of more distal tumours remains to be determined.

Treatment and prognosis

Good long-term survival may result if diagnosis is early and the tumour is resectable. Of the 29 patients cited above, 14 were progressing well after surgery at the time of the report and of these, seven had survived over 2 years and two, over 17 years.

Malignancy in other gluten-sensitive groups

Dermatitis herpetiformis

The majority of patients with dermatitis herpetiformis (DH) have abnormalities in the small intestinal biopsy which are similar to those found in CD, while others may have early [101] or latent mucosal lesions [102]. In view of this, an increased frequency of malignancy might be expected and this has indeed been reported on many occasions [103]. A retrospective survey of 109 patients followed at one centre from 1969 to the end of 1981 found that seven had developed malignant tumours of which three were lymphomas, giving a relative risk of 100 [104]. It is important that all patients with DH are referred for small intestinal biopsy and receive a gluten-free diet to improve general health, benefit the rash [105] and guard against the development of malignancy [20].

Relatives of patients with CD

CD is a familial condition in which about 10–15% of first degree relatives are affected [106,107]. A survey of 1329 relatives of 139 coeliac patients revealed an overall increase in cancer deaths [108] (Table 5.5). If relatives with undiagnosed CD are dying of malignancy then an excess number due to lymphoma and oesophageal carcinoma might be expected. An excess of deaths in men attributable to cancer of the oesophagus, bladder and brain was indeed found and also in women, an increase from carcinoma of the breast. Four deaths from

Table 5.5 Deaths from cancer in relatives of patients with CD [108]

Relatives of coeliac patients	Number of deaths due to cancer		Probability
	Expected	Observed	
Total	113.56	149	<0.001
Male	58.80	72	NS
Oesophagus	2.23	9	<0.001
Bladder	2.21	7	<0.01
Brain	0.24	4	<0.001
Female	54.68	77	<0.01
Breast	10.79	22	<0.01

lymphoma occurred in two men and two women, but these frequencies were not statistically significant. Studies of this type have limitations and while no firm conclusions can be drawn, CD occurring in family members should nevertheless be actively sought so that the benefits of treatment can be offered.

Non-specific chronic ulceration (jejunoileitis) of the small intestine

This is an uncommon complication of CD characterized by chronic ulcers, which are found in the jejunum, occasionally in the ileum, and rarely in the colon. Symptoms such as fever, weight loss, anorexia, abdominal pain and diarrhoea may occur in a patient previously well-controlled on a gluten-free diet. Patients are usually very unwell with anaemia and a low serum albumin resulting from protein-losing enteropathy. Barium studies of the small bowel will reveal ulceration and stricture formation which is often extensive (Fig. 5.15). The ulcers may bleed, perforate, or cause strictures in the bowel, which are often presenting features, bringing the patient to diagnosis by laparotomy.

With the onset of ulceration, the response to a gluten-free diet is lost. Treatment with steroids and azathioprine may induce remission, but in some cases, resection of an ulcerated segment of bowel, especially if stenotic, is necessary [109]. In general the outlook is poor, for out of 33 patients in one series, 24 died, 16 of these within 7 months of developing symptoms referable to bowel ulceration [110].

The clinical features of chronic ulceration and lymphoma are similar and both tend to develop in middle life, making definitive diagnosis a problem. A further difficulty is that both conditions may coexist in the same patient and sometimes ulceration will be diagnosed before intestinal lymphoma becomes apparent [18,109,110]. Isaacson *et al.* [62,111] have made a case for believing that ulceration is a precursor of malignant lymphoma due to neoplastic T cells which may, or may not, be identified in the lesions (Fig. 5.16).

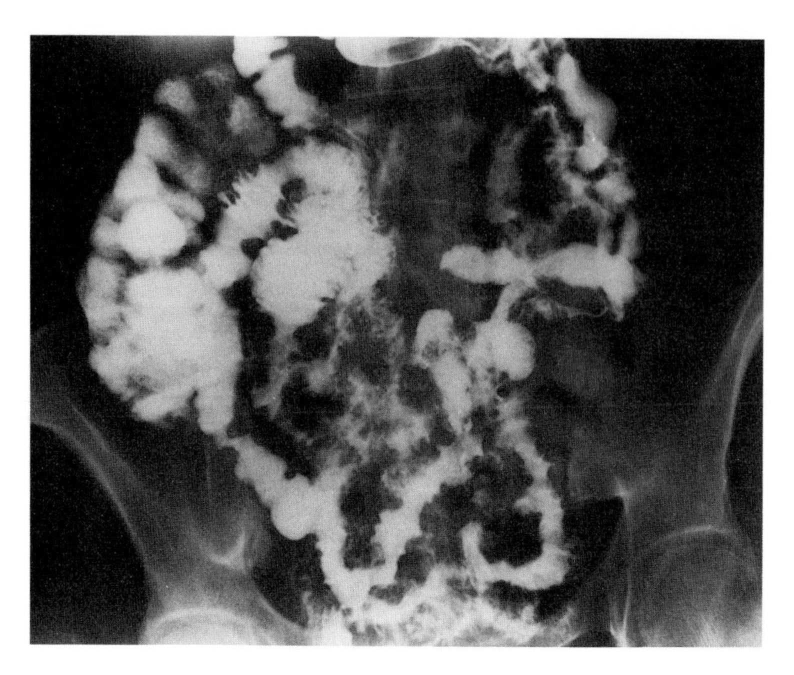

Fig. 5.15 Non-specific chronic ulceration of the small intestine in CD. This radiograph shows diffuse disease of the entire small intestine, with mucosal effacement and multiple irregular strictures.

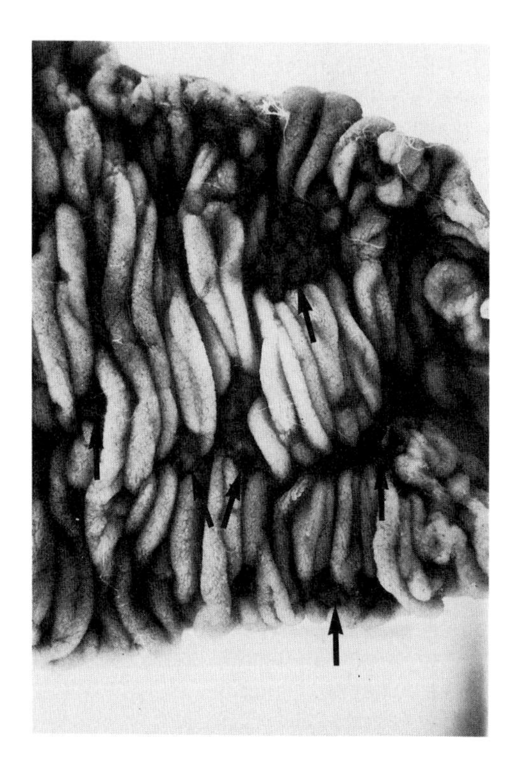

Fig. 5.16 Non-specific ulceration (arrows) of the jejunum complicating CD. There was no evidence of ulceration in the ileum or of lymphoma when this affected jejunal segment was resected and carefully examined histologically. Seven years later the patient presented with a bowel perforation through lymphoma in the ileum. (Courtesy of H. Thompson, D.H. Wright, P.G. Isaacson, E.L. Jones.)

It should be remembered that intestinal ulceration in CD may, very rarely, be caused by conditions such as coexistent Crohn's disease, polyarteritis nodosa, cytomegalic inclusion body disease, opportunistic fungal infections, ischaemia and radiation. We have encountered examples of all these in our patients, but usually as single examples. Other features of these conditions may be present which suggest that they be considered as the cause of ulceration, such as inflammatory bowel disease, polyarteritis nodosa or ischaemia. An enquiry about previous irradiation should always be made.

Relationship between flat mucosa and malignancy

Consideration must be given to those patients who present with malignancy, have a flat small intestinal biopsy and die shortly afterwards. Some claim that these patients do not have CD [112–114] and one investigation appears to support this contention [115]. In this study 93% of coeliac patients without complications had raised levels of antigliadin antibody, whereas these were not found in any of 16 patients with a flat biopsy and T cell lymphoma. The precise diagnosis of these patients, however, has been challenged [116]. Among the 16 patients with lymphoma were three with symptoms originating from childhood, whilst another had a 30-year history of diarrhoea, suggesting that some of these cases really did have CD complicated by malignancy, simply because it is quite unrealistic to attribute such long histories to lymphoma. This would be in keeping with a report [63] of a 58-year-old man who developed a T cell lymphoma 25 years after CD had been diagnosed on the basis of steatorrhoea and a flat jejunal biopsy. He responded clinically to a gluten-free diet, and the morphology of the intestinal mucosa also improved. He remained healthy until symptoms of cancer appeared about 1 year before death. Furthermore, it is not known what changes occur in antibody levels when a patient subsequently develops T cell lymphoma. It may well be that the emergence of lymphoma inhibits the ability to mount a humoral response to α-gliadin, so that in reality, there are not two distinct forms of enteropathy. Clearly, absence of α-gliadin antibodies in the setting of EATL cannot, at present, be accepted as stringent proof that such patients do not have CD.

While there may be uncertainty about the diagnosis in this group there is strong evidence which indicates that most, if not all patients, have CD which is complicated by lymphoma. Patients with a flat biopsy and lymphoma have a similar human leucocyte antigen (HLA) profile [17,22], a similar frequency of hyposplenism or splenic atrophy [117,118] and similar changes in intraepithelial T cell subsets [119] to patients with uncomplicated CD. While the development of malignancy often precipitates symptomatic CD, patients usually give a long history compatible with this diagnosis [19] although some have very short histories or no symptoms which could be attributed to gluten sensitivity. It is known from family studies that asymptomatic patients do occur [107] and in these individuals events such as surgery, enteric infection or pregnancy may be required to provoke overt disease. It is reasonable to add to this list the onset of malignancy as a causative factor (see Fig. 6.14).

The appearance of jejunal biopsies taken from patients with cancer does not support the view that cancer is responsible for producing a flat mucosa [120–123]. It is also pertinent to this argument that patients in remission on a gluten-free diet, who then go on to develop lymphoma, do not show any deterioration in jejunal morphology [30,124].

Does gluten restriction prevent malignancy?

It is clear that the early diagnosis of malignancy in CD still poses formidable problems which are unlikely to be surmounted in the near future. The question then arises as to whether this complication can be prevented by strict adherence to a gluten-free diet. Some considerations suggest that this may be so.

The jejunal mucosa in CD has features of pre-malignancy with regard both to carcinoma [80] and lymphoma [13]. These include increased mitotic activity in the crypts and lymphoid cells, and also irregularity and increased basophilia of the surface epithelium. Carcinogens might penetrate more easily the damaged mucosa which may be deficient in carcinogen-detoxifying enzymes [125]. A gluten-free diet substantially restores the architecture of the mucosa towards normal, and may therefore reduce the malignant potential. An early study did not show that a gluten-free diet was protective, which is not particularly surprising if protection is dependent on duration and strictness of the diet, since the average time on diet was only 7.5 years [19]. The same series of patients was therefore kept under surveillance for a further 11 years with the particular aim of assessing the effect of diet on malignancy after this period [20]. This analysis suggested that a gluten-free diet does influence the subsequent development of malignancy.

In patients who had taken a strict gluten-free diet for 5 or more consecutive years the overall cancer risk was not significantly increased, while there was a significantly increased risk among patients on a normal or reduced gluten-free diet (Table 5.6). Two lymphomas occurred in the strict gluten-free diet group which may indicate that in such patients the relatively short time on diet was insufficient to reverse the effects of previous exposure to an oncogenic stimulus, which had been operative for many years, probably from birth. Alternatively, in some cases, factors other than gluten may influence the development

Table 5.6 Cancer morbidity in CD by diet group [20]

Site	Diet group	Numbers (groups)	Observed numbers	Expected numbers	Observed : expected numbers of tumours	Probability
All sites	1	108	14	9.06	1.5	NS
	2	102	17	6.42	2.6	<0.001
Mouth, pharynx,	1	108	1	0.33	3.0	NS
oesophagus	2	102	5	0.22	22.7	<0.001
Non-Hodgkin's	1	108	2	0.12	16.7	<0.01
lymphoma	2	102	7	0.09	77.8	<0.001
Remainder	1	108	11	8.61	1.3	NS
	2	102	5	6.11	0.8	NS

Group 1, gluten-free diet group.
Group 2, normal or reduced gluten diet group.

of malignancy. When the two diet groups (strict gluten-free diet groups for 5 years or more vs the gluten-ingesting group) were compared with regard to cancers of the mouth, pharynx, oesophagus and lymphoma combined, a significant difference emerged. Excess morbidity was also computed as observed-minus-expected numbers of tumours divided by person–years at risk. Excess morbidity was clearly related to the amount of gluten ingested, with a significant decreasing trend in this index relative to increased elimination of gluten from the diet (Table 5.7) being observed.

These results support a protective role for a gluten-free diet against the development of malignancy as a complication of CD, and strengthen the view that all patients should be advised to adhere to a strict gluten-free diet for life. While there are no other detailed studies, anecdotal evidence from Galway also supports this contention [126].

Table 5.7 Cancer morbidity in CD by three diet groups in mouth, pharynx, oesophagus and lymphoma [20]

Group	Numbers (groups)	Observed numbers	Expected numbers	Observed : expected numbers of tumours	Probability	Excess morbidity rate
Normal diet	46	7	0.19	36.8	<0.001	10.7
Reduced gluten	56	5	0.12	41.7	<0.001	5.0
Strict gluten-free diet	108	3	0.46	6.5	<0.05	1.2

Excess morbidity rate is calculated as observed-minus-expected tumours divided by person–years at risk for each of the groups. The decreasing trend in the rate over increasing adherence to gluten-free diet was significant ($p<0.01$) [20].

Aetiology of malignancy in CD

Why patients with CD have an increased risk of developing malignancy is unknown, although several mechanisms might be involved. The lesion in the jejunal mucosa has features of pre-malignancy [80,13] and lymphoid cell hyperplasia might also give rise to malignancy, in that the more mitoses that occur, the greater the chance of malignancy arising [14]. These local factors may help to explain why tumours in CD are particularly likely to affect the proximal intestine, which is true for both lymphoma [127] and adenocarcinoma [79]. While the distribution of carcinoma in the small bowel in CD is similar to that for primary carcinoma, in CD it is the second most common invasive malignancy after lymphoma [17]. Primary small intestinal lymphoma is differently distributed in that it involves the ileum in most patients [128].

More general mechanisms, however, must also be considered because coeliac malignancy is not confined to the bowel. Carcinogens may gain access through the damaged intestinal mucosa, which in addition, because of enzyme deficiencies, may be unable to detoxify potentially damaging substances. Tissue antigen phenotypes predispose to neoplasia both in animals and humans [129–131]. In CD the HLA status differs from that found in the general population and thus could be another factor in the initiation of malignancy [132].

An abnormally developed or altered immune system may predispose to the development of malignancy. For example, patients with hypogammaglobulinaemia have a five-fold increase of cancer due mainly to excesses of stomach cancer (47-fold) and lymphomas (30-fold) [133]. In ataxia telangiectasia many varieties of malignancy may develop [134] and non-Hodgkin's lymphoma occurs in the Wiskott–Aldrich syndrome [135].

Patients receiving immunosuppressive drugs, particularly for renal transplantation, have a higher frequency of lymphomas and sarcomas [136]. In addition, in disorders with a likely immunological aetiology, an increased incidence of malignancy is observed as in Sjögren's syndrome, dermatomyositis, systemic lupus erythematosus and sarcoidosis [137]. Similar considerations may be relevant to the origins of malignancy in CD, since a variety of immunological disturbances occurs in this disorder, which might impede or otherwise influence, the elimination of malignant cells, and so allow tumour development. Lymphoma associated with human T cell leukaemia/lymphoma virus (HTLV-1), human immunodeficiency virus (HIV) and Epstein–Barr virus (EBV) are well-recognized and EBV has also been incriminated in the genesis of nasopharyngeal carcinoma (138–140). The immunological disturbances found in CD might yet be found to provide an environment for the replication of oncogenic viruses.

References

1 Cooke WT, Holmes GKT. Malignancy. In: Cooke WT, Holmes GKT, eds. *Coeliac Disease*. Edinburgh: Churchill Livingstone, 1984:172–96.

2 Lehmkuhl H. Ein fall von gleichmassigem diffusem lymphosarkom des Dunndarms. *Virchows Arch [A]* 1927;264:39–44.

3 Golden R. The small intestine and diarrhoea. *Am J Roentgenol* 1936;36:892–901.

4 Fairley NH, Mackie FP. The clinical and biochemical syndrome in lymphadenoma and allied diseases involving the mesenteric glands. *Br Med J* 1937;1:375–80.

5 Salvesen HA, Kobro M. Symptomatic sprue. *Acta Med Scand* 1939;102:277–94.

6 Harrison HE, Harrison HC, Tompsett RR, Barr DP. Potassium deficiency in a case of lymphosarcoma with the sprue syndrome. *Am J Med* 1947;2:131–43.

7 Oehler VV. Sprue. *Gastroenterologia* 1953; 79:257–82.

8 Friedlander PH, Gorvy V. Steatorrhoea. *Br Med J* 1955;2:809–12.

9 French JM, Hawkins CF. The gluten free diet in idiopathic steatorrhoea. *Med Clin North Am* 1957;41:1585–96.

10 Upshaw CB, Pollard HM. The sprue syndrome associated with intraabdominal lymphoblastoma. *Gastroenterology* 1957;33: 104–12.

11 Best CN, Cook PB. Case of mesenteric reticulosarcoma associated with gluten-sensitive steatorrhoea. *Br Med J* 1961;2: 496–8.

12 Scudamore HH. Observations on secondary malabsorption syndrome of intestinal origin. *Ann Intern Med* 1961;55:433–47.

13 Gough KR, Read AE, Naish JM. Intestinal reticulosis as a complication of idiopathic steatorrhoea. *Gut* 1962;3:232–9.

14 Austad WI, Cornes JS, Gough KR, McCarthy CF, Read AE. Steatorrhoea and malignant lymphoma. The relationship of malignant tumours of lymphoid tissue and coeliac disease. *Am J Dig Dis* 1967;12:475–90.

15 Harris OD, Cooke WT, Thompson H, Waterhouse JAH. Malignancy in adult coeliac disease and idiopathic steatorrhoea. *Am J Med* 1967;42:899–912.

16 Case records of the Massachusetts General Hospital. *New Engl J Med* 1958;259:491–5.

17 Swinson CM, Slavin G, Coles EC, Booth CC. Coeliac disease and malignancy. *Lancet* 1983;i:111–15.

18 Freeman HJ, Weinstein WM, Shnitka TK, Piercy JRA, Wensel RH. Primary abdominal lymphoma. Presenting manifestations of coeliac sprue, or complicating dermatitis herpetiformis. *Am J Med* 1977;63:585–94.

19 Holmes GKT, Stokes PL, Sorahan TM, Prior P, Waterhouse JAH, Cooke WT. Coeliac disease, gluten free diet and malignancy. *Gut* 1976;17:612–19.

20 Holmes GKT, Prior P, Lane MR, Pope RN, Allan RN. Malignancy in coeliac disease — effect of a gluten free diet. *Gut* 1989;30: 333–8.

21 Brandt L, Hagander B, Norden A, Stenstam M. Lymphoma of the small intestine in adult coeliac disease. *Acta Med Scand* 1978;204:467–70.

22 O'Driscoll BRC, Stevens FM, O'Gorman TA *et al.* HLA type of patients with coeliac disease and malignancy in the West of Ireland. *Gut* 1982;23:662–5.

23 Selby WS, Gallagher ND. Malignancy in a 19 year experience of adult coeliac disease. *Dig Dis Sci* 1979;24:684–8.

24 Nielsen OH, Jacobsen O, Pedersen ER *et al.* Non-tropical sprue. Malignant disease and mortality rate. *Scand J Gastroenterol* 1985; 20:13–18.

25 Logan RFA, Rifkind EA, Turner ID, Ferguson A. Mortality in coeliac disease. *Gastroenterology* 1989;97:265–71.

26 Whorwell PJ, Foster KJ, Alderson MR, Wright R. Death from ischaemic heart disease and malignancy in adult coeliac disease. *Lancet* 1976;ii:113–14.

27 Arnaud-Battandier F, Schmitz J, Ricour C, Rey J. Intestinal malignant lymphoma in a child with familial coeliac disease. *J Pediatr Gastroenterol Nutr* 1983;2:320–3.

28 McCrae WM, Eastwood MA, Martin MR, Sircus W. Neglected coeliac disease. *Lancet* 1975;i:187–90.

29 Cooper BT, Holmes GKT, Ferguson R, Cooke WT. Coeliac disease and malignancy. *Medicine* 1980;59:249–61.

30 Cooper BT, Read AE. Small intestinal lymphoma. *World J Surg* 1985;9:930–7.

31 Cooke WT, Holmes GKT. Definition and epidemiology. In: Cooke WT, Holmes GKT, eds. *Coeliac Disease*. Edinburgh: Churchill Livingstone, 1984:11–22.

32 Prineas JW, Mason AS, Henson RA. Myo-

pathy in metabolic bone disease. *Br J Med* 1965;1:1034–6.
33 Cooke WT, Smith WT. Neurological disorders associated with adult coeliac disease. *Brain* 1966;89:683–722.
34 Finan PJ, Thompson MR. Surgical presentation of small bowel lymphoma in coeliac disease. *Postgrad Med J* 1980;56:859–61.
35 Cooke WT, Peeney ALP, Hawkins CF. Symptoms, signs and diagnostic features of steatorrhoea. *Q J Med* 1953;22:59–77.
36 Benson GD, Kowlessar OD, Sleisenger MH. Adult coeliac disease with emphasis on response to gluten free diet. *Medicine* 1964; 43:1–40.
37 Barry RE, Baker P, Read AE. The clinical presentation. *Clin Gastroenterol* 1974; 3:55–69.
38 Coulson IH, Sanderson KV. T-cell lymphoma presenting as tumour d'emblee mycosis fungoides associated with coeliac disease. *J R Soc Med* 1985;78(Suppl. 11): 23–4.
39 Cooper BT, Holmes GKT, Cooke WT. Lymphoma risk in coeliac disease of later life. *Digestion* 1982;22:89–92.
40 Asquith P, Thompson RA, Cooke WT. Serum immunoglobulins in adult coeliac disease. *Lancet* 1969;ii:129–31.
41 Hodges JR, Isaacson PG, Eade OE, Wright R. histiocytosis of the intestine. *Gut* 1979; 20:854–7.
42 Cooper BT, Ukabam SO, Barry RE, Read AE. Serum lysozyme activity in coeliac disease: a possible aid to the diagnosis of malignant change? *J Clin Path* 1981;34: 1358–60.
43 Bourke MA, McLoughlin DM, Stevens FM, McCarthy CF. Serum lysozyme: is it a useful marker of malignant lymphoma in coeliac disease. *Ir J Med Sci* 1983;152: 125–8.
44 Stenstam M, Brandt L, Hallberg T. Subnormal responses of blood lymphocytes to phytohaemagglutinin in adult coeliac disease complicated by intestinal lymphoma. *Scand J Gastroenterol* 1983;18:777–81.
45 Holmes GKT, Bratt PM, Ling NR, Cooke WT. DNA-synthesizing cells in the blood in coeliac disease and inflammatory bowel disease. *Clin Exp Immunol* 1977;28: 484–9.
46 Ferguson R, Asquith P, Cooke WT. The jejunal cellular infiltrate in coeliac disease complicated by lymphoma. *Gut* 1974;15: 458–61.
47 Tucker WFG, Leonard JN, Fry L. Increased risk of lymphomas in dermatitis herpetiformis. *J R Soc Med* 1983;76:95–7.
48 Barry RE, Read AE. Coeliac disease and malignancy. *Q J Med* 1973;42:665–75.
49 Isaacson P. Malignant histiocytosis of the intestine: the early histological lesion. *Gut* 1980;21:381–6.
50 Achkar E, Carey WD, Petras R, Sivak MV, Revta R. Comparison of suction capsule and endoscopic biopsy of small bowel mucosa. *Gastrointest Endosc* 1986;32:278–81.
51 Dandalides SM, Carey WD, Petras R, Achkar E. Endoscopic small bowel biopsy: a controlled trial evaluating forceps size and biopsy location in the diagnosis of normal and abnormal mucosal architecture. *Gastrointest Endosc* 1989;35:197–200.
52 Roehrkasse RL, Roberts IM, Wald A, Talamo TS, Mendelow H. Coeliac sprue complicated by lymphoma presenting with multiple gastric ulcers. *Gastroenterology* 1986;91: 740–5.
53 Hall MJ, Cooper BT, Rooney N, Thompson H, Read AE. Coeliac disease and malignancy of the duodenum: diagnosis by endoscopy, successful treatment of the malignancy, and response to a gluten free diet. *Gut* 1991;32: 90–2.
54 Jones B, Bayless TM, Fishman EK, Siegelman SS. Lymphadenopathy in coeliac disease: computed tomographic observations. *Am J Roentgenol* 1984;142:1127–32.
55 Nicholson DA. Unusual presentation of non-Hodgkin's lymphoma of the small bowel. *Br J Radiol* 1990;63:814–16.
56 Holmes GKT. Mesenteric lymph node cavitation in coeliac disease. *Gut* 1986;27: 728–33.
57 Taylor CR. An immunological study of follicular lymphoma, reticulum cell sarcoma and Hodgkin's disease. *Eur J Cancer* 1976; 12:61–75.
58 Henry K, Farrer Brown G. Primary lymphomas of the gastrointestinal tract. 1. Plasma cell tumours. *Histopathology* 1977;1:53–76.
59 Isaacson PG, Wright DH. Malignant histiocytosis of the intestine. Its relationship to malabsorption and ulcerative jejunitis. *Hum Pathol* 1978;9:661–77.
60 Isaacson PG, Jones DB, Millward-Sadler GH, Judd MA, Payne S. Alpha-1-antitrypsin in human macrophages. *J Clin Pathol* 1981; 34:382–90.
61 Isaacson PG, Jones DB, Sworn MJ, Wright

DH. Malignant histiocytosis of the intestine: report of three cases with immunological and cytochemical analysis. *J Clin Pathol* 1982;35:510–16.

62 Isaacson PG, O'Connor NTJ, Spencer J *et al.* Malignant histiocytosis of the intestine: A T-cell lymphoma. *Lancet* 1985;ii: 688–91.

63 Loughran TP, Kadin ME, Deeg J. T-cell intestinal lymphoma associated with coeliac sprue. *Ann Intern Med* 1986;104:44–7.

64 Salter DM, Krajewski AS, Dewar AE. Immunophenotype analysis of malignant histiocytosis of the intestine. *J Clin Pathol* 1986;39:8–15.

65 Ferguson A. Models of immunologically-driven small intestinal damage. In: Marsh MN, ed. *Immunopathology of the Small Intestine.* Chichester: Wiley, 1987:225–52.

66 Goudie RB, Lee FD. Does occult monoclonal proliferation of non-malignant T cells cause secondary immunopathological disorders? *J Pathol* 1989;158:91–2.

67 Isaacson PG, Cerf-Bensussan N, Jarry A, Brousse N, Krajewski AS, Spencer J. Enteropathy-associated T cell lymphoma (malignant histiocytosis of the intestine) is derived from intraepithelial T cells. *J Pathol* 1987;152:217A.

68 Spencer J, Cerf-Bensussan N, Jarry A, Guy-Grand D, Krajewski AS, Isaacson PG. Enteropathy-associated T cell lymphoma (malignant histiocytosis of the intestine) is recognized by a monoclonal antibody (HML-1) that defines a membrane molecule on human mucosal lymphocytes. *Am J Pathol* 1988;132:1–5.

69 Stein H, Dienemann D, Sperling M, Zeitz M, Riecken EO. Identification of a T cell lymphoma category derived from intestinal-mucosa-associated T cells. *Lancet* 1988;2: 1053–4.

70 Cerf-Bensussan N, Jarry A, Brousse N, Lisowska-Grospierre B, Guy-Grand D, Griscelli C. A monoclonal antibody (HML-1) defining a novel membrane molecule present on human intestinal lymphocytes. *Eur J Immunol* 1987;17:1279–85.

71 Alfsen GC, Beiske K, Bell H, Martin PF. Low-grade intestinal lymphoma of intraepithelial T lymphocytes with concomitant enteropathy-associated T cell lymphoma: case report suggesting a possible histogenic relationship. *Hum Pathol* 1989;20:909–13.

72 Foucar K, Foucar E, Mitros F, Clamon G, Goeken J, Crossett J. Epitheliotropic lymphoma of the small bowel. Report of a fatal case with cytotoxic/suppressor T-cell immunotype. *Cancer* 1984;54:54–60.

73 Pallesen G, Hamilton-Dutoit SJ. Monoclonal antibody (HML-1) labelling of T-cell lymphomas. *Lancet* 1989;i:223.

74 Whitehead R. Primary lymphadenopathy complicating idiopathic steatorrhoea. *Gut* 1968;9:569–75.

75 Paulley JW. Observations on the aetiology of idiopathic steatorrhoea. Jejunal and lymph node biopsies. *Br Med J* 1954;2:1318–21.

76 Simmonds JP, Rosenthal FD. Lymphadenopathy in coeliac disease. *Gut* 1981;22: 756–8.

77 Kavin H. Coeliac disease complicated by chronic nongranulomatous ulcerative enterocolitis-nodular lymphoid hyperplasia, and disseminated intravascular coagulation. *Dig Dis Sci* 1981;26:73–80.

78 Horowitz A, Shiner M. The recognition of premalignant change in jejunal mucosal biopsies of patients with malabsorption. *J Submicrosc Cytol Pathol* 1981;13: 423–43.

79 Holmes GKT, Dunn GI, Cockel R, Brookes VS. Adenocarcinoma of the small bowel complicating coeliac disease. *Gut* 1980;21: 1010–16.

80 Joske RA. Primary carcinoma of the jejunum with atrophic jejunitis and intestinal malabsorption. *Gastroenterology* 1960;38: 810–16.

81 Blackwell JB. Two cases of carcinoma of the small bowel with malabsorption. *Gut* 1961;2:377.

82 Girdwood RH, Delamore IW, Williams AW. Jejunal biopsy in malabsorption disorder of the adult. *Br Med J* 1961;1:319–23.

83 Shearman DJC, Girdwood RH, Williams WA, Delamore IW. A study with electron microscope of the jejunal epithelium in primary malabsorptive disease. *Gut* 1961;3: 16–25.

84 Moertel CG, Hargreaves MM. Coexistence of adenocarcinoma of the jejunum and non-tropical sprue. *JAMA* 1961;176:612–14.

85 Fric P, Bednar B, Niederie B, Lepsik J. Jejunal adenocarcinoma in a woman with non-tropical sprue. *Gastroenterology* 1972; 44:330–4.

86 Brzechwa-Ajdukiewicz A, McCarthy CF, Austad W, Cornes J, Harrison WJ, Read AE. Carcinoma, villous atrophy and steatorrhoea. *Gut* 1966;7:572–7.

87 Shiner M. Effect of a gluten free diet in 17

patients with idiopathic steatorrhoea. *Am J Dig Dis* 1963;8:969–83.
88 Lee FD. Nature of the mucosal changes associated with malignant neoplasms in the small intestine. *Gut* 1966;7:361–7.
89 Asch T, Seaman WB. Idiopathic steatorrhoea and small bowel cancer. *Radiology* 1971; 100:217–25.
90 Barry RE, Morris JS, Kenwright S, Read AE. Coeliac disease and malignancy. The possible importance of familial involvement. *Scand J Gastroenterol* 1971;6:205–7.
91 Kenwright S. Coeliac disease and small bowel carcinoma. *Postgrad Med J* 1972;48: 673–7.
92 Petreshock EP, Pessah M, Menachemi E. Adenocarcinoma of the jejunum associated with non-tropical sprue. *Am J Dig Dis* 1975; 20:796–802.
93 Collins SM, Hamilton JD, Lewis TD, Laufer I. Small bowel malabsorption and gastrointestinal malignancy. *Radiology* 1978;126: 693–9.
94 Javier J, Lukie B. Duodenal adenocarcinoma complicating coeliac disease. *Dig Dis Sci* 1980;25:150–3.
95 O'Brien CJ, Saverymuttu S, Hodgson HJF, Evans DJ. Coeliac disease, adenocarcinoma of jejunum and *in situ* squamous carcinoma of oesophagus. *J Clin Pathol* 1983;36:62–7.
96 Magnussen PA, Grant JW. Perforation of a jejunal adenocarcinoma complicating coeliac disease. *J R Soc Med* 1986;79: 114–15.
97 Levine ML, Dorf BS, Bank S. Adenocarcinoma of the duodenum in a patient with non-tropical sprue. *Am J Gastroenterol* 1986;81:800–2.
98 Nielsen SNJ, Wold LE. Adenocarcinoma of jejunum in association with non-tropical sprue. *Arch Pathol Lab Med* 1986;110: 822–4.
99 Straker J, Gunasekaran S, Brady PG. Adenocarcinoma of the jejunum in association with coeliac sprue. *J Clin Gastroenterol* 1989;11:320–3.
100 Gostout CJ, Schroeder KW, Burton DD. Small bowel enteroscopy: an early experience in gastrointestinal bleeding of unknown origin. *Gastrointest Endosc* 1991; 37:5–8.
101 Fry L, Seah PP, Harper PG, Hoffbrand AV, McMinn RMH. The small bowel in dermatitis herpetiformis. *J Clin Pathol* 1974;27: 817–24.
102 Weinstein WM. Latent coeliac disease. *Gastroenterology* 1974;66:489–93.
103 Jenkins D, Lynde CW, Stewart WD. Histiocytic lymphoma occurring in a patient with dermatitis herpetiformis. *J Am Acad Dermatol* 1983;9:252–6.
104 Leonard JN, Tucker WFG, Fry JS *et al.* Increased incidence of malignancy in dermatitis herpetiformis. *Br Med J* 1983;1:16–18.
105 Cooke WT, Holmes GKT. Skin manifestations and dermatitis herpetiformis. In: Cooke WT, Holmes GKT, eds. *Coeliac Disease*. Edinburgh: Churchill Livingstone, 1984;214–24.
106 MacDonald WC, Dobbins WO, Rubin CE. Studies of the familial nature of coeliac sprue using biopsy of the small intestine. *New Engl J Med* 1965;272:448–56.
107 Stokes PL, Ferguson R, Holmes GKT, Cooke WT. Familial aspects of coeliac disease. *Q J Med* 1976;45:567–82.
108 Stokes PL, Prior P, Sorahan TM, McWalter RJ, Waterhouse JAH, Cooke WT. Malignancy in relatives of patients with coeliac disease. *Br J Prev Soc Med* 1976;30:12–21.
109 Baer AN, Bayless TM, Yardley JH. Intestinal ulceration and malabsorption syndromes. *Gastroenterology* 1980;79:754–65.
110 Bayless TM, Yardley JH, Baer A, Hendrix TR. Intestinal ulceration, flat mucosa and malabsorption. Report of registry of 33 patients. In: McNichol B, McCarthy CF, Fottrell PF, eds. *Perspectives in Coeliac Disease*. Lancaster: MTP Press, 1978: 311–12.
111 Isaacson PG. Malignant histiocytosis of the intestine: the early lesion. *Gut* 1980;21: 381–6.
112 Brunt PW, Sircus W, MacLean N. Neoplasia and the coeliac syndrome in adults. *Lancet* 1969;i:180–4.
113 Hourihane DO'B, Weir DG. Malignant coeliac syndrome. Report of two cases with malabsorption and microscopic foci of intestinal lymphoma. *Gastroenterology* 1970; 59:130–9.
114 Barry RE, Read AE. Coeliac disease and malignancy. *Q J Med* 1973;42:665–75.
115 O'Farrelly C, Feighery C, O'Briain DS *et al.* Humoral response to wheat protein in patients with coeliac disease and enteropathy associated T cell lymphoma. *Br Med J* 1986;293:908–10.
116 Loft DE, Marsh MN. Humoral response to wheat protein in patients with coeliac disease and enteropathy associated T cell lymphoma. *Br Med J* 1986;293:1439.

117 Robertson DAF, Swinson CM, Hall R, Losowsky MS. Coeliac disease, splenic function and malignancy. *Gut* 1982;23: 666–9.

118 O'Grady JG, Stevens FM, McCarthy CF. Coeliac disease: Does hyposplenism predispose to the development of malignant disease? *Am J Gastroenterol* 1985;80:27–9.

119 Spencer J, MacDonald TT, Diss TC, Walker-Smith JA, Ciclitira PJ, Isaacson PG. Changes in intraepithelial lymphocyte subpopulations in coeliac disease and enteropathy associated T cell lymphoma (malignant histiocytosis of the intestine). *Gut* 1989;30: 339–46.

120 Girdwood RH. Malignancy and the small intestinal mucosa. *Br Med J* 1964;2:1592.

121 Deller DJ, Murrell TGC, Blowes R. Jejunal biopsy in malignant disease. *Aust Ann Med* 1967;16:236–41.

122 Klipstein FA, Smarth G. Intestinal structure and function in neoplastic disease. *Am J Dig Dis* 1969;14:887–99.

123 Gilat T, Fischel B, Danon J, Loewenthal M. Morphology of small bowel mucosa in malignancy. *Digestion* 1972;7:147–55.

124 Cooke WT, Thompson H, Williams JA. Malignancy and adult coeliac disease. *Gut* 1969;10:108–11.

125 Wattenberg LW. Carcinogen detoxifying mechanisms in the gastrointestinal tract. *Gastroenterology* 1966;51:932–5.

126 McCarthy CF. Coeliac disease. *Ir J Coll Phys Surg* 1990;19:45–7.

127 Read AE. Malignant disease and steatorrhoea. *Mod Trends Gastroent* 1970;4: 180–97.

128 Rachmilewitz D, Okon E. In: Berk JE, ed. *Bockus Gastroenterology*. Philadelphia: WB Saunders, 1985:1865–73.

129 Zervas, JD, Delamore IW, Israels MCG. Leucocyte phenotypes in Hodgkin's disease. *Lancet* 1970;ii:634–5.

130 Chapius B, Von Fliedner VE, Jeannet M *et al*. Increased frequency of DR2 in patients with aplastic anaemia and increased DR sharing in their parents. *Br J Haematol* 1986;63:51–7.

131 Festenstein H. The biological consequences of altered MHC expression on tumours. *Br Med Bull* 1987;43:217–27.

132 Kagnoff MF. Understanding the molecular basis of coeliac disease. *Gut* 1990;31: 497–9.

133 Kinlen LJ, Webster DB, Bird AG *et al*. Prospective study of cancer in patients with hypogammaglobulinaemia. *Lancet* 1985;i: 263–6.

134 Swift M, Reitnauer P, Morrell D, Chase CL. Breast and other cancers in families with ataxia-telangiectasia. *New Engl J Med* 1987; 316:1289–94.

135 Frizzera G, Rosai J, Dehner LP, Spector BD, Kersey JH. Lymphoreticular disorders in primary immunodeficiencies: new findings based on an up-to-date histologic classification of 35 cases. *Cancer* 1980;46:692–9.

136 Matas AJ, Hertel BF, Rosai J, Simmons RL, Najarian JS. Post-transplant malignant lymphomas. Distinctive morphologic features related to its pathogenesis. *Am J Med* 1976;61:716–20.

137 Kassan SS, Thomas TL, Moutsopoulos HM *et al*. Increased risk of lymphoma in sicca syndrome. *Ann Intern Med* 1978;89:888–92.

138 Henle W, Henle G. Epstein–Barr virus and human malignancies. *Adv Viral Oncol* 1985;5:201–38.

139 Knowles DM, Chamulak GA, Subar M *et al*. Lymphoid neoplasia associated with the acquired immunodeficiency syndrome (AIDS). *Ann Intern Med* 1988;108:744–53.

140 Devita VT, Jaffe ES, Mauch P, Longo DL. Lymphocytic lymphomas. In: Devita VT, Hellman S, Rosenberg SA, eds. *Cancer, Principles and Practice of Oncology*. Philadelphia: JB Lippincott, 1989:1741–92.

Chapter 6/Mucosal pathology in gluten sensitivity

MICHAEL N. MARSH

During the 30 years since the peroral technique of jejunal biopsy was introduced into gastroenterological practice, it has been customary to define coeliac disease (CD) in terms of a mucosal lesion which is invariably associated with malabsorption and improves with dietary gluten withdrawal [1–4]. Within the same period, the mucosal abnormalities in CD have traditionally been described in terms of so-called 'villous atrophy' [5,6]. This system of terminology nowadays can be seen to be meaningless, outmoded and inappropriate to current needs, while its widespread usage continues to thwart full elucidation of the underlying basis of the local mucosal lesions [7,8]. It is as though the terminology itself defined the pathology; this state of affairs can no longer be allowed to persist.

Another reason for continuing uncertainty about the mechanisms of gluten-induced mucosal damage stems from undue concern with the flat lesion, and a failure to recognize the presence, and importance, of other more subtle manifestations of gluten-induced changes in mucosal architecture [9]. The basis of this approach seems to have arisen historically from the use of histological [10], cytochemical [11–14] and electron microscopic techniques [15–17] aimed primarily at the enterocyte, rather than at other facets of the accompanying trans-mural damage. The results of such observations were consequently interpreted solely in terms of Frazer's well-articulated proposals regarding deficiency of 'peptidase' enzyme in the coeliac enterocyte [18].

There next followed an era during which enterocyte damage was attributed to immunological phenomena, either T cell-mediated or antibody-dependent cytolysis, or antigen–antibody complex deposition in the region of the basal lamina [19–24]. In a further attempt at pathogenesis, it was proposed that coeliac enterocytes may express an abnormal receptor reactive with gliadin in a lectin-like manner [25]. This proposal is unnecessary to explain the initiation of mucosal pathology via the enterocyte, since current evidence indicates that gliadin activity resides in small oligopeptides which are entirely lacking in carbohydrate (i.e. 'lectin-like') side-chains (see Chapter 11) [8].

Thus, despite the interesting and ingenious approaches raised by these studies, they are flawed either in conceptual terms or by technical problems [26], so that none can any longer be considered effective answers to mucosal pathology associated with gluten sensitivity [26,27].

Mucosal immunopathology in gluten sensitivity

A more acceptable solution to these problems has come with other detailed analyses of the coeliac lesion by immunopathological techniques, and from correlations derived from experimental work in graft transplantation. It is these latter studies which have so greatly contributed to our knowledge and understanding of the varied, although stereotyped ways in which the intestinal mucosa responds to cell mediated, or T lymphocyte-dependent influences.

Such work, initially commenced in the 1960s and 1970s, provided the first demonstration of villous effacement and of crypt hyperplasia and hypertrophy. It was also shown that such lesions were less easy to reproduce in either neonatally thymectomized or nude animals. These experiments established two important principles: (1) that competent T lymphocytes, probably acting via lymphokine secretion, are necessary, for the initiation and progress of graft-versus-host (GVH) reactions; and (2) that T lymphocytes are capable of modulating the established villous-crypt architecture of the small intestine in the mature animal [28,29].

The various published models of GVH provide an important series of parallels by which the group of enteropathies with similar mucosal morphological alterations, such as gluten sensitivity; tropical sprue and tropical enteropathy; giardiasis; and infantile reactions to dietary food antigens can most usefully be evaluated [7,8,28–31].

In other recent experimental approaches to GVH, mucosal changes of a less florid degree have been brought about which reveal more varied and subtle effects of T cell-mediated influences on mucosal architecture than was appreciated heretofore [32,33]. It is pertinent that some of these lesions closely resemble mucosal lesions seen in patients with dermatitis herpetiformis (DH), and among relatives of known CD patients.

At this point, it is necessary to recall that the classic textbook description of CD, with its flat avillous mucosa and associated syndromes of diarrhoea and malabsorption stems from the earliest studies when the first operative [34] and peroral biopsies [5,6,10] revealed the typical advanced mucosal lesion. On the other hand, additional types of reversible, gluten-induced lesions, such as those already alluded to in DH, have been described. Together they form the wider context of what should now be termed, and recognized as, the gluten-sensitivity spectrum. This distinction is important, not purely for academic reasons, but because of its clinical relevance simply because it is becoming increasingly apparent that symptomatic coeliac malabsorption probably

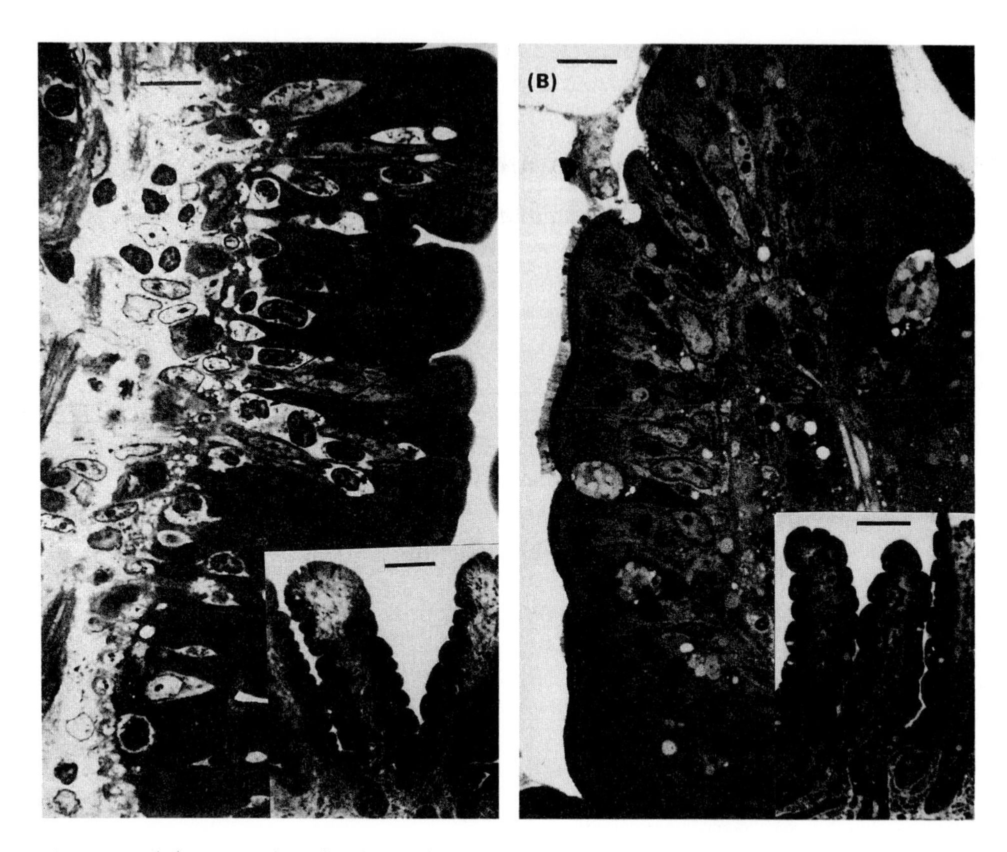

Fig. 6.1 Each large panel in this figure depicts the typical range of 'infiltrative' (Type 1) mucosal lesions associated with gluten sensitivity. Note normal villous pattern, non-enlargement of crypts and infiltration of villous epithelium by variable numbers of uniformly small lymphocytes (long arrows). (A) untreated DH. (B) treated patient, specimen obtained 12 hours following oral challenge with 3 g FF3.

accounts for only 30% of the entire disease spectrum. Therefore, in order that the fundamental immunopathological basis of gluten sensitivity be understood, it is now becoming necessary that the range of mucosal lesions seen across this spectrum will be both acknowledged and assimilated into clinical practice [7,8].

Patterns of gluten-induced mucosal change

Three major, distinctive, and dynamically interrelated patterns of mucosal change are present across the gluten-sensitivity spectrum which, in parallel with GVH disease, may be arbitrarily termed the infiltrative, hyperplastic and destructive (flat) lesions [7,8,35–37].

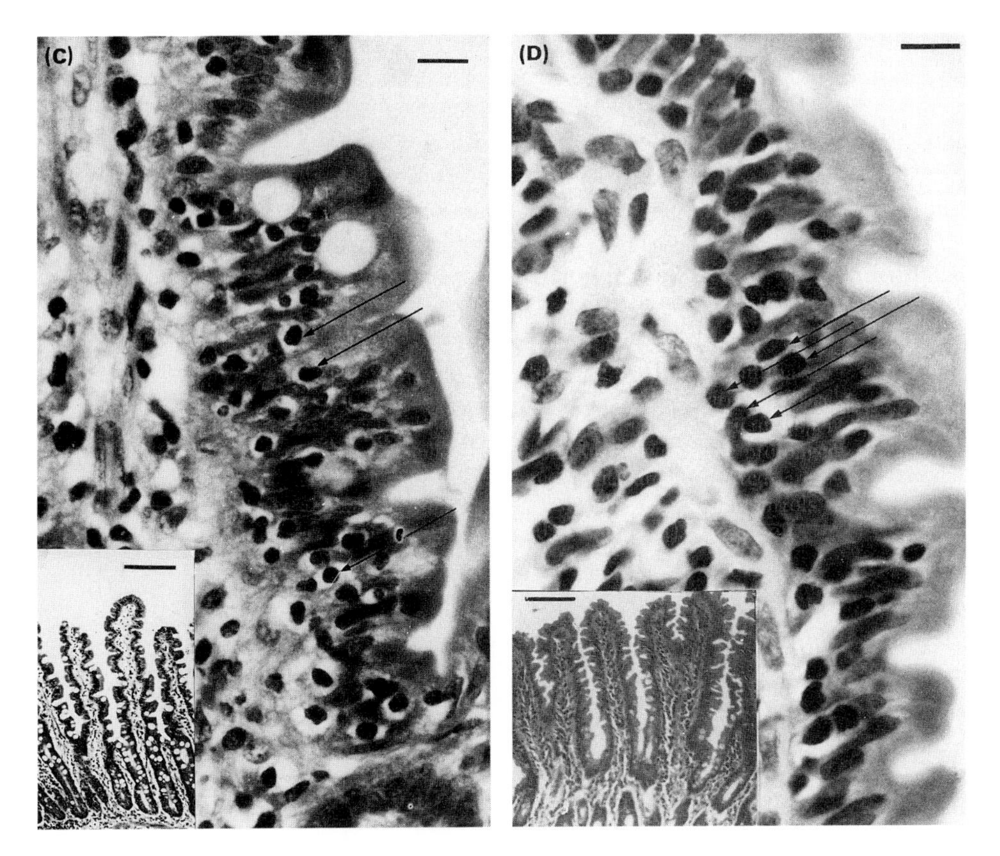

Fig. 6.1 *continued.* (C) first degree relative of known CD subject. (D) this section represents the first biopsy obtained from a patient whose jejunal mucosa was subsequently observed to become flat over the ensuing 2 years [98]: the flat (Type 3) lesion is illustrated in Fig. 6.3. The computerized morphometric analysis of all the specimens obtained from this patient are illustrated in Fig. 6.12; there the first specimen (7/78) and third specimen (3/81) refer to Figs 6.1D and 6.3, respectively. (Magnification bars, 10 μm; insets, 100 μm.)

The infiltrative (Type 1) lesion

This lesion comprises normal mucosal architecture in which the villous epithelium carries a variable infiltrate of small, non-mitotic lymphocytes. There are three circumstances in which this lesion has been defined and recognized (Fig. 6.1).

1 Most importantly, it is the classic lesion of DH as first described by Fry and his colleagues in London [38,39]. That the infiltrate of small lymphocytes into villous epithelium [40] is gluten dependent is evidenced by their decline following dietary gluten restriction. This lesion (Fig. 6.1) is present in about 40% of DH patients presenting to clinic.

2 Secondly, an identical mucosal lesion was identified in 25% of first degree relatives of known CD cases, drawn from the Manchester and Merseyside regions of northwest England [41]. During the conduct of this study, all relatives with flat lesions (incidence ~15%) were excluded thus leaving only mucosae with reasonably normal villous architecture (Fig. 6.1). This lesion was not associated with any gastrointestinal symptomatology, malabsorption, or abnormal permeance to ^{51}Cr-EDTA, thus suggesting that a presumptive genetic trait for increased permeability [42] is not an increased risk factor for gluten sensitivity.

3 Thirdly, oral gluten challenge of treated coeliac patients [43–47] causes a lymphoid infiltrative lesion (Fig. 6.1). In a study from our laboratory [44] patients were challenged with Frazer's fraction 3 (FF3) [48] in a series of graded doses per challenge, ranging through 0.1–12.0 g. The response, quantitated by computerized image analysis, revealed a dose-dependent, time-related infiltration of small lymphocytes into villous epithelium [44] maximal at around 12 hours post-challenge. This was an antigen-specific response in the gluten-sensitive patients alone, since they did not respond to a 500 mg oral challenge with β-lactoglobulin (βLG), while controls showed no response to either immunogen [49].

The hyperplastic (Type 2) lesion

This lesion is virtually identical to the infiltrative lesion, but with the addition of hypertrophic crypts, whose epithelium may also be infiltrated by lymphocytes (Fig. 6.2). This is seen in about 20% of untreated DH patients [40] and is inducible with moderate dose oral challenge (3–6 g) FF3.

The hyperplastic lesion is important, and was first described in a neonatal murine model of GVH [32]. While this lesion is recognized to be another manifestation of a pure T cell-mediated response by intestinal mucosa, it must also be seen to reflect an important early effect of T cell activation on mucosal architecture, i.e. enlargement of crypts without any simultaneous reduction in villous height.

In our Manchester series of published DH cases [40], the infiltrative and hyperplastic lesions together accounted for approximately one-half of the 32 mucosae analysed.

The destructive (Type 3) lesion

This lesion is characterized by the established 'flat' mucosa of classic CD, which has been the object of most research concerned with gluten sensitivity. It typifies criteria of a fully developed cell-mediated mucosal immune response (Table 6.1), which in architectural terms encompasses hypertrophic crypts, lamina propria swelling and a flattened surface

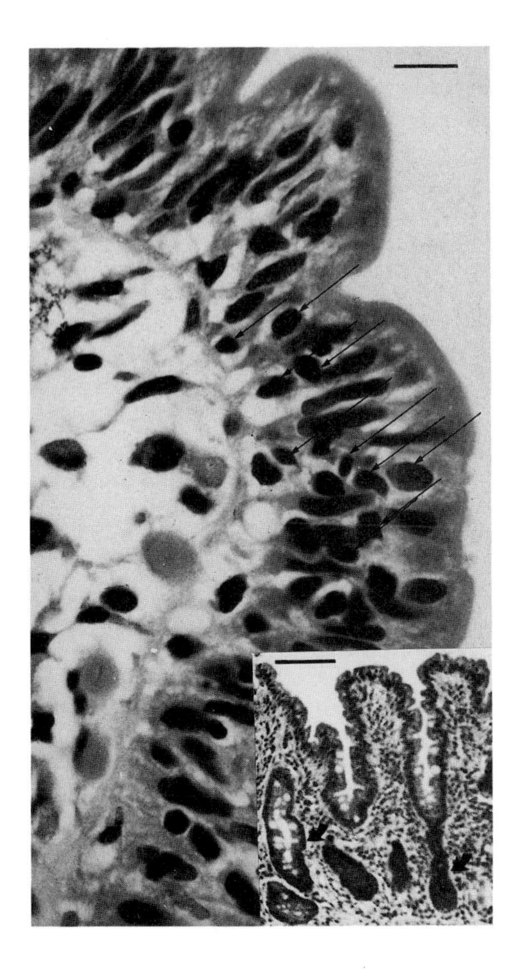

Fig. 6.2 An infiltrative-hyperplastic (Type 2) lesion demonstrating enlarged crypts (curved arrows, inset) in addition to normal villi whose epithelium is infiltrated by small lymphocytes (long arrows). (Magnification bar, 10 μm; inset, 100 μm.)

Table 6.1 Features of advanced cell-mediated immunological inflammation in small intestinal mucosa

Increased microvascular hyperpermeability	Increased rate of cell division
Increased cell populations	Increased rate of cell migration
Plasma cells	Goblet cell hyperplasia
Neutrophils	Altered differentiation profile of brush border
Eosinophils	Membrane hydrolases
Basophils	Increased permeability
Mast cells	Increased fluid secretion
Elaboration of inflammatory cytokines/ mediators	Reduced fluid absorption
	Lymphocyte infiltration
	Surface epithelium
	Crypt epithelium
	Up-regulation of MHC class 2 expression and secretory component expression

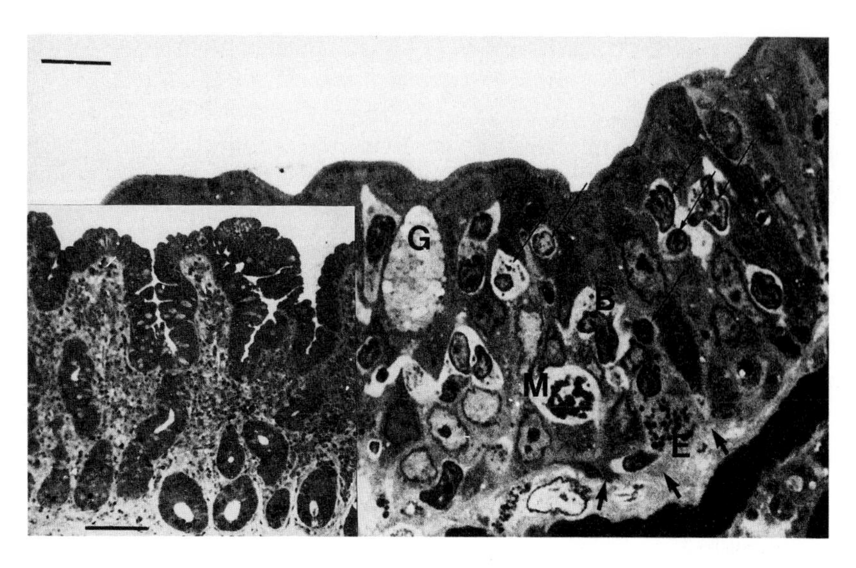

Fig. 6.3 This micrograph illustrates classical flat, or destructive (Type 3) lesion of classical CD. Epithelium now contains a heterogeneous population of IEL (arrowed) with expanded cytoplasm, heterochromatic nuclei, and of variable size including mitotic (M) and 'blast-like' (B) examples. Beneath basal lamina (thick arrows) lies dilated capillary containing sludged, distorted erythrocytes. G, goblet cell; E, enterochromaffin cell. (Magnification bar, 10 μm; inset, 100 μm.)

epithelium (Fig. 6.3). Such changes are not exclusive to gluten sensitivity, but occur in tropical sprue, and some cases of giardiasis and short-term food sensitivities in infants [50], in addition to experimental allograft rejection and GVH disease [31,35,37,51–53]. Similar pathology is also observed in some forms of immunodeficiency [54], and in immunoproliferative disease of the small intestine [55].

We know that a flat (Type 3) destructive lesion occurs in only about 40% of DH patients, and in 10–20% first degree coeliac relatives. In the former, and approximately 50% of the latter, such an advanced lesion evidently lies dormant so that these individuals are virtually asymptomatic. From this it seems likely that overt coeliac malabsorption with a flat lesion affects only 30–40% genetically susceptible individuals, and that in the remainder the mucosal lesion, of whatever type, remains subclinical or 'latent'. This consideration is of some practical clinical importance, because CD is usually defined as malabsorption occurring in the context of a flat lesion which must respond to a gluten-free diet [1–3]; clearly, if this definition only applies to the characteristic presentation of approximately one-third of all subjects, its validity needs to be seriously questioned, since it obviously fails to embrace all gluten-sensitive individuals. What is becoming obvious is the need to redefine gluten sensitivity, perhaps in terms of molecular markers (major histocompatibility complex (MHC) structural polymorphisms, T cell receptor polymorphisms, and so on) rather than in morphological imaging which, as is evident here, is too variable for a uniform approach. Furthermore, because of extensive clinical latency, the identification of persons (especially those with quiescent flat lesions) who should nevertheless benefit from gluten restriction, is unlikely to occur.

The pre-infiltrative (Type 0) lesion

In various large series of DH patients a small proportion (~5%) of patients, although gluten sensitized by virtue of granular IgA deposits in papillary dermis, have intestinal mucosal biopsies that are indistinguishable from normal [56–59].

In recent studies of one such group of DH patients in Edinburgh [58], intestinal secretions were demonstrated to contain anti-α-gliadin antibodies of sIgA and sIgM type in equivalent titre to those typical of untreated coeliac patients with destructive (Type 3) flattened lesions. Compared with a control group, anti-α-gliadin IgM secretory antibodies proved to be most discriminating. This type of mucosal response, with its associated systemic sensitization to gluten, might be termed the pre-infiltrative (Type 0) lesion (Fig. 6.4).

There are other parallels to this phenomenon, such as the M2 antigen that (rarely) appears in primary biliary cirrhosis long before the bile ducts and hepatic lobules are subject to lymphocytic infiltration, piecemeal necrosis and eventual end-stage cirrhosis [60]; and the circulating 64 kDa [61] anti-β-cell antibody that arises before the islets are invaded and destroyed by T lymphocytes both in humans [62] and

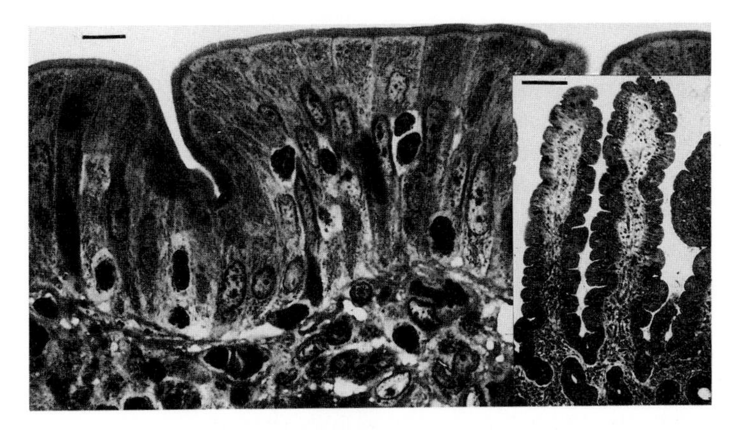

Fig. 6.4 Jejunal biopsy from untreated DH patient showing normal villous architecture, normal epithelium and scanty infiltrate of IEL; such appearances typify the 'pre-infiltrative' (Type 0) lesion of gluten sensitivity. (Magnification bar, 10 μm; inset, 100 μm.)

in the NOD mouse model of insulin-dependent diabetes mellitus (IDDM) [63]. In this context, it should be noted that in diabetic twins, the presence of antibodies and activated (DR^+) T cells regresses within 5 years if the second twin has not developed hyperglycaemia by that time [64]. Similar events occur in the NOD mouse; pancreatic infiltration by lymphocytes occurs within a fairly tight age-span and recedes by the 30th week of life. By that time, only 20% of the male, and 70% of the female animals will develop symptomatic disease [65].

The transient immunological phenomena in IDDM may also pertain to gluten sensitivity. At present, however, we do not know whether the pre-infiltrative lesion, or the infiltrative (Types 1 and 2) lesions always progress, remain static (and for how long), or ultimately regress in some individuals. Unlike DH patients [58] who have a ready skin marker of systemic sensitization to dietary gluten, the identification of other individuals within the gluten-sensitivity spectrum will be difficult, unless 'at-risk' individuals are sought, such as close family relatives. Nevertheless, it can be seen that data of this kind are now necessary in order to provide numerical estimates of the extent of this condition and to enhance our perception of the natural history of gluten sensitivity, an area about which there still remains considerable ignorance.

The hypoplastic/atrophic (Type 4) lesion

At the other end of the spectrum are some gluten-sensitive individuals who become antigen unresponsive, develop patchy or diffuse jejuno-ileitis [66–68], intestinal ulceration [69], or the coeliac-associated lymphoma (enteropathy-associated T cell lymphoma (EATL)) [70]. In this small fraction of patients ill-health may persist for years in the presence of a continuing flat lesion that cannot naively be attributed to occasional dietary indiscretions. In others, complication arise *de novo* from the onset of the complicating lesion; gluten sensitivity in this setting is presumed to have remained latent during former years of these patients' lives. Usually patients with this type of presentation are middle-aged or beyond and have malabsorption that responds poorly, or transiently, to steroids, a strict (hospital-enforced) gluten-, and even milk-free diet, with or without additional parenteral supplementation [71–73]. Alternatively, the presentation may be abrupt, with recurrent severe diarrhoea, abdominal pain and masses in an hitherto well-treated coeliac [72], or with acute bleeding, perforation or intestinal obstruction due to tumour masses, stricture formation or mucosal ulceration and fissuring. Ulcers are invariably the site of microfoci of EATL [69,74–77].

Considerable confusion about the categorization of such cases has been generated by earlier definitions of 'CD' which demanded evidence of mucosal regeneration as proof of gluten sensitivity [1–4]. However, throughout the literature there are important clues that attest to the true, gluten-driven basis of this part of the spectrum, like atrophy of the spleen [66,68,78,79] which is a highly discriminatory index of gluten sensitivity: a typical proximal flat (Type 3) lesion [68,69]; human leucocyte antigen (HLA) background or childhood history [69,70,78,80]; and that a strict gluten-free diet defers onset of EATL [81].

Some difficulties have arisen in the past because either the lymphoma has arisen *de novo* or a typical proximal mucosal lesion could not be [79], or was not demonstrated. However, it is now evidently clear that gluten sensitivity may remain latent for several years, and present initially in the later years of life [71]. It is very likely that subtle lesions associated with gluten sensitivity will either have been overlooked, not recognized for what they are, or merely dismissed as representing non-specific inflammatory change; proximal gluten challenge may also be necessary to demonstrate the sensitivity [82]. In this context, it is to be noted that EATL patients with either a pure coeliac syndrome, or DH, tend to demonstrate a reduced population of lymphoplasmacytic elements within epithelium and lamina propria [83,84]; further evidence of specific unresponsiveness is demonstrated by low levels of anti-α-gliadin antibody in such individuals [70]. This is often associated with widespread depletion of intestinal lymphoid tissue [85], mesenteric lymph node cavitation with hyalinization of T cell territory [79,86] and splenic atrophy [79,87–89].

The unresponsiveness may be related to the development of suppressor clones, as is evident in other chronic T cell-mediated conditions [90–92], and which may be MHC class 2 directed [91,93]; or alternatively to the tumour itself, which could lead to a syndrome analogous to chronic GVH resulting in progressive wasting, cachexia, lymphoid hypoplasia and immunosuppression [37,94].

Overall, there is overwhelming evidence to indicate that gluten sensitivity is the most common preceding event that leads to EATL/chronic jejunoileitis [69,70,79,82,95]. This facet of the gluten-sensitive spectrum appears to arise from the multifocal origin of clone(s) of malignant T cells within the intestinal tract whose effects render the mucosal unresponsive to further antigen withdrawal, resulting in a true hypoplasia and progressive atrophy of the entire mucosal lining of the intestinal wall [72,79,95,96]. The evolution of this hypoplastic/atrophic (Type 4) lesion demands recognition of a presumptive T cell-mediated end-stage lesion in some people with undoubted gluten sensitivity. This process is analogous to immunologically mediated destruction of thyroid in myxoedema, liver in chronic active cirrhosis or primary biliary cirrhosis; pancreatic islets in IDDM and gastric wall in pernicious anaemia (PA) [8], as well as in experimental GVH disease [31,35,37] (Table 6.2).

Table 6.2 Suggested causes of end-stage (irreversible) intestinal failure

Presumptive immune-mediated	Non-immune causes
Unresponsive gluten sensitivity	Ischaemia
Protracted diarrhoea of infancy (immunological variant)	Radiation enteritis/fibrosis
Scleroderma	Inflammatory (diffuse cicatrizing Crohn's disease)
Diffuse intestinal lymphoma	
Graft-versus-host disease	
Marasmus/Kwashiorkor/persistent diarrhoea syndrome	

Interrelationships of defined lesions: gluten challenge

From the beginning, it could be argued that the description of each mucosal lesion represents a series of self-contained vignettes that bear no dynamic relationship to one another. However, some clue to their interrelationship is provided by observations on the structural features and epithelial lymphoid infiltrates of a large series of DH patients studied in Manchester by computerized image analysis (Fig. 6.5). When arrayed in descending values of surface epithelial volume (V_{SE}), it can be seen (Fig. 6.6) that a doubling of crypt epithelial volume (V_{CR}) accompanied by lymphoid infiltration occurs before V_{SE} moves below the reference range established for control (volunteer) villi. Crypt epithelial volumes continue to increase as V_{SE} entered the range for untreated, flat coeliac mucosa [40]. At this stage crypt epithelial lymphoid infiltrates ($N_{V(CR)}$) are maintained at high level, while total surface epithelial lymphocytes ($N_{V(SE)}$) fall into control range.

Nevertheless, this display lacks dynamic relationships, since each mucosal specimen represents a separate event. One way of overcoming this impasse is by gluten challenge of well-treated coeliac patients in remission. A considerable amount of work concerned with the effects of gluten challenge has been published which can be categorized into (1) diagnostic challenge, and (2) approaches concerned with mechanisms of flattening, damage and mucosal inflammation. Those mechanisms have yet to be fully characterized, while on the other hand, the natural evolution of a typical flat lesion has only been recorded on rare occasions [97,98].

The sedate view, generally offered by most text books holds that '...the mucosa gradually is infiltrated by lymphocytes and plasma cells while surface enterocytes, being damaged directly by the "toxicity" of gluten causes progressive effacement of villi until flattening occurs. To compensate, crypt hypertrophy occurs with an increase in the rate and speed of cell division and of cell transit upwards to the surface'

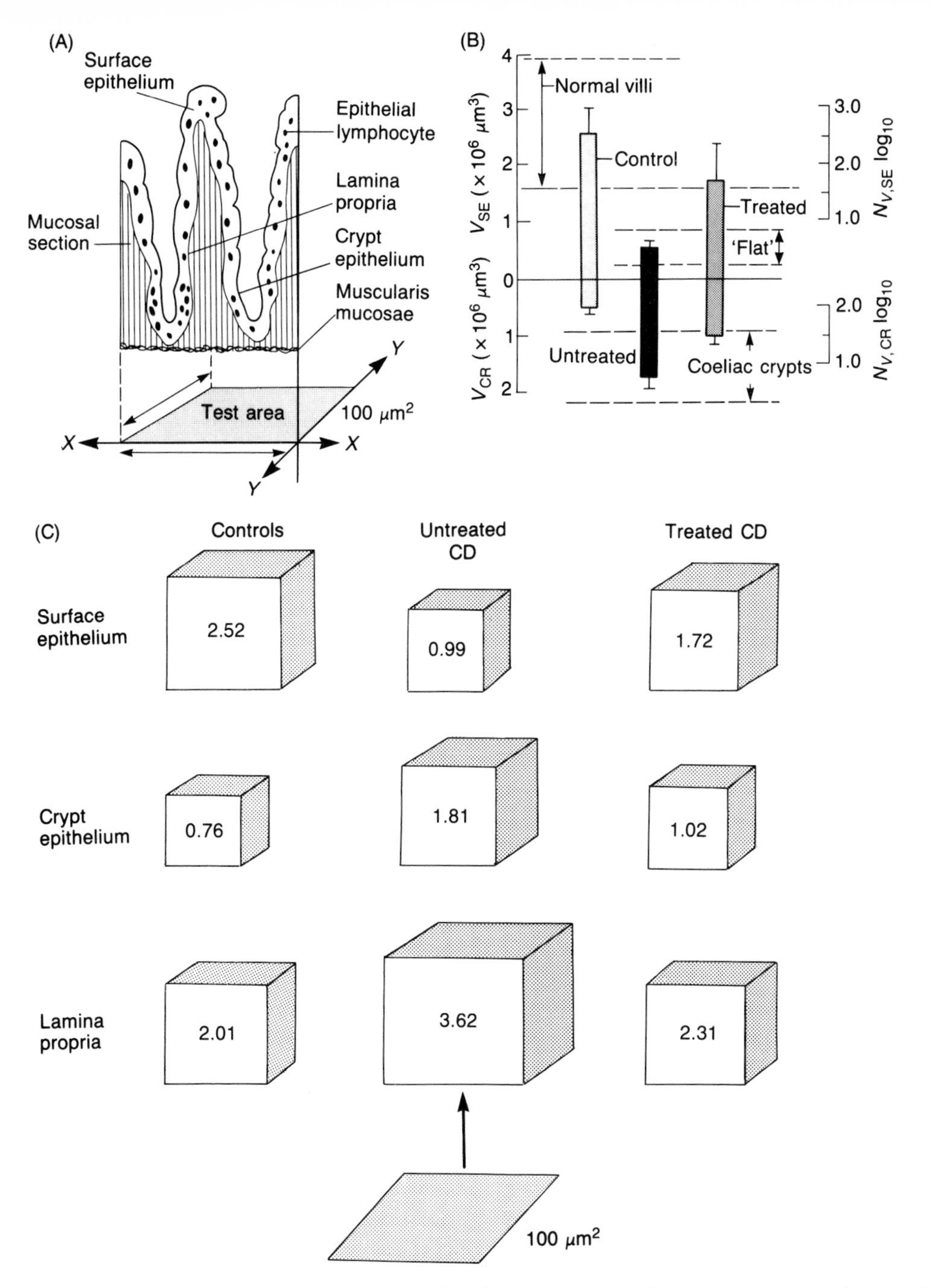

Fig. 6.5 Computerized image analysis is employed to quantitate and compare any type of mucosal lesion. Volumes of epithelium (surface, V_{SE}; crypt, V_{CR}) and lamina propria (V_{LP}) are determined with reference to a constant (100 μm^2) test square (XY) of muscularis mucosae (A). The volumes obtained can be displayed either as (B) or (C). (B) displays linear values on the ordinates V_{SE} or V_{CR}, respectively. Arrows and horizontal dashed lines indicate reference ranges for (a) normal villi (b) coeliac mucosae and (c) coeliac crypts. In addition, relevant measurements of the absolute number of IEL per mucosal compartment (i.e. in surface epithelium, $N_{V,SE}$ and in crypt epithelium, $N_{V,CR}$) can be displayed on the right hand upper and lower logarithmic scales. (C) displays cubes of equivalent volume, such that their cross-sectional (areal) faces can be drawn to scale in a semiquantitative manner.

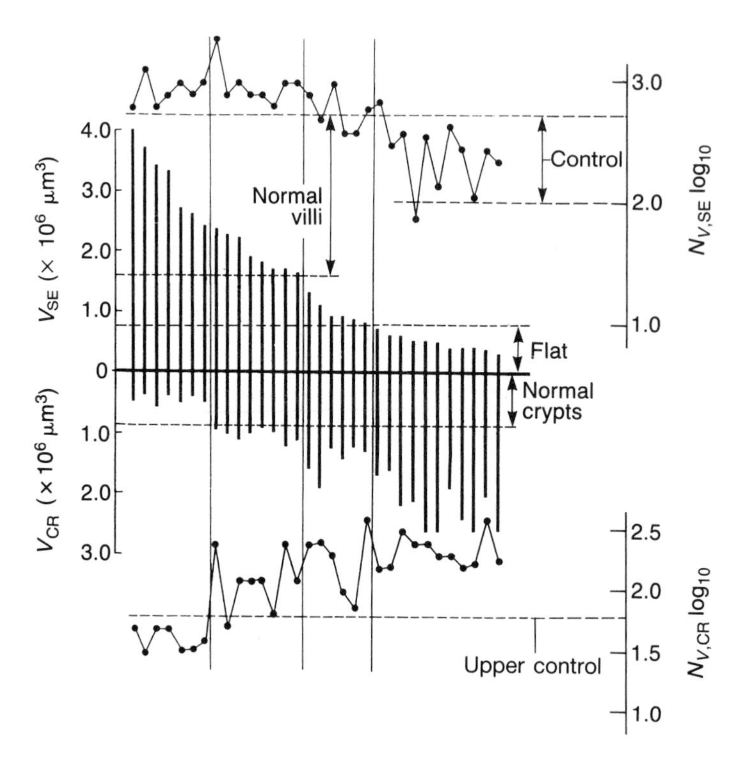

Fig. 6.6 The principles described in Fig. 6.5 are here illustrated for mucosae obtained from 32 patients with untreated DH (non-gluten-free diet). Values for V_{SE} are displayed in descending order (left to right) and those for crypt epithelial volume (V_{CR}) underneath, and corresponding IEL populations for each compartment displayed on right hand log axes. Dashed horizontal lines and arrows define relevant reference ranges. The first seven mucosae illustrate 'infiltrative' (Type 1) lesions, followed by eight with crypt enlargement ('hyperplastic' Type 2 lesions). The 11 mucosae to the extreme right are all examples of flat 'destructive' (Type 3) lesions. Note infiltration of crypt epithelium by cIEL at point of crypt hypertrophy. There is a progressive reduction in surface IEL as mucosae flatten, while crypt infiltrates remain high throughout the series.

[99,100]. This view generally fulfils the 'haemolytic' model of mucosal damage in which crypt hypertrophy is seen purely as a response to the increased rate of desquamation of enterocytes from the flattened mucosal surface, in much the same way that marrow hypertrophy compensates for increased peripheral erythrocyte losses in haemolytic anaemias [71,101,102].

In our laboratory it was thought desirable to approach the problem of flattening systematically, since it was argued that if the coeliac lesions were due to cell-mediated immunopathological influences, then a graded series of challenges (analogous to the performance of a Mantoux reaction for tuberculin sensitivity) would reveal detailed information about the sequence of changes reflecting the transition from a villous-bearing mucosa to the classic flat (Type 3) lesion. In

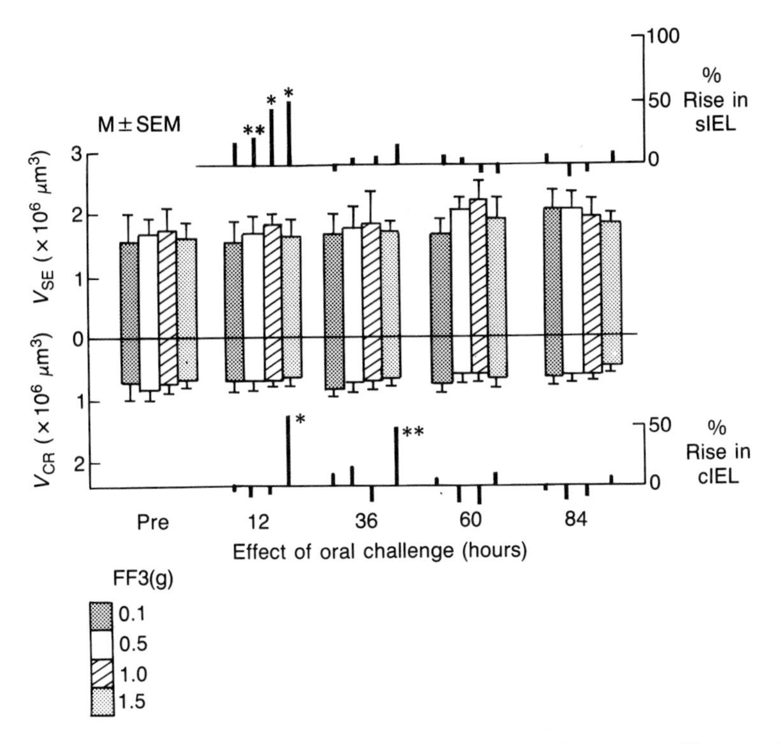

Fig. 6.7 The effect of oral challenge with FF3 on treated mucosae of known gluten-sensitive individuals. Note dose-dependent increment in villous IEL (as percentage rise in sIEL on pre-challenge value) at 12 hours post-challenge, while the first detectable alteration in crypt IEL (cIEL) occurs with 1.5 g FF3 challenge. During each set of four dose challenges, mucosal architecture remained unaffected. (*$p \leq 0.01$; **$p < 0.05$).

adopting this approach we selected small groups of treated coeliac patients and challenged separate individuals with a varying oral dose of FF3, comprising either 0.1, 0.5, 1.0, 1.5, 3, 6 or 12 g. Before each challenge a control biopsy was performed, together with four further biopsies (at 12, 36, 60 and 84 hours) post-challenge; the control protein was 0.5 g β-lactoglobulin (βLG). Other non-coeliac volunteers underwent similar challenges with either FF3 or βLG; only the coeliac patients responded to FF3, and the experimental design permitted observations of dose responses, and time responses.

With small oral challenges (0.1–1.0 g FF3) a dose-dependent increment of intraepithelial lymphocytes (IEL) within villous surface epithelium (sIEL) was observed, unaccompanied by architectural changes in either V_{SE} and V_{CR} [44]. With 1.5 g FF3, the dose response of sIEL continued, but infiltration of crypt epithelium (cIEL) also occurred, both of which peaked at 12 hours post-challenge (Fig. 6.7).

With 3 g FF3, villous architecture remained unchanged despite continuing infiltration by sIEL, although there was now an increase in

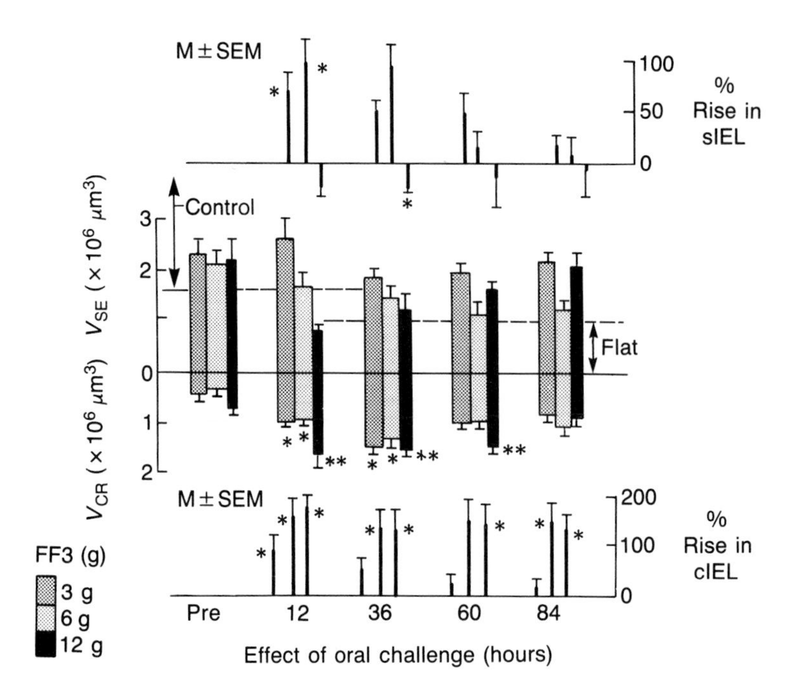

Fig. 6.8 With higher dose (FF3) challenges, there are continued increases in sIEL and cIEL; note that increases in cIEL persist throughout challenges with both 6 and 12 g FF3, whereas sIEL fail to rise with 12 g FF3, presumably due to mucosal flattening which is evident by 12 hours post-challenge. With 3 g challenge, crypt hypertrophy occurs in the absence of any significant loss of villous epithelial volumes (i.e. reduction in villous height) ($*p<0.01$; $**p<0.02$).

crypt epithelial volume (V_{CR}) which, exceeding by a factor of two, pre-challenge values came now to lie within the reference range for coeliac crypts [103]. Furthermore, at this dose cIEL remained elevated throughout the challenge, while sIEL peaked only at 12 hours and waned thereafter (Fig. 6.8).

With 6 g FF3, crypt hypertrophy persisted throughout the challenge series (12–84 hours) accompanied by a sustained rise in cIEL (Figs 6.8, 6.9). Between 12 and 36 hours post-challenge sIEL were increased, but between 60 and 84 hours post-challenge, as villous flattening set in, there was a parallel fall in sIEL. Villous flattening occurred by 12 hours following a 12 g FF3 challenge, and at this stage there was no further dose-responsive increase in sIEL, which remained low (Fig. 6.8). On the other hand, crypt hypertrophy was again evident by 12 hours and persisted through 84 hours, accompanied by a persistent and sustained rise in cIEL throughout [103]. During these challenges, the percentage of granular IEL also increased [104].

It should be evident from the foregoing that this extensive series of experiments have established the patterns of mucosal change associated with eventual mucosal flattening. Importantly, it has been shown in a

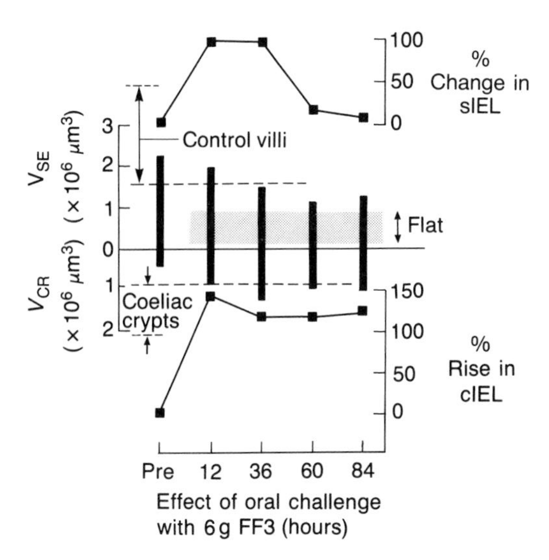

Fig. 6.9 Mucosal responses to 6 g FF3 challenge from the same patient observed over 5 days. They illustrate change from normal (first pre-challenge specimen) to infiltrative and infiltrative-hyperplastic lesions (second (12 hour) to third (36 hour post-challenge) specimens) followed by flattening (last two specimens at 60 and 84 hour post-challenge) in which sIEL fall, but cIEL are maintained at high level. This time-chart illustrates dynamic sequence and relationship between infiltrative, (crypt) hyperplastic and flat lesions.

dynamic setting that the lesions described above (Types 1–3) are sequential, interrelated phases in the evolution of the classic flat lesion (Fig. 6.9). There is first infiltration of villous epithelium and then of crypt epithelium, followed by crypt hypertrophy which represents the first architectural change in mucosal structure. It should be noted that crypt hypertrophy occurs despite the presence of normally structured villi, although both villous and crypt epithelium are subject to infiltrates by small lymphocytes. As progressive increases in crypt size occurred with larger challenges, villous flattening was seen to slowly follow (Figs 6.10, 6.11).

These results firmly establish that crypt hypertrophy with epithelial lymphoid infiltration is an early and important phase in the initiation of mucosal flattening. The early challenge appearances are similar to mucosae seen in first degree coeliac relatives [41], patients with DH [40] and in the T cell-mediated model of neonatal [32] and adult [31,35] GVH in experimental animals. Secondly, it is evident that gluten challenge does not damage surface (villous) enterocytes as an initial phase in mucosal flattening and conversely that crypt hypertrophy cannot solely be a response to such mucosal flattening; clearly, the 'haemolytic' model of mucosal flattening is no longer a tenable or rational explanation of the observed phenomena [6,101,102]. Thirdly, the evolving series of changes documented is similar to the natural

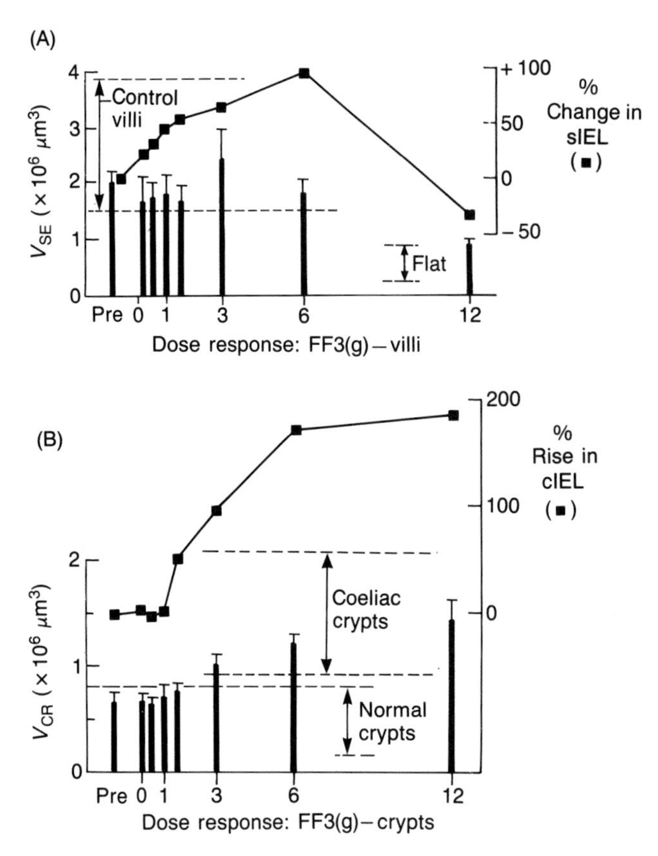

Fig. 6.10 The method of challenge employed, together with quantitative technique of computerized image analysis permits construction of dose-response curves, both for surface epithelium (A) and crypt epithelium (B). Illustrated are composite data at 12 hour post-challenge with each of the seven doses of FF3. Note that at this time point, crypt hypertrophy occurs (with 3 and 6 g FF3) before villous flattening becomes evident (12 g FF3), while crypt epithelium is infiltrated by IEL (1.5 g) before hypertrophy (3 g) is evident. Infiltration of surface epithelium occurs in advance of crypt epithelium; furthermore the incremental rise is considerably less than that observed in crypts, and is not sustained as villous flattening is brought about by 12 g dose challenge.

evolution of mucosal changes (Fig. 6.12) followed in a patient over a 3-year period [98].

Together, these observations are consistent with a progressive model (Fig. 6.13) of identifiable, cell-mediated mucosal reactions to gluten. In a wider context, the recognition of distinct, yet dynamically interrelated developmental phases in the evolution of a flat mucosa places in perspective the morphological changes described in allied conditions, such as tropical mucosal reactions, giardiasis and other childhood food protein hypersensitivities in which one, or more, of the observed pat-

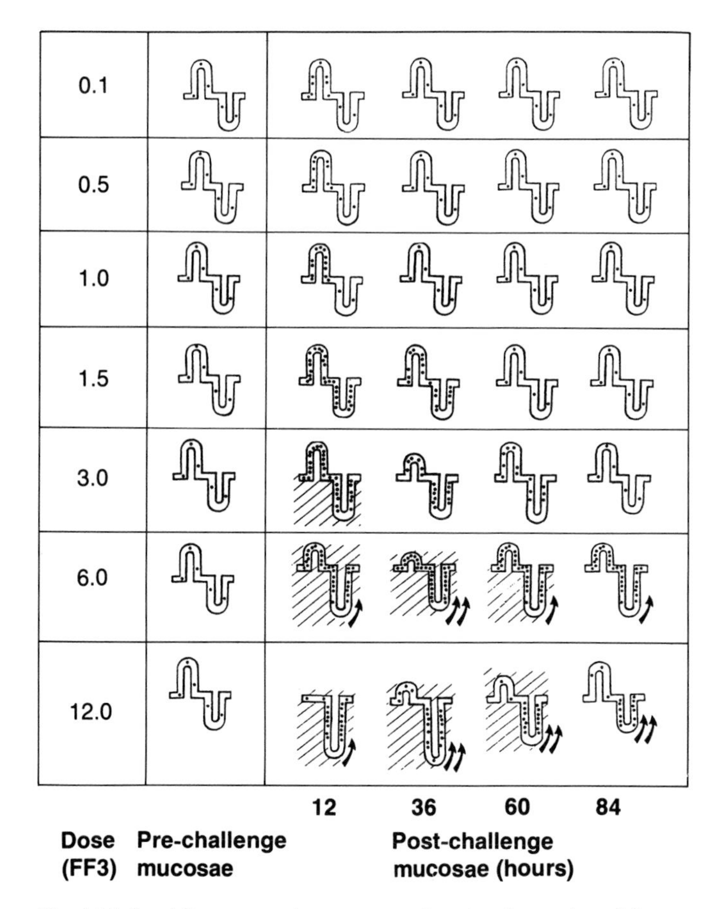

Fig. 6.11 Semidiagrammatic representation, in chequerboard format, of dose/time responses of coeliac mucosae to gluten challenge. Cross-hatching indicates architectural changes to crypts and/or villi. Arrows indicate changes in crypt cell mitotic activity. The dose-response for crypts and for villi at 12 hour post-challenge, for example, is illustrated in Fig. 6.10. (Format of diagram is based on Ferguson [31].)

terns has been variously described (Fig. 6.13). Together, they likewise suggest that the underlying mechanism may be that of a cell-mediated immune response to these varied environmental immunogens. Despite such varied reactions, recognition of their pathology permits a reasonable classification on the basis outlined above, and elsewhere [7–9,31, 35,36,49,50,53,105].

Latent gluten sensitivity

The term latent, as applied to gluten sensitivity, was probably used first by Weinstein [106], who showed that mild lesions in DH could be converted to flat lesions by additional oral feeding of gluten. This

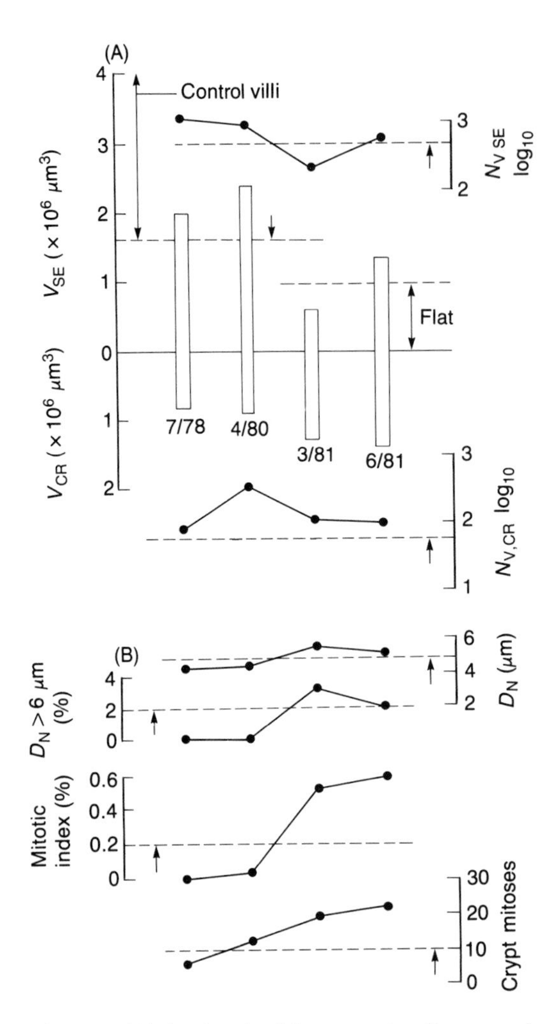

Fig. 6.12 (A) the data in this composite diagram refer to four mucosal specimens obtained from one patient between July 1978 and June 1981 during which their appearances progressed from an infiltrative-hyperplastic lesion (see Fig. 6.1D) to a flat destructive lesion (see Fig. 6.3) by March 1981. The final mucosa shows villous regrowth following 6 months gluten restriction by this patient. Note that sIEL fall ($N_{V,SE}$) when mucosa flattens (3/81), although cIEL ($N_{V,CR}$) remain elevated above upper reference ranges (horizontal dotted lines and arrowheads). Arrowheads indicate upper reference range for IEL in surface epithelium, and upper reference range for crypt epithelium. (B) illustrates the other expected changes accompanying a flat (Type 3) lesion, such as increase in the size (D_N) and percentage of 'blast-like' IEL (D_N >6 μm diameter) and their mitotic index (>0.2%), together with a marked increase in crypt cell mitotic activity. Arrowheads indicate upper reference ranges. (From Marsh [98].)

usage of the term is very restricted, and clearly has no relevance to the more important concept of clinical latency.

Since then it has become evident that individuals who are indubi-

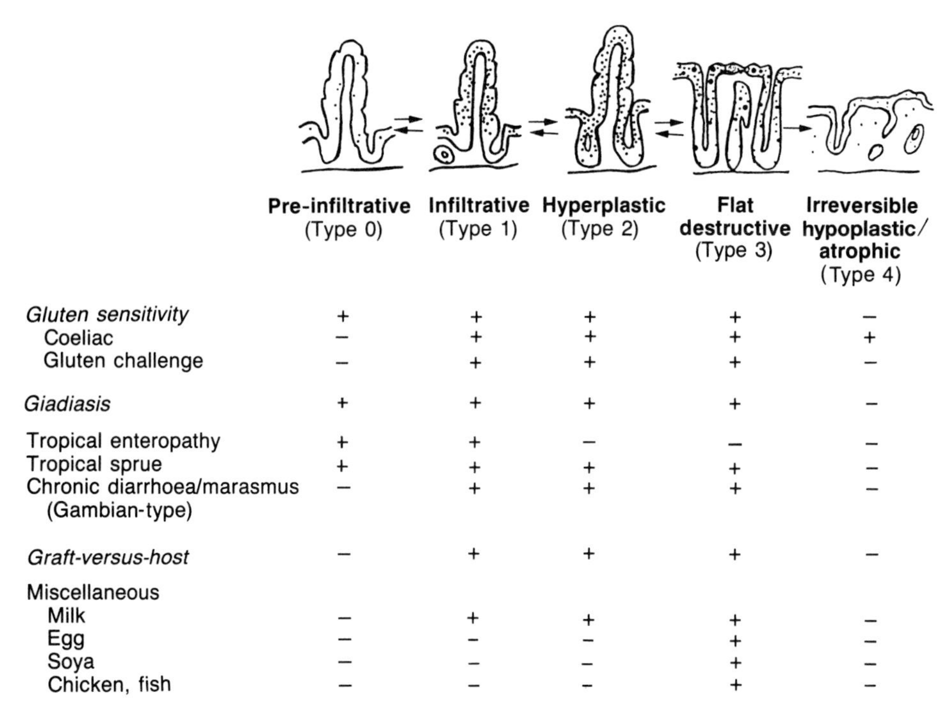

	Pre-infiltrative (Type 0)	**Infiltrative** (Type 1)	**Hyperplastic** (Type 2)	**Flat destructive** (Type 3)	**Irreversible hypoplastic/ atrophic** (Type 4)
Gluten sensitivity	+	+	+	+	–
Coeliac	–	+	+	+	+
Gluten challenge	–	+	+	+	–
Giadiasis	+	+	+	+	–
Tropical enteropathy	+	+	–	–	–
Tropical sprue	+	+	+	+	–
Chronic diarrhoea/marasmus (Gambian-type)	–	+	+	+	–
Graft-versus-host	–	+	+	+	–
Miscellaneous					
Milk	–	+	+	+	–
Egg	–	–	–	+	–
Soya	–	–	–	+	–
Chicken, fish	–	–	–	+	–

Fig. 6.13 Various patterns of mucosal immunopathology occur throughout the gluten-sensitivity spectrum: these include the pre-infiltrative, infiltrative, hyperplastic, flat-destructive, and irreversible hypoplastic/atrophic types, as described in text. Similar pathological changes are also seen in tropical enteropathy and tropical sprue which obviously represent extreme ends of the host response to one, or many, microbial (? cross-reactive) epitopes. Analogous changes are seen in giardiasis in which most individuals react with an infiltrative/hyperplastic response and only rarely with a flat-destructive lesion. Food-based host responses seem to be based on similar host-directed forms of mucosal immunopathology. Malignant (lymphomatous) transformation, invariably seen in the setting of an end-stage, irreversible, and hence truly atrophic lesion, only appears to occur in gluten-sensitive individuals.

tably sensitized to gluten may develop any lesion (Types 0–4) and yet be entirely asymptomatic, as indicated above. It thus follows that clinically latent mucosal lesions are only likely to be uncovered by (1) the presence of skin blistering in DH [58], (2) acute complications of EATL, chronic inflammation or jejunoileitis such as perforation, bleeding, intestinal obstruction, abdominal pain or fairly rapid onset of diarrhoea [66–69,71–77,79,82], (3) a systematic investigational follow-up of family relatives of known coeliac subjects [107] or (4) by performing a jejunal biopsy in suspicious clinical circumstances, such as progressive ill-health, lack of energy, recurrent unresponsive iron deficiency or growth deficiency [108–111].

The extent of latent (subclinical) gluten sensitivity is seemingly large, and numerically probably represents 60–70% of all gluten-sensitive subjects. For example, ~40% DH patients have a Type 3 lesion that is usually quiescent. In first degree coeliac relatives, about 10% have a silent Type 1 infiltrative lesion, while 15% have a flat lesion among which 50% are asymptomatic. It is also evident from smaller series of coeliac-associated lymphoma, that a severe and often progressive (Type 4 atrophic) lesion is present in some cases before clinical complications set in and bring the condition to light, while from studies in DH [58], some patients have a normal biopsy morphologically despite local production of high titre anti-α-gliadin antibodies. If a similar set of circumstances obtains in coeliac individuals, then the difficulty in recognition can be readily appreciated, unless other tests are employed in addition to mucosal biopsy to expose the underlying sensitivity. It has been estimated that a truer prevalence figure throughout northern Europe might be 1:300 [112].

This leads to further aspects of latent gluten sensitivity that must be appreciated. There is now an ever-expanding literature describing children [97,107,108,113,114] and adults [58,98,107,109,110] in whom suspicions of gluten sensitization were not evidently confirmed by the presence of a damaged mucosa. In some cases, a typical flat mucosa could be identified, but only after the lapse of several years. Nevertheless, despite the presence of a 'normal' biopsy there were earlier systemic manifestations of gluten sensitization-like blisters [58], growth retardation, iron deficiency, and elevated local anti-α-gliadin antibody production [58,97,107,111].

It should also be appreciated that although concordance for disease (flat mucosa!) in identical twins is estimated to be high at 70% [111], there is a long interval between onset of disease in either twin that can be as long as 8 years [113,114]. Therefore, unlike IDDM where the second twin usually develops symptomatic hyperglycaemia within 5 years if he or she is destined also to develop IDDM, the situation in gluten sensitivity is different and emphasizes the important role of environmental factors in revealing the nascent predisposition. It is also evident that the earliest lesions (Type 0) will lack a lymphoid infiltrate of villous epithelium.

Given the genetic background, and the evidence that gluten is necessary, what factors are necessary to induce flattening, cause symptoms and lead to an apparent fall in incidence in Eire, UK, Israel and Finland, but not in neighbouring Sweden? Clearly, the role of environment is important and includes:

1 age of weaning;
2 period of breast feeding;
3 birth order;
4 concurrent infection;
5 additional metabolic stresses (operative surgery, pregnancy, delivery);
6 neoplastic transformation.

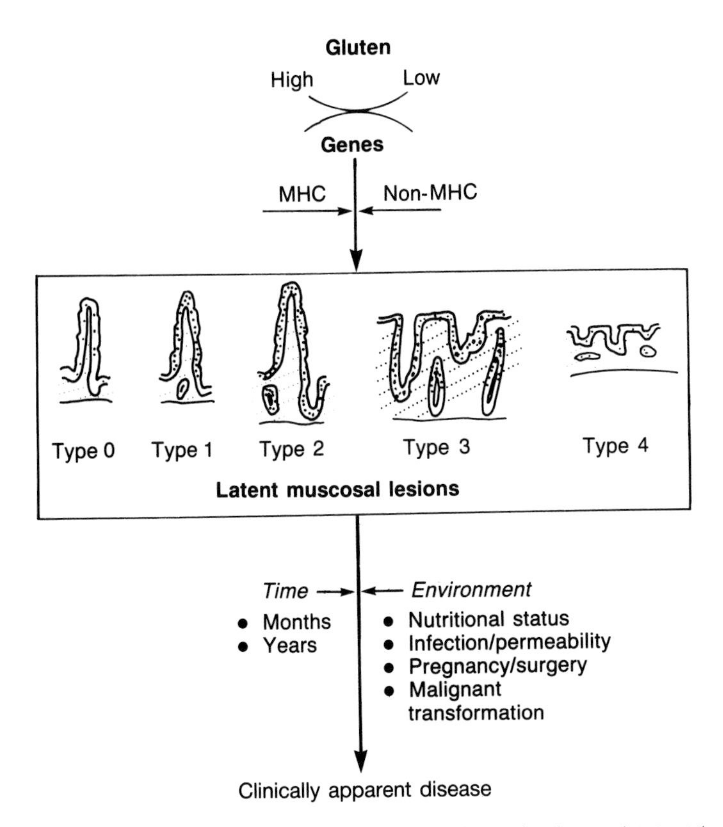

Fig. 6.14 In the presence of a certain MHC class 2 haplotype ('DQw2') together with other undoubted genes and gluten ingestion, a state of gluten sensitivity develops in which five different types of mucosal lesion are evident. These may remain latent, or be awakened by impact from a variety of environmental stimuli at any time throughout the patient's lifespan. The literature firmly attests to the fact that the majority of gluten-sensitized patients, despite whatever lesion they may have, are asymptomatic (i.e. latent). Those who develop symptomatic coeliac-sprue disease with classical symptoms of diarrhoea, weight loss or nutrient malabsorption (~30% of entire spectrum) invariably have a flat (Type 3) lesion.

Presumably, many of these factors amplify existing inflammatory lesions within the mucosa which hitherto remained chronically dormant and thus latent. Indeed, it can be advanced, provocatively, that gluten sensitivity, whatever the underlying type of lesion developed, is essentially an asymptomatic condition that is manifested, at any age, by the influence of a variety of environmental stimuli and insults (Fig. 6.14).

The lamina propria

One of the major, although often forgotten, aspects of the gluten-induced mucosal lesion is that it is transmural. Those who doubt (or are surprised by) this statement should re-read Paulley's original description of full-thickness biopsies obtained at laparotomy in patients with idiopathic steatorrhoea [34]. The same holds true for rectal tissue [115]; in this location, the use of grab forceps invariably provides submucosal tissue in addition to mucous membrane. This is not the case for jejunal biopsies, unfortunately, which only comprise mucous membrane proper (epithelium, lamina propria and muscularis mucosae); as a result little thought or consideration is (or has ever been) given to the role and involvement of subepithelial tissues in the disease process. Past coeliac research has been directed solely at mucosal architectural changes, altered epithelial cell dynamics and IEL, although there are scarcely any hard data for a major primary role for epithelium, or individual enterocytes, as initiators of mucosal pathology. Furthermore, it is very hard to see how the entire intestinal wall could be involved, if the major (or singular event) occurs only above the basement membrane. On the other hand, there is good evidence that mucosal architectural changes wrought by activated lamina propria T lymphocytes are important in GVH [30,116,117] and in models employing cultured foetal intestinal explants [118,119]. Is there evidence that mucosal T cells could similarly be involved in the immunopathology of gluten sensitivity?

Indirectly, the occurrence of gluten sensitivity in individuals with IgA deficiency [54,120] or panhypogammaglobulinaemia [121] suggests a central role for T cells. Further evidence indicates that humoral responses in coeliac patients are essentially secondary bystander events [122,123], and that locally produced high-titre antibodies are unable to cause mucosal damage [58].

In vitro work with peripheral blood mononuclear cells with the lymphocyte migration inhibition assay (LMIF), or macrophage procoagulant assay (MPCA), indicate that there is cellular hypersensitivity to gliadin-derived peptides [124–130]. MPCA depends on activated macrophages which develop a membrane-associated procoagulant mechanism of fibrin formation which restricts their mobility, e.g. from capillary tubes [131–133]. MPCA is a sensitive, antigen-specific measure of cell-mediated immunity.

In translating these observations to the mucosa, it is likely that lamina propria (DR^+) macrophages are activated and hence able to present pathogenic gliadin oligopeptides that have traversed the hyperpermeant epithelial barrier to $CD4^+$ T lymphocytes. Pure T cell-mediated reactions result in fibrin formation [134] and in untreated coeliac mucosa, fibrinogen extravasates from the hyperpermeable vasculature [27] and is thus available to be converted to fibrin. Furthermore, the identification of antigen-specific upregulation of interleukin 2 receptors (IL2-R) in circulating blood implies activation not only of mucosal lymphocytes via oral antigenic challenge [135,136] but also those of

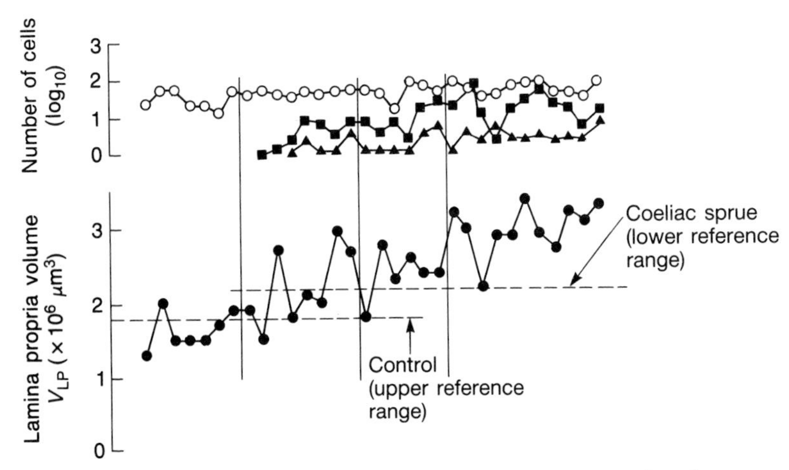

Fig. 6.15 This diagram illustrates lamina propria volumes (× 10^6 μm^3) as determined by computerized image analysis for 32 DH patients on normal diet (compare with Fig. 6.6). Lamina propria volumes begin to increase at the stage of crypt hypertrophy, a process accompanied by the appearance of neutrophils (■) and scanty basophils (▲) into the mesenchyme, presumably emigrating via local microvasculature. There is no material change in mast cell (○) content as the mucosae progressively flatten. (From Marsh [40].)

the predominantly $CD4^+$ population within the lamina propria [137].

Thus, there appears to be good evidence for an antigen-driven cascade, via macrophage and lymphocyte activation, leading to IL2-R production. Following this, further phlogistic reactions take place, possibly via proinflammatory $CD4^+$ cells, analogous to Th1 murine cells concerned in delayed-type hypersensitivity (DTH) reactions [138], which directly or indirectly cause accumulation of neutrophils, mast cells and basophils [139,140] activation of eosinophils and neutrophils [141,142], degranulation of mast cells [143], and the production of lipoxygenase-derived inflammatory products 15-HETE [144], prostaglandin secretion [145], microvascular hyperpermeability [115] and complement activation [146].

In a series of 32 untreated DH patients [40] progressive swelling of the lamina propria, and infiltration by neutrophils, mast cells and basophils was noted as mucosae evolved through Type 1, 2 and 3 stages to become flat (Fig. 6.15). It is noteworthy that swelling and early neutrophilic infiltration of lamina propria had occurred well before any marked change in villous morphology was apparent (Fig. 6.6). Rapid swelling of lamina propria with extravascular leakage of fibrinogen was also a prominent feature of our detailed study of gluten challenge of rectal coeliac mucosa [115].

What is still unclear is the nature of the phenomena that in GVH disease, gluten-sensitive enteropathy and allied cell-mediated reactions lead to the characteristic evolution of villous flattening, when a similar cascade of inflammatory mediators seen in Crohn's jejunitis fails to bring about the same kind of architectural remodelling which occurs in GVH disease. Further insights have come from some ingenious studies with explanted human foetal gut [118,119] in which crypt hypertrophy was shown to be a rapid response to activation of lamina propria lymphocytes (note that IEL are *absent* from this model) by anti-CD3 monoclonal antibody. This treatment not only evoked expression of CD25, but also resulted in epithelial infiltration by $CD3^{+}$ lymphocytes. Since such explants do not suffer the additional complication of infiltration by blood-borne cells, it is evident that local differentiation, mitotic expansion and migration of lamina propria T cells can contribute directly to the size of the IEL lymphocyte pool, as well as modulate mucosal architecture.

Here then is further, albeit indirect, evidence that activation of the lamina propria does influence and modulate epithelial behaviour, and lymphocyte populations therein. Nevertheless, the factors responsible for rapid crypt hypertrophy in these explants, on stimulation, is still unknown. These thoughts should be tempered by the results of a study of AIDS enteropathy in which depletion of CD4 cells could be the reason why crypt hypertrophy failed to materialize in some specimens [147].

The enterocyte in gluten sensitivity

The reason for the impaired vitality of surface enterocytes that typically characterize the flat, destructive (Type 3) lesion in this condition is not understood. As stated in the introduction to this chapter, early work in coeliac disease was directed solely at the enterocyte, rather than the whole mucosa, an event historically propelled by Frazer's powerfully articulated views regarding the so-called 'peptidase' deficiency [18]. Even subsequent attempts to explain cell damage were similarly biased toward the enterocyte, although many of these theories lacked substantiating evidence and can be safely dismissed. On the other hand, it should now be firmly appreciated that a similar appearance of surface enterocytes and an increased IEL density is seen in other flat lesions associated with tropical sprue [148], immunodeficiency [54], giardiasis, coccidiosis and immunoproliferative small intestinal disease (IPSID) [55]. It should also be remembered that with Type 1 and 2 lesions (in which there is substantial lymphoid infiltration of epithelium), enterocyte dimensions are normal.

Thus, it is evident that it is something intrinsic to the actual process of flattening, or being flat, that appears to result in changes in cell size, function, reduced vitality and premature death of surface enterocytes. What factor, or factors, are operative in this process is entirely unknown.

The shape of polarized epithelial cells depends on adjacent connections via terminal web and basal lamina and in their absence, individual cells tend to round up and become spherical [149,150]. Signals derived through such attachments provide for correct orientation and organization of the cytoskeleton which, in turn, determines cell shape, height and orientation.

Connections with basal lamina, and its components may be critical here, since when dispersed cells come into contact with such material, they organize and form regular epithelial monolayers. The basal lamina, since it derives from epithelium as well as lamina propria mesenchymal cells [151,152], may therefore be abnormally structured if one important contributor, like epithelium, is damaged.

Observations on gluten-damaged jejunal [27] and rectal [115] tissues from this laboratory suggest that basal lamina remains structurally intact, since immunoreactive fibrinogen and complement [153], escaping from locally damaged hyperpermeable microvasculature, are confined to the lamina propria and do not penetrate the interepithelial cell spaces. Such observations do not, however, preclude the possibility of molecular damage to basal lamina resulting from the discharge of enzymes and other bioactive material from activated inflammatory cells [154] thereby causing disruption of connections important for maintaining cell shape and physiological integrity. This observation is probably in keeping with recent data indicating that basal lamina (e.g. laminin) is a long-lasting structure [155] and is not turned over synchronously with the upwardly mobile column of migrating epithelial cells, as previously suggested [156,157].

The other possibility depends on the availability of oxygen and other vital metabolites that are critical from the subepithelial capillaries which, in the flattened lesion are probably subject to inflammatory damage.

Any reduction or loss of capillary blood flow exceeding more than 1–2 minutes is likely to cause anoxic damage leading to the formation of hypoxanthine and the rapid formation via xanthine oxidase of hydrogen peroxide and the superoxide anion ($O_2^{\bullet -}$) [158]; this could be a self-perpetuating circuit [159]. Furthermore, the extensive remodelling of the microvascular bed, attendant on mucosal flattening, could be another factor capable of endangering the vitality of surface and upper crypt cells compared with those of the mid/basal crypt regions which are supplied by larger, intercryptal vessels derived from submucosal vasculature. The mucosal microvasculature is directly involved in cell-mediated reactions, e.g. in the skin during the pure T lymphocyte response to intradermal tuberculin [134,160], or in the rectal [115] and jejunal mucosa [139,161] in coeliac sprue disease. Such observations, although descriptive in nature, include hypertrophy both of endothelial cells and pericytes and the margination, adherence and extravasation of inflammatory cells (lymphocytes, neutrophils, eosinophils and basophils) and of plasma proteins leading to tissue oedema [160,162]. Activation of the endothelium by inflammatory mediators and other cytokines could result in platelet activation, formation of microthrombi, and hence focal ischaemia of surface enterocytes. Interestingly, the ultrastructural features of damaged surface coeliac enterocytes, which comprise microvillar irregularities, mitochondrial swelling, dilatation of endoplasmic reticulum, and prominence and rupture of lysosomes [163–165] are identical to those induced in small intestinal enterocytes as a result of experimental ischaemia [161,166].

Scant attention has been paid to the vasculature of the lamina propria, yet it is probably the most important factor in directing function, and controlling the metabolic integrity of the intestinal mucosa. It is difficult to think of any circumstance in which vessel growth together with supporting mesenchymal elements is not critical either to embryonic development and growth, tissue healing and repair, or neoplastic transformation. The failure of a coeliac mucosa to respond, and regrow villi, must ultimately depend on a parallel failure of microvessels to initiate that repair process. The discovery of those factors which inhibit neovascularization could contribute greatly to our understanding of the processes of mucosal remodelling that accompany cell-mediated enteropathies.

Intraepithelial lymphocytes

This is a curious population of mucosal lymphocytes which probably comprises one of the largest collections of lymphoid tissue within the adult intestine. IEL have been closely related to gluten sensitivity from the earliest times when their density in surface epithelium was first shown to be elevated. Paradoxically, in the flat destructive lesion, the actual population of IEL, in absolute terms, is markedly increased ($\times 5$) within crypt epithelium [167] unlike surface epithelium in which numbers are in the low normal range [168,169] (Fig. 6.16). This disparity may be due to the high rate of desquamation of enterocytes from the surface epithelium, with consequent losses of IEL to lumen; the extent to which this is a physiologically determined process is unknown. It should also be noted that in the Type 1 and Type 2 lesions, there are real increases of IEL within the villi, despite intact preservation of the epithelial layer [40,41] in these lesions.

Despite intensive investigation over 20 years, it has still not been possible to glimpse into the function of these cells or to perceive what particular role, if any, they play in the mucosal lesions associated with gluten sensitivity [170]. It is evident that some IEL, especially those that are $CD8^+$, are attracted within epithelium by gluten (spontaneously by diet, or by experimental challenge); conversely, a gluten-free diet causes these infiltrates to regress.

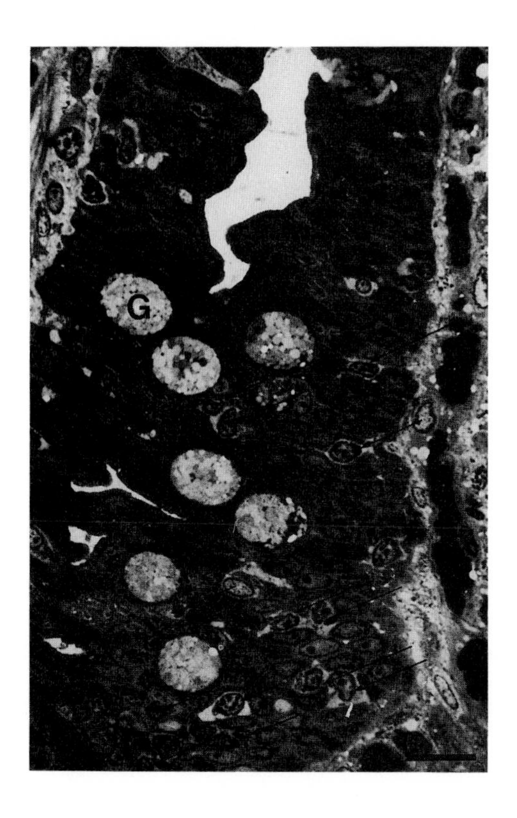

Fig. 6.16 Detail from untreated coeliac (flat, destructive lesion) illustrating marked increase in population of IEL (arrows) within crypt epithelium. G, Goblet cells. (Magnification bar, 100 μm.)

As the mucosal lesion deteriorates (Types 1–3) the IEL become larger, show morphological evidence of 'activation', and begin to increase their rate of mitosis (Figs 6.12, 6.16–6.18). The mechanism behind this change is unknown [168,170,171], but the increase in mitotic figures among IEL in flat mucosae is a useful way to distinguish flat coeliac sprue mucosae from non-gluten-induced flat mucosae [171–173]. The presence of large IEL in flat mucosae remains unexplained and does not appear to be a manifestation of antigen (gluten)-induced lymphocytic blast transformation since it is not seen among the heavy gluten-induced infiltrates that characterize Type 1 and Type 2 'infiltrative' lesions [40,41,170] (Fig. 6.1).

In humans, the majority of IEL are $CD3^+$ $CD8^+$ [174–176] while in untreated coeliac sprue cases, there is an expanded population (~30%) of $CD3^+$ $CD4^-$ $CD8^-$ (double negative) lymphocytes [95]. In regard to the former subsets ($CD3^+$ $CD8^+$) the majority, both in control and coeliac subjects, are CD45 RA^- [177]. However, an expanded population of $CD3^+$ (70%) and $CD8^+$ (62%) express the 180 kDa isoform CD45 RO compared with ~50% for both populations in controls. All $CD3^+$ IEL express varying amounts of CD45 RB, often reciprocally in relation to RO. All IEL (controls and coeliacs) of the $CD4^+$ subset (~5%) are also CD45 RO^{high}. Thus, in untreated coeliac patients there is an accumulation of CD45 RO^{high} RB^{low} IEL in the mucosa, regressing

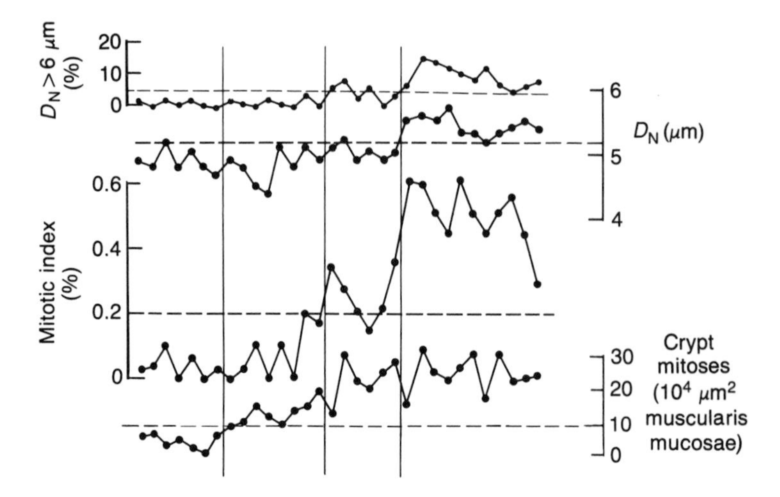

Fig. 6.17 Additional quantitative data for 32 DH mucosae (see Figs 6.6, 6.15). In this diagram, the progressive increases in the size (mean IEL nuclear diameter, D_N) and percentage of blast-like IEL with large heterochromatic nuclei and expanded cytoplasm (D_N >6 μm) together with evidence of their rising mitotic activity within epithelium (mitotic index) are illustrated. In this series, note that mitotic activity of IEL increases before detectable increases in size of IEL, and percentage of 'blasts' take place. Lower graph shows progressive rises in crypt epithelial cell mitotic activity across the whole series (Fig. 6.6) as mucosal flattening occurs. (From Marsh [40].)

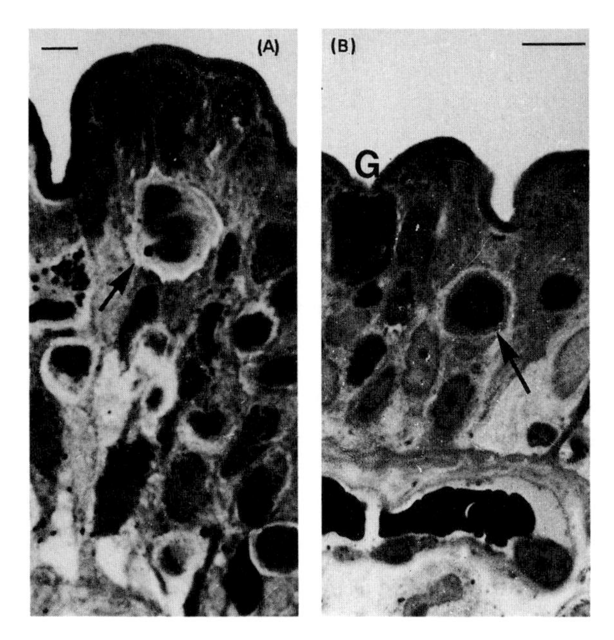

Fig. 6.18 Details from surface epithelium of flat destructive (Type 3) gluten-induced mucosal lesions illustrating mitotic (A, arrows) and 'blast-like' (B, arrows) IEL. G, goblet cells. (Magnification bars, 10 μm.) (From Marsh [168].)

after treatment [178]. Since CD45 RA^+ cells (~5% IEL) are naïve or unprimed T cells, it is clear that the majority of $CD3^+$ IEL in untreated coeliacs are memory, or primed, lymphocytes [179,180]. The reason for this, and the way in which, and in what site, those cells acquire memory in the intestinal mucosa require further analysis.

It is also of interest that such cells (CD45 RA^- RO^+) are more sensitive to antigen stimulation and recall, and secrete IFNγ (γ-type interferon) when stimulated [181]. Other evidence indicates that elaboration of IFNγ by IEL results in upregulation and more extensive expression of MHC class 2 allospecificities among surface and crypt enterocytes [182] and is consistent with the observed relationship between MHC expression and IEL territory [183,184].

At present data are scant, and it seems likely that some of the changes described are not exclusive to gluten sensitivity, but may also be seen in other enteropathies in which architectural remodelling is a major feature [178]. It is also odd that if such cells are antigen-primed, they do not seem to be responding to gluten antigen in the conventional manner [185]; this may be simply due to the fact that the majority of IEL is $CD8^+$. Clearly, much more needs to be learned about these cells, their response to gluten challenge and withdrawal and their subsequent activation (cytokine) pathways dependent on the particular CD45 isoform expressed.

Recent excitement has been generated by the observation that in some species, a relatively high proportion of IEL express not the conventional α/β T cell receptor (TCR 2) but the γ/δ type (TCR 1). It is generally agreed that in the normal human intestine, about 90% IEL are TCR 2 (α/β) cells, while only about 10% carry TCR 2 (γ/δ) receptors [186–189]. A large proportion of γ/δ IEL (~60%) characterize the expanded (~30% of $CD3^+$ IEL) population of $CD3^+$ double negative ($CD3^+$ $CD4^-$ $CD8^-$) cells seen in coeliac sprue mucosae, while the remainder are $CD3^+$ CD8 $\alpha^+\beta^-$; i.e. they express only the α-chain of the expressed CD8 cell surface heterodimer. It is possible that the α-chain expressed in such cells is induced by epithelium [186]. Up to 45% $CD3^+$ $CD8^+$ IEL expresses only one-half of this molecule.

Of the γ/δ subset, ~50% express V9 (Ti.A) gene products in association with V2, while the remainder express Vγ1/Vδ1 δTCS-1^+ [190]. In untreated coeliac sprue patients with Type 3 lesions, the Vγ1/Vδ1 subset is increased, together with the $CD3^+$ $CD4^-$ $CD8^-$ subset (of which they comprise the majority) to upwards of 30% [95,187,189]. Interestingly, this subset remains elevated despite gluten withdrawal, suggesting that they may have nothing to do with gluten sensitivity in general, or with the evolution of mucosal immunopathology in particular. Although it has been suggested that γ/δ cells may develop cytotoxicity towards enterocytes in the presence of gluten [187] it is still not explained how such activity would, or could be, selectively delivered to surface enterocytes alone, while those similar γ/δ gluten-activated IEL within crypt epithelium remain impotent.

The presence of an elevated population of γ/δ^+ IEL in gluten sensitivity may be of help in population surveillance programmes seeking potential gluten-sensitive individuals, especially that large group of gluten-sensitized individuals hinted at earlier in this chapter which is asymptomatic, irrespective of the type of lesion. Finally, it should be noted that mucosal flattening can be brought about by activated lamina propria cells that are TCR α/β [118,119] and that in experimental GVH, in which mucosal flattening again can be brought about solely by $CD4^+$ cells, the increase natural-killer associated cytotoxicity appears to play no major role in the evolution of mucosal pathology [30,35,37].

Gluten sensitivity: the rectal mucosa

Preoccupation with the effect of gluten on jejunal mucosa, and particularly the jejunal enterocyte as prime suspect in the pathogenesis of gluten sensitivity, has certainly obscured the view that in sensitized individuals gluten and other prolamins may be expected to damage any mucosal surface broadly within gut-associated lymphoid tissue (GALT) [191]. In recent years this principle seems to have been entirely forgotten, despite earlier observations from Rubin's laboratory in Seattle, Washington, on ileal and rectal responses to gluten infusion. Of the two studies published [192,193], approximately 5% of coeliac subjects were thought, from subjective observations, to have an abnormal rectal mucosa, and thus to be showing some kind of local response to gluten.

Only two other papers relate to this topic. The first was a retrospective review of 438 coeliac patients in whom diarrhoea was a major presenting complaint. Of 42 rectal biopsies taken 14 were abnormal, 11 revealed 'proctitic' features and the remaining three had the typical features of ulcerative colitis [194]. In the second study [195], 21 rectal biopsies from 135 coeliac patients were reviewed retrospectively, of which seven were abnormal; two were compatible with 'acute colitis' and five revealed features of 'microscopic lymphocytic colitis'. The retrospective, unselected nature of these data sheds very little light on the quest for a coeliac-induced proctocolitis. On the contrary the rare, but proven, coexistence of ulcerative colitis and CD is well known [196,197]. Since these earlier reports, a further 25 examples have been published [198–209]; there is also a demonstrable increased risk factor for ulcerative colitis among first degree coeliac relatives, estimated to be 5–15 fold [210,211].

Thus there appears to be more than a chance association between CD and an inflammatory colitis but whether the latter is a self-limiting, gluten-sensitive phenomenon, or part of a spectrum of distal large bowel inflammation which progresses from mild changes (microscopic) to overt ulcerative colitis is uncertain [212].

Normal colonic mucosa comprises a single layer of epithelium, interspersed with numerous goblet cells which line the flat luminal surface together with crypts which in section, are aligned parallel to each other and penetrate the lamina propria tissues. The lamina propria contains a sparse population of lymphocytes, plasma cells and eosinophils; neutrophils and basophils are absent, their presence being viewed as an index of mucosal inflammation. Normally, colonic epithelial cells do not express MHC class 2 alloantigen [213] and the majority of IEL are $CD8^+$; approximately one-third also expresses the 'activation' surface marker CD7; Leu11, CD16 cells (NK) are extremely rare. In the lamina, $CD4^+$ lymphocytes are present in a ratio of 3 : 1 over $CD8^+$ cells.

In the original work on rectal gluten challenge [193] cereal enemas were instilled into coeliac patients, including 50 g wheat in four subjects, and rectal biopsies obtained before and after challenge. Two patients developed systemic symptoms following such enormous challenges accompanied by a haemorrhagic macroscopic colitis. Histologically, there was rapid and intense infiltration by neutrophils of epithelium, lamina propria and submucosa, with occasional microabscesses within the surface epithelium.

Work from our laboratory [115,212,214] was designed to reevaluate this literary and experimental background in order (1) to determine whether untreated coeliac patients do have a self-limited gluten-dependent proctitis, (2) to evaluate afresh the immunopathological response of rectal mucosa to controlled gluten challenge and (3) to assess the possibility of whether rectal mucosa could be employed as an avenue for diagnosis, especially in individuals where a conventional jejunal biopsy might be difficult, as in small infants, pregnant women, or the elderly.

Comparison between control, disease control and coeliac rectal mucosa

This study was based on a computerized, morphometric analysis of rectal biopsies from six volunteer control, 15 gastrointestinal disease control and 23 coeliac patients, nine of which were untreated. The results of this detailed study revealed that there were no architectural differences between all controls or untreated and treated coeliacs, in terms of volumes of surface and crypt epithelium or lamina propria (Fig. 6.19). In untreated coeliacs, there was a 10-fold increase in plasma cells ($p<0.025$) which normalized on gluten restriction (Fig. 6.20); the mast cells were also elevated ($p<0.05$) and remained elevated during dietary treatment ($p<0.025$) (Fig. 6.21). There were no significant alter-

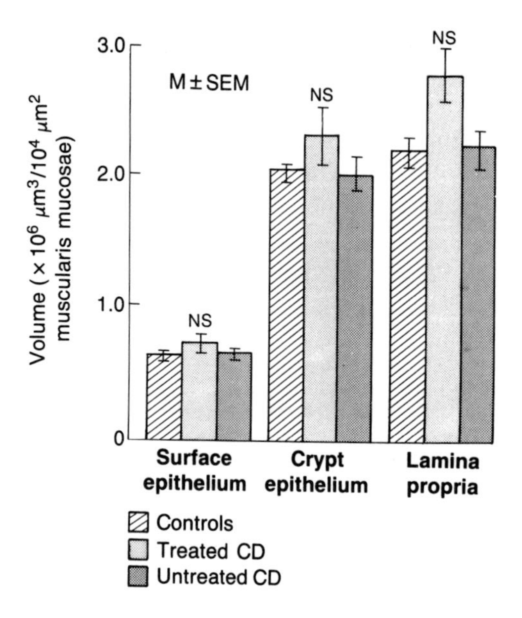

Fig. 6.19 Computerized image analysis of rectal mucosa reveals no significant differences in volumes of surface and crypt epithelium, or of lamina propria between control and untreated or treated gluten-sensitive individuals.

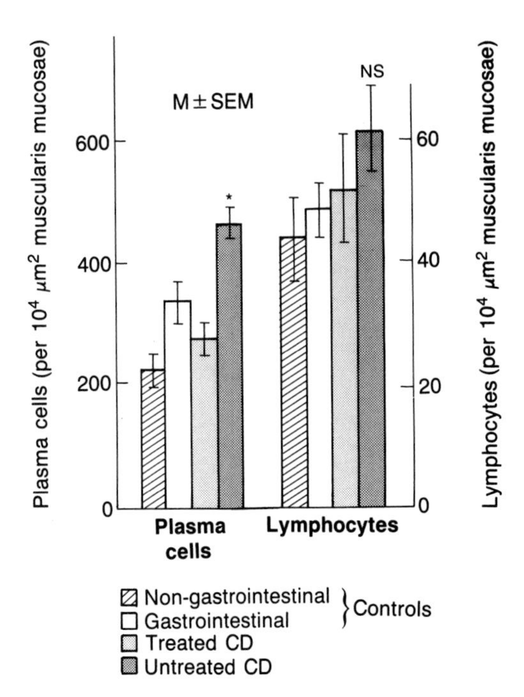

Fig. 6.20 Plasma cell populations are significantly elevated in rectal mucosae of untreated gluten-sensitive patients, compared with post-treatment values, whereas no significant difference was detected in lymphocyte populations as a result of treatment ($*p<0.025$).

ations in lymphocyte populations (Fig. 6.22) either within epithelium or lamina propria (Fig. 6.20), while numbers of neutrophils, eosinophils or basophils were too small for any meaningful comment [212].

Thus in untreated coeliac patients with established flat (Type 3) jejunal lesions, there is a mild chronic inflammatory cell infiltrate

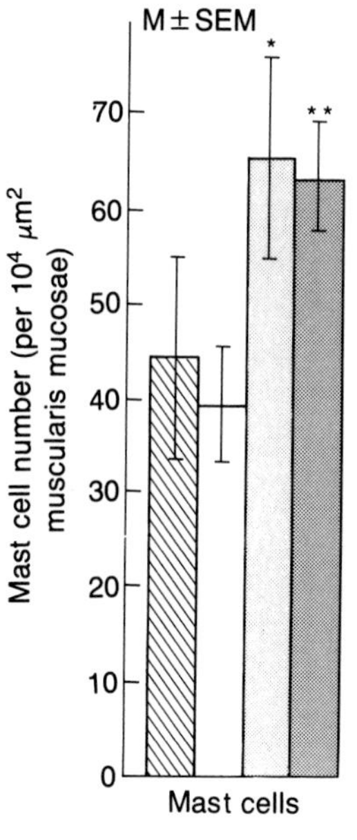

Fig. 6.21 In contrast to plasma cells and lymphocytes in lamina propria (Fig. 6.20) mast cell populations appeared to remain elevated in gluten-sensitized individuals during treatment with a gluten-free diet (*$p<0.05$; **p0.025). (See key on Fig. 6.20.)

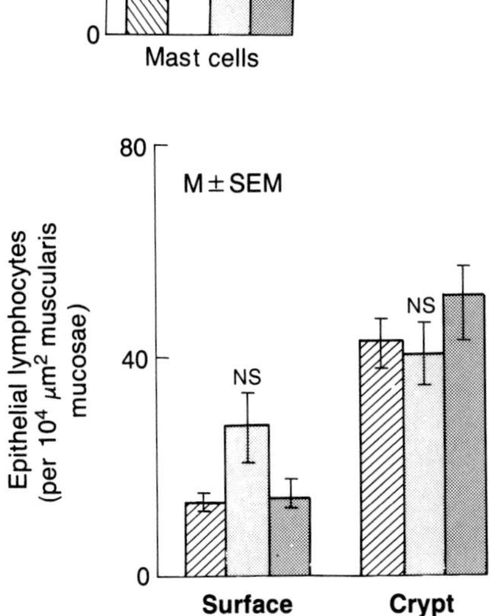

Fig. 6.22 No significant alteration in IEL (either in surface or crypt epithelium of rectal mucosa) was observed between control individuals, and untreated or treated gluten-sensitive patients. (See key on Fig. 6.19.)

within lamina propria which, excepting mast cells, resolves with gluten restriction. Despite that, lamina propria volumes were not increased, indicating absence of an inflammatory reaction, increased microvascular involvement or extravasation of circulating fluid and plasma proteins.

Response of coeliac rectum to gluten challenge

Following challenge with a standard dose of 2 g FF3, there was a biphasic response in lamina propria, the initial changes occurring by 6–8 hours, and the second through 36–96 hours post-challenge (Figs 6.23, 6.24).

During the initial phase there was rapid tissue swelling due to increased microvascular hyperpermeability, extravasation of immunoreactive fibrinogen (Fig. 6.25) and a rapid (50%) fall in granulated mucosal mast cells (Fig. 6.26) followed by a fairly swift influx of neutrophils (Fig. 6.27). During this time, neutrophils were plentiful within the vessels, together with eosinophils, basophils and lymphocytes, both in the superficial and deep vessels, including the submucosa, indicating that the intestinal response to gluten is *transmural*, as was initially shown by Paulley in operative specimens of jejunum [34] (Fig. 6.28).

The second phase of mucosal swelling was more prolonged and could have been related to the influx of basophils that peaked at around 36 hours. Microvascular changes were also prominent at this time, comprising hypertrophied pericytes and endothelial cells whose nuclei bulged into the vessel lumina (Fig. 6.29). Through the challenge, there was no alteration in surface or crypt epithelial volume.

There was a progressive decrease in rectal potential difference from −48 to −41 mV which was significant 12 hours after a 4 g FF3 challenge ($p<0.05$) as measured by the rectal bag diagnosis technique [215] (Fig. 6.30). During the same period net Na^+ and Cl^- absorption fell (5.2–3.5 : 6.8–5.4 μmol/hour per cm^2, respectively) but not to demonstrably significant levels, while water and K^+ fluxes remained unchanged. Analogous phenomena did not occur in any of the disease control subjects.

These observations show that in coeliac patients the evolving inflammatory response evokes a small increase in mucosal conductance and hence ionic permeability of the surface epithelium, thus explaining the observed reductions in net Na^+ and Cl^- absorption. These changes are far less marked than those associated with fulminant ulcerative colitis [216,217] in which NaCl absorption is virtually ablated, transmucosal conductance increased, and potential difference reduced. Nevertheless, with the severe haemorrhagic proctitis induced by high dose gluten challenge [193] similar changes in mucosal transport could be expected to occur.

There were progressive increases in mucosal lymphocytes, with a peak of IEL (Fig. 6.31) at 6–8 hours post-challenge; these were predominantly of $CD8^+$ type. IEL did not show any increase in size, or mitotic activity, during the evolution of the inflammatory reaction.

Although in many studies of gluten challenge attention has been directed solely towards surface epithelium, its expression of MHC class 2 antigen and infiltration by IEL, other studies have revealed that jejunum reacts rapidly within a few hours of contact with gluten with an acute inflammatory response which, like rectum, involves lamina propria swelling and oedema, neutrophilic infiltration, complement utilization, and ultrastructural changes in basal lamina and

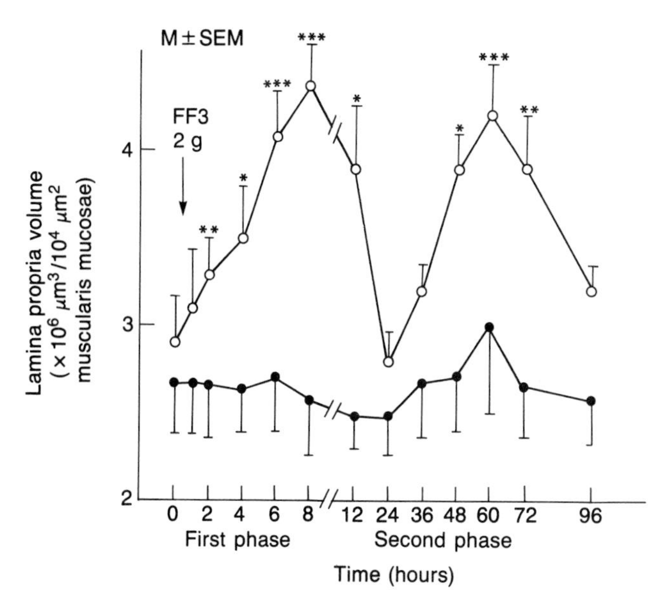

Fig. 6.23 Following 2 g rectal challenge with FF3, biphasic swelling of lamina propria volume (expressed on vertical axis $\times$ $10^6\mu m^3/10^4\mu m^2$ muscularis mucosae) was observed. The initial rapid response peaked at 8 hours in coeliac patients (open symbols) but not controls (closed symbols). The second phase was more prolonged (36–96 hours post-challenge). Time-point significance values are illustrated; areas-under-curves for both peaks (Wilcoxon signed rank test) coeliacs versus controls were significantly different ($p<0.01$; $*p<0.05$; $**p0.02$; $***p<0.01$). (From Loft *et al.* [115].)

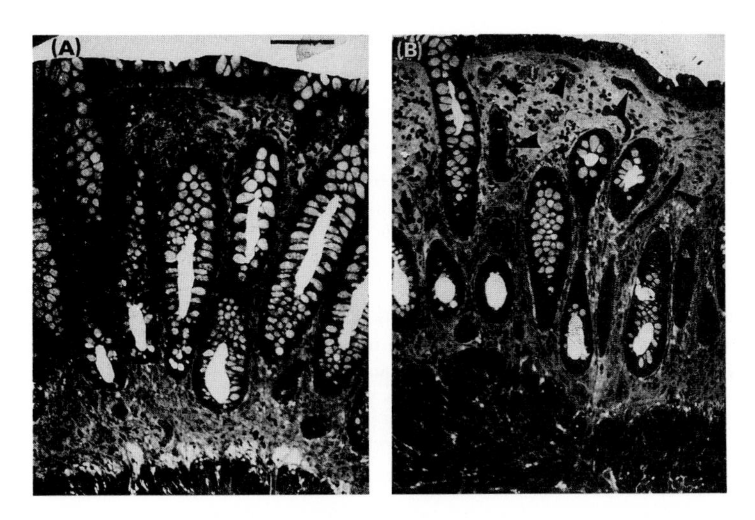

Fig. 6.24 These 1 μm toluidine blue-stained micrographs illustrate typical appearances of rectal mucosa before (A) and at 12 hour post-challenge with 2 g FF3 (B). In latter note oedema of upper subepithelial region and marked inflammatory dilatation (arrow heads) of microvasculature. (Magnification bar, 100 μm.)

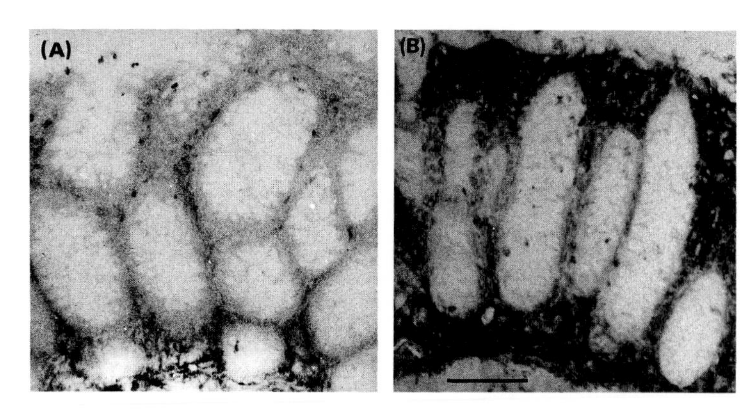

Fig. 6.25 These two micrographs are frozen sections of rectal mucosa before (A) and 1 hour after (B) challenge with 2 g FF3, following use of antifibrinogen monoclonal antibody. Note acute appearances of immunoreactive fibrinogen throughout lamina propria (but not epithelium) as rapidly as 1 hour after gluten contacts the rectal mucosa. (Magnification bar, 10 μm.)

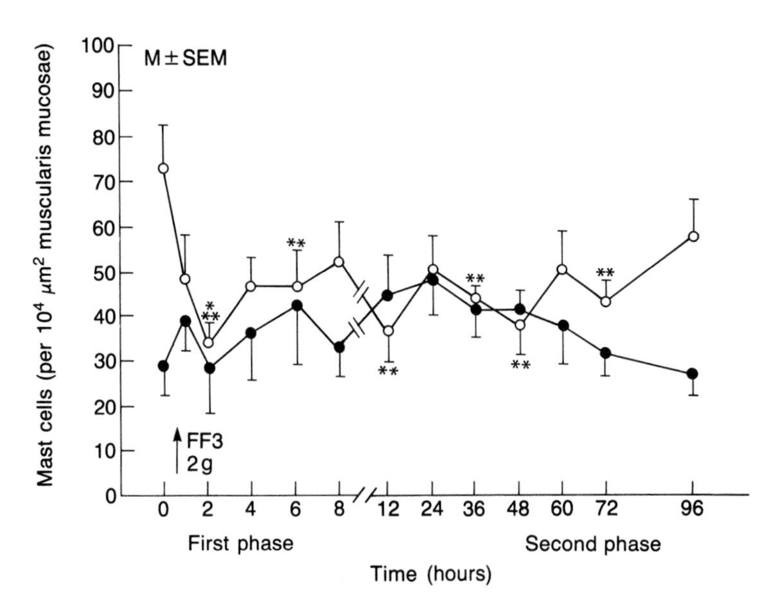

Fig. 6.26 The absolute number of identifiable (i.e. granulated) tissue mast cells, in coeliac tissue (○), at each time point per specimen are shown on left hand vertical axis, relative to $10^4 \mu m^2$ test area of muscularis mucosae. Note rapid fall (~50%) within 2 hours of challenge with 2 g FF3. No significant changes were observed in mast cell content of challenged rectal mucosae of control subjects (●) (**$p \pm 0.02$; ***$p < 0.01$).

microvasculature [21,218,219]. Our findings [115] are directly analogous to the pure T cell-mediated dermal reaction to tuberculin protein, comprising early mobilization of lymphocytes, increased microvascular

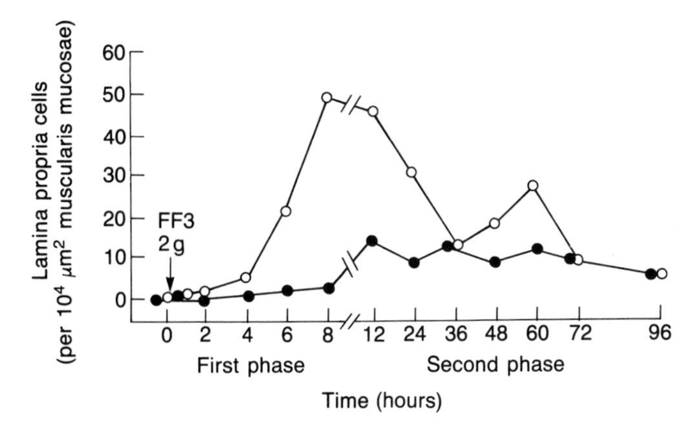

Fig. 6.27 Time course of neutrophilic (○) and basophilic (●) infiltrates into lamina propria of challenged rectal mucosae of coeliac patients. There was rapid influx of neutrophils peaking at 8 hour post-challenge, followed by a lesser, and more sustained rise in tissue basophils.

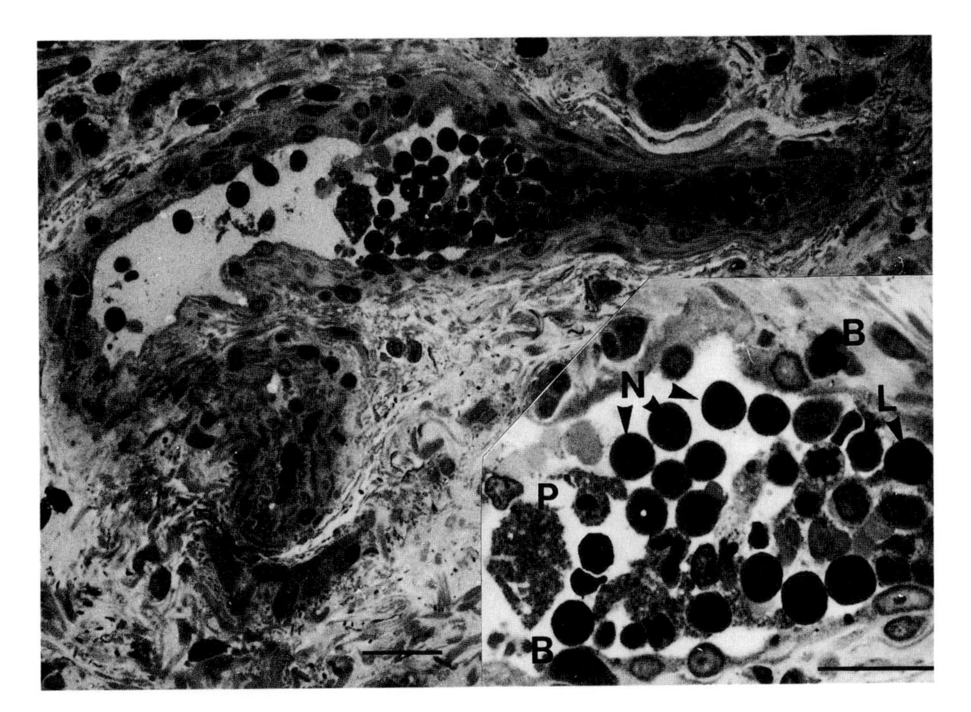

Fig. 6.28 A 1 μm toluidine blue-stained section of a large submucosal vein deep within rectal mucosa which is virtually choked with a variety of inflammatory cells destined to emigrate into tissue spaces, 6 hour post-challenge. Inset reveals neutrophils (N), lymphocytes (L), and two basophils, (B) the latter which lie immediately adjacent to external wall of vessel. P denotes intravascular platelet aggregate. (Magnification bar, 10 μm.)

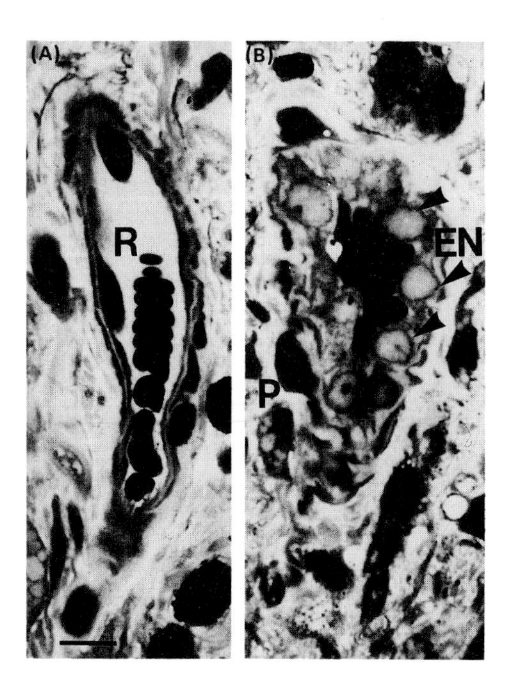

Fig. 6.29 Effects of gluten-induced inflammatory change on the microvasculature is illustrated in (B) from a late (72 hour post-challenge) rectal biopsy. There is marked hypertrophy and prominence of pericytes, (P) and endothelial cells, (EN) whose nuclei bulge into lumen of capillary to engage clump of distorted erythrocytes. These appearances contrast with pre-challenge mucosa (A) in which endothelial cells are fusiform in appearance and lack features of activated cells; furthermore, the intraluminal erythrocytes (R) remain suspended in plasma and are not subject to distortion (see also Fig. 6.3). (Magnification bar, 10 μm.)

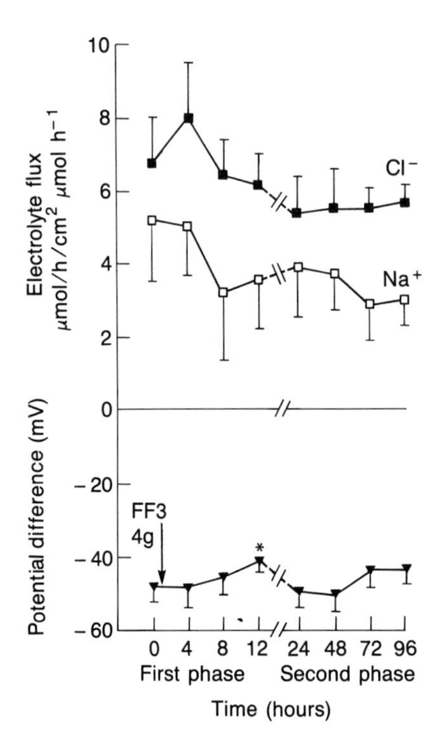

Fig. 6.30 Changes in electrolyte fluxes and potential difference were monitored by an intrarectal dialysis bag technique throughout challenges with 4 g FF3. Note significant rise in rectal potential difference at 12 hour post-challenge, while changes in Na^+ and Cl^- secretion did not achieve statistically significant values (*p0.05).

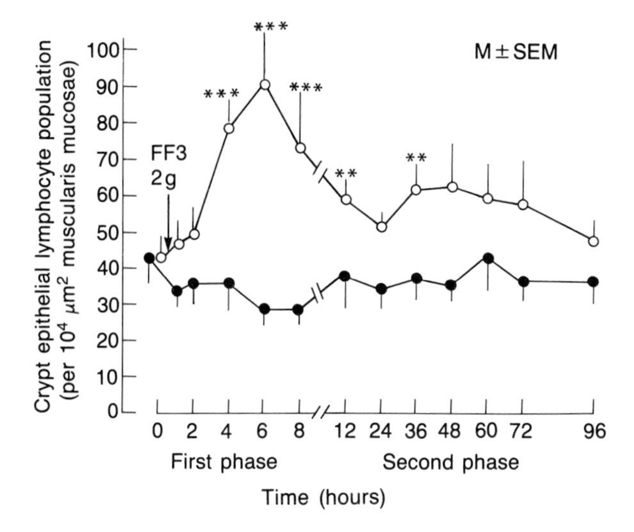

Fig. 6.31 The increase in total IEL in rectal mucosae following 2 g challenge with FF3 are recorded on vertical axis (as mean absolute population size per 10^4 μm^2 test area of muscularis mucosae). IEL peaked around 4–8 hour post-challenge and waned thereafter in gluten-sensitized subjects (○); disease controls showed no response (●). Probability values relate to comparisons with pre-challenge data for coeliac group only ($**p<0.025$; $***p<0.01$).

permeability with extravasation of fibrinogen, discharge and degranulation of mast cells, infiltration by basophils and later alterations to the microvessels and their attendant connective tissue elements [160, 162]. Moreover, the biphasic early and late reactions to antigen in skin are reminiscent of those documented in rectal mucosa, as also in murine dermal reactivity to dinitrochlorobenzene. Here, the early response appeared due to a T lymphocyte-derived IgE-like factor (of M_r 70 000) that armed local mast cells for antigen-specific mediator release [220,221].

In summary, the evidence locates the origin of the immunological response to gluten within the lamina propria and submucosal tissues of distal colon. The role subserved by lymphocytic infiltration of intestinal epithelium, although a marker of a local cell-mediated immune response [32,50], does not necessarily imply mucosal damage or destruction [38,44,50,148,167]. Nevertheless, despite continuing uncertainties regarding their role in mucosal cell-mediated immunity, the 6 hour rectal response of IEL was viewed as the basis of a rapid, convenient and prospective test of gluten sensitivity.

Diagnostic potential of gluten challenge

Analysis of the previous data showed that if the 6 hour post-challenge peak in IEL was expressed as a percentage of the pre-challenge value, then a +10% increment would have 100% sensitivity for gluten sensitivity. Our aim in setting up this study [214] was firstly to assess, prospectively, the validity of this index on a series of consecutive individuals referred to our unit for jejunal biopsy. Secondly, the aim was to investigate the response of untreated coeliac patients, the diagnostic criterion (of gluten sensitivity) being the presence of a Type 3 flat upper jejunal lesion. The study was performed with a 2 g dose of FF3 instilled into the rectum of 44 subjects, comprising 21 disease controls and 23 coeliac patients (of whom nine were untreated).

All coeliac patients responded at 6 hours, in terms of an increase in IEL (medians: untreated; +63% ($p<0.0001$) Mann Whitney U test: treated; +61% ($p<0.0001$) against disease controls; −4% (NS response)) (Fig. 6.32). These results yielded a mean diagnostic sensitivity for all coeliac patients of 89% (*conf* limits; 78–93%), and specificity of 91%; there were two false positives and two false negatives (Fig. 6.33).

There is no doubt, therefore, that rectal gluten challenge offers a simple, quick and reliable test for gluten sensitivity that is both highly sensitive and specific and which compares extremely well with other antibody tests currently advocated for prospective diagnosis [214]. Its wider diagnostic potential, in terms of family or population surveys, or in the investigation of other cell-mediated intestinal reactions (e.g. giardiasis or other dietary sensitivities) has yet to be realized. It is also an alternative to those subjects who are unable to tolerate oral intubation procedures and in whom a diagnosis of CD may be difficult to confirm with accuracy.

In our formal study [115] we showed by computerized image analysis that mucosal volume compartments did not change. Therefore, regarding rectal diagnostic challenge, the two specimens obtained before and after challenge can be read with respect to changes in IEL by

Table 6.3 Comparison of IEL (expressed as densities and absolute number) in rectal mucosae of control, and untreated or treated gluten-sensitive individuals

	Density (IEL/enterocyte)			Absolute number (IEL/10^4 μm^2 muscularis mucosae)		
	Surface epithelium	Crypt epithelium	Total	Surface epithelium	Crypt epithelium	Total
Control subjects	26	23	49	15	45	60
Gluten sensitized						
Untreated	38	20	58	25	47	72
Treated	29	26	55	17	51	67

This tabulation shows that density of crypt IEL (cIEL) is less than the density of surface IEL (sIEL) in each group of subjects. Despite increased densities, the absolute number of sIEL is far *less* than comparable numbers for cIEL (right hand panel). It should therefore be appreciated that with such small numbers of cells, sIEL in rectal mucosa are far more prone to analytical error than cIEL.

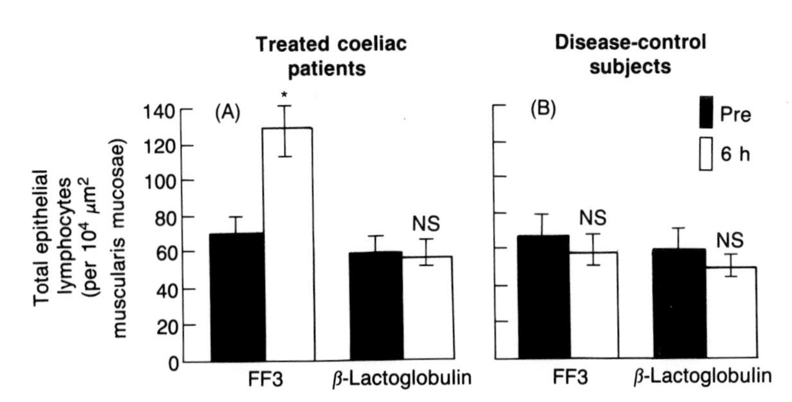

Fig. 6.32 The 6 hour prospective diagnostic test for gluten sensitivity. Here it can be seen that in gluten-sensitive subjects (A) alone there is a significant rise in the absolute number of IEL (per 10^4 μm^2 muscularis mucosae) following challenge with gluten (FF3) but not to the control protein challenge with β-lactoglobulin. Note that disease-control subjects (B) showed no response to either immunogen ($*p<0.05$).

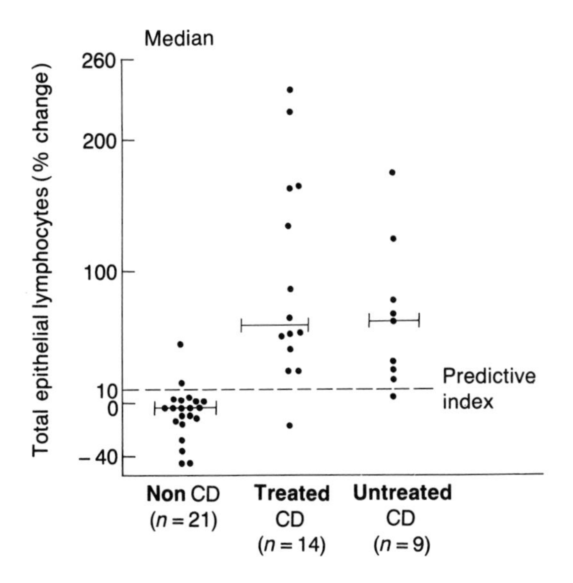

Fig. 6.33 Percentage change (0–6 hours) in epithelial lymphocyte populations. In terms of percentage change, it can be seen that the +10% predictive index allowed prospective diagnosis to be made on all, except two, gluten-sensitized patients. There were also two false-positives among the non-CD control group ($p<0.0001$). (From Loft, Marsh [214].)

simply relating lymphocyte 'counts' to a constant length of muscularis mucosae; there is no requirement to adjust for alterations in size of lymphocytes or in volumes of epithelium, or for specialized equipment.

It is important, however, that IEL are expressed in absolute terms, and not as densities, otherwise (Table 6.3) completely different results will be obtained. This is the problem with a recent [222] retrospective study of material derived from a different study [193] in which IEL were counted per 100 epithelial cells. The results suggested that surface IEL in treated coeliac patients were higher than in controls, while crypt epithelial lymphocyte densities were said to be less than those of control mucosae (computerized image analysis says the opposite). The second flaw in Austin's paper [222] was statistical in that the number of biopsies, rather than patients, was used in the calculations, i.e. 14 specimens from five controls were compared with 17 specimens from seven treated patients. When analysed correctly, however, the difference in IEL hardly reaches any useful significance level ($p = 0.03$; Wilcoxon's rank sum test) in comparison with the original authors' p value of <0.01, which is clearly untenable. As our data show for colonic mucosae, crypt IEL >surface IEL and it is therefore important that the outcome of the way in which results are expressed is understood. Although there are fewer IEL in surface epithelium compared with crypts, their densities are apparently higher, and thus are more subject to analytic error when evaluated solely in terms of ratios to epithelial cells [212].

Gluten sensitivity; the gastric mucosa

In recent times, investigators appear to have lost sight of the fact that chronic exposure to gluten may damage the structure and the function of gastric mucosa in gluten-sensitive individuals. This omission seems to have originated from the 1960s when, with the introduction of the peroral biopsy technique, research progressively became focused on the small intestinal lesion and in particular on the damaged enterocyte and the quest for the absent peptidase.

However, seen within its wider context, it is evident that damage to the intestinal tract in gluten sensitivity is not confined to, or expressly concerned with, the jejunal enterocyte whatsoever, but reflects a host-directed response towards gluten exposure at any mucosal site, including stomach and rectum (and perhaps other gut-associated mucosal surfaces as well). That the stomach is involved in adult CD ('idiopathic steatorrhoea') and tropical sprue had not escaped the clinician-scientists of the early decades of this century who investigated gastric acid production as a routine work-up of megaloblastic anaemias, especially to aid differentiation from Addisonian pernicious anaemia (PA) [223–229]. Despite technical limitations imposed by their period of office, those physicians nevertheless had shown defects in gastric emptying and secretion resulting in achlorhydria (alcohol- or histamine-fast),hypochlorhydria, and low output of 'intrinsic factor' (IF) [228,229]. It was also known that in cases of recovered sprue, unlike true Addisonian anaemia, there might be recovery of secretion of acid and of the gastric 'IF' [229].

With the later advent of gastric biopsy, and tests individually capable

Table 6.4 Studies on gastric acid production in tropical sprue, CD and DH

	Series of cases	Achlorhydria	Hypochlorhydria	Total
Tropical sprue				
Fairley, Mackie [224]	26	7	8	15
Holmes, Starr [225]	5	1	–	1
Fairley [227]	44	14	11	25
Castle *et al.* [229]	92	20	–	20
Baker [232]	30	5	10	15
Floch *et al.* [235]	18	10	–	10
Vaish *et al.* [237]	30	9	5	14
Moshal *et al.* [239]	24	3	11	14
Total	269	69	45	114
Percentage		(26)	(17)	(43)
CD				
Blumgart [223]	3	1	1	2
Bennett *et al.* [256]	12	2	–	2
Hanes, McBryde [226]	9	1	5	6
Snell [257]	33	8	2	10
Badenoch [230]	26	7	12	19
Friedlander, Gorvy [231]	10	2	4	6
Doig, Girdwood [233]	29	5	–	5
Girdwood *et al.* [234]	9	2	–	2
Hansky, Shiner [236]	10	4	–	4
Cooke [238]	120	48	–	48
Fausa *et al.* [245]	32	2	7	9
Total	293	82	31	113
Percentage		(28)	(11)	(39)
DH				
Cream, Scott [240]	43	1	2	3
Andersson [241,242]	11	4	6	10
Heading *et al.* [243]	22	4	8	22
Fausa [244]	25	7	12	19
Fausa *et al.* [245]	37	14	7	21
O'Donoghue *et al.* [247]	33	7	8	15
Stockbrugger *et al.* [246]	17	7	5	12
Thune *et al.* [248]	62	25	11	36
Gillberg *et al.* [249]	116	30	48	78
Total	366	99	107	206
Percentage		(25)	(31)	(56)
Overview	928	250	183	433
		(27)	(20)	(47)

of assessing absorption of pteroylmonoglutamate and vitamin B_{12}, it became evident that in a substantial proportion of coeliac and tropical sprue cases there was atrophic gastritis or gastric atrophy, absorption of vitamin B_{12} was often decreased, and excretion of urinary pepsinogen reduced [230–239].

The prevalence of histamine-fast achlorhydria (HFA) in untreated CD is probably ~30%, with hypochlorhydria increasing that figure by another 10–15%. These figures compare with crude estimates in tropical sprue and in DH [240–249] of around 30% and 20%, respectively. Overall, approximately 40–50% with these types of enteropathy suffer some degree of impaired acid secretion, with chronic (atrophic) gastritis (Table 6.4). However, it is clear that in CD and DH, chronic atrophic gastritis may be present although acid output is normal [236,247], a phenomenon also observed throughout the spectrum of PA [250]. Thus, the gastric lesion may be patchy, and islands of functional tissue that are missed on biopsy may remain [251]. Furthermore, it would appear that in general, acid output ceases before IF production stops [250,252–255]. In 120 adult cases of CD Cooke [238] stated that gastric atrophy/atrophic gastritis was not rare and was likely to be present in >20% patients with an HFA.

Antibodies to GPC (gastric parietal cell) are seen principally in DH, and reflect gastric atrophy; the presence of IF antibodies either in DH or CD only arises with coexisting Addisonian PA [244,247,258] and is a rare phenomenon.

Far less is known of the immunohistological changes in gastric mucosa in untreated gluten sensitivity than its functional deficiencies; the latter having mostly been performed before the advent of the flexible gastric biopsy technique introduced by Wood. In one study [236] of 15 subjects, nine had normal gastric biopsies, while six showed chronic atrophic gastritis : gastric atrophy. IF output was not studied, and in four subjects with a low serum B_{12} level, use of an external source of IF did not improve absorption of a test dose of radioactive B_{12}; two of them were also on a gluten-free diet. Analogous findings were seen in (Caribbean) tropical sprue [235], with diffuse atrophic gastritis persisting for at least 1 year after treatment, despite the return of acid secretion in some cases.

The nature of the severe gastric atrophy in CD and DH (or tropical sprue) is uncertain, but is obviously akin to the development of an analogous lesion in PA [259], and other related familial conditions such as iron deficiency anaemia, thyroid disorders and diabetes mellitus [250]. Furthermore, serial studies reveal all these lesions to be persistent, even though some function may return in the 'sprue' syndrome, although never in Addisonian PA. Thus the sprue lesion is not a manifestation of the latter, even though the diagnoses may be confused inter alia, especially if diarrhoea is not a major symptom of the patient with malabsorption [256,257].

It is evident, then, that the gastric lesion is related to gluten ingestion (or in tropical sprue to the effects, perhaps, of chronic exposure to intestinal microbes). It is tempting to suggest that such lesions are, like those in PA, due to T cell-mediated tissue destruction, rather than to the presence of (auto)antibodies. The few studies relevant to immunohistological features of the mucosa [260,261] fail to address this question adequately, so that it is not possible to advance knowledge any further. Nevertheless, the observation stands that in 30–50% patients with gluten sensitivity, gastric atrophy and achlorhydria do occur, and that during the lifelong natural evolution of gluten sensitivity, the stomach is vulnerable to attack in addition to the small intestine. It is likely that the reduced acid secretion in such individuals predisposes them to recurrent intestinal infections, and hence to the acute clinical unmasking of the underlying (latent) sensitivity (Fig. 6.10).

The recent descriptions of lymphocytic gastritis [262] add another dimension to these considerations. In a prospective study of 4840 patients by Haot *et al.* [263], 1.4% or 66 had a 'varioliform gastritis' comprising swollen folds bearing umbilicated lesions often capped by aphthoid ulceration, which histologically revealed infiltration of superficial (body) epithelium and pits by numerous small lymphocytes. Conversely, 20% of the biopsies revealing lymphocytic gastritis were not associated with gross lesions visible by gastroscopy — although follow-up gastroscopies suggest that surface lesions do not persist indefinitely, thus perhaps accounting for this disparity. In another study [264], the T lymphocytic infiltrate was associated in ~40% patients with Helicobacter pylori-positive biopsies, and in ~80% patients when tested serologically. Finally, in a somewhat poorly controlled retrospective evaluation of patients with 'sprue and sprue-like intestinal lesions' [265], just under 50% showed lymphoid infiltrates of gastric epithelium.

Generally, in each of these three series, the age ranges tended to lie in the fourth and fifth decades, often with male predominance. However, the (earlier) natural history of this lesion remains unknown; furthermore, the infiltration is not associated with gastric atrophy [262] while function studies (acid output) have yet to be carried out. Whether lymphocytic gastritis does represent an immunological response to local antigenic stimulation (gluten or otherwise) has not been proven either, and in this regard, further tightly controlled and structured follow-up studies will be necessary.

References

1 Pink IJ, Creamer B. Response to a gluten-free diet of patients with coeliac syndrome. *Lancet* 1967;i:300–4.
2 Rubin CE, Eidelman S, Weinstein WM. Sprue by any other name. *Gastroenterology* 1970;58:409–13.
3 Booth CC. Enterocyte in coeliac disease. *Br Med J* 1970;iii:725–31.
4 Cooke WT, Asquith P. Introduction and definition. In: Cooke WT, Asquith P, eds. *Coeliac Disease. Clinics in Gastroenterology*. London: WB Saunders, 1974: 3–10.
5 Doniach I, Shiner M. Duodenal and jejunal biopsies. II. Histology. *Gastroenterology* 1957;33:71–86.
6 Shiner M, Doniach I. Histopathologic studies in steatorrhoea. *Gastroenterology* 1960;38:419–40.
7 Marsh MN. The morphology and immunopathology of the jejunal lesion in gluten-sensitivity. *Eur J Gastroenterol Hepatol*

1991;3:163–8.

8 Marsh MN. Gluten, MHC and the small intestine: A molecular and immunobiologic approach to the spectrum of gluten-sensitivity ('celiac sprue'). *Gastroenterology* 1992:102:330–54.

9 Marsh MN. The immunopathology of the small intestinal reaction in gluten-sensitivity. *Immunol Invest* 1989;18: 509–31.

10 Rubin CE, Brandborg LL, Phelps PC, Taylor HC. Studies of celiac disease. I. The apparent identical and specific nature of the duodenal and proximal jejunal lesion in celiac disease and idiopathic steatorrhoea. *Gastroenterology* 1960;38:28–49.

11 Padykula HA, Strauss EW, Ladman AJ. A morphological and histochemical analysis of the human jejunal epithelium in non-tropical sprue. *Gastroenterology* 1961;40: 735–65.

12 Spiro HM, Filipe MI, Stewart JS, Pearse AGE. Functional histochemistry of the small bowel mucosa in malabsorptive syndromes. *Gut* 1964;5:145–54.

13 Samloff IM, Davis JS, Schenk EA. A clinical and histochemical study of celiac disease before and during a gluten-free diet. *Gastroenterology* 1965;48:155–72.

14 Riecken EO. Histochemical findings in some intestinal abnormalities in relation to structure compared with the changes in idiopathic steatorrhoea. In: Booth CC, Dowling RH, eds. *Coeliac Disease*. London: Churchill Livingstone, 1970:174–85.

15 Curran RC, Creamer B. Ultrastructural changes in some disorders of the small intestine associated with malabsorption. *J Pathol Bact* 1963;86:1–8.

16 Rubin W, Ross L, Sleisenger MH, Weser E. An electron microscopic study of adult celiac disease. *Lab Invest* 1966;15:1720–47.

17 Shiner M. Electron microscopy of jejunal mucosa. In: Cooke WT, Asquith P, eds. *Coeliac Disease. Clinics in Gastroenterology*. London: WB Saunders, 1974:33–53.

18 Frazer AC. Pathogenetic concepts of the malabsorption syndrome. *Gastroenterology* 1960;38:389–98.

19 Flores AF, Winter HS, Bhan AK. *In vitro* models to assess immunoregulatory T lymphocyte subsets in gluten-sensitive enteropathy. *Gastroenterology* 1983;82:A1058.

20 Ezeoke A, Ferguson O, Fakhri W, Hekkens W, Hobbs JR. Antibodies in the sera of coeliac patients which can co-opt K-cells to attack gluten-labelled targets. In: Hekkens W, Pena AS, eds. *Coeliac Disease*. Leiden: Stenfert Kroese, 1975:176–86.

21 Anand BS, Piris J, Jerrome DW, Offord RE, Truelove SC. The timing of histological damage following a single challenge with gluten in treated coeliac disease. *Q J Med* 1981;197:83–94.

22 Doe WF, Booth CC, Brown DL. Evidence for complement-binding immune complexes in adult coeliac disease, Crohn's disease and ulcerative colitis. *Lancet* 1973;i:402–4.

23 Shiner M. Ultrastructural changes suggestive reactions in the jejunal mucosa of coeliac children following gluten challenge. *Gut* 1973;14:1–12.

24 Shiner M, Ballard J. Antigen-antibody reactions in jejunal mucosa in childhood coeliac disease after gluten challenge. *Lancet* 1972;i:1202–5.

25 Weiser MM, Douglas AP. An alternative mechanism for gluten toxicity in coeliac disease. *Lancet* 1976;i:567–9.

26 Strober W. Gluten-sensitive enteropathy — an abnormal immunologic response of the gastrointestinal tract to a dietary protein. In: Shorter RG, Kirsner JB, eds. *Gastrointestinal Immunity for the Clinician*. New York: Grune and Stratton, 1985:75–112.

27 Marsh MN. Immunocytes, enterocytes and the lamina propria: an immunopathologic framework of coeliac disease. *J R Coll Physicians Lond* 1983;17:205–12.

28 Ferguson A, Parrott DMV. Histopathology and time-course of rejection of allografts of mouse small intestine. *Transplantation* 1973;15:546–54.

29 Ferguson A, Jarrett EEE. Hypersensitivity reactions in the small intestine. I. Thymus dependence of experimental partial villous atrophy. *Gut* 1975;16:114–17.

30 Ferguson A. Immunological reactions in the small intestine. *J Clin Nutr Gastroenterol* 1988;3:109–13.

31 Ferguson A. Models of immunologically-driven small intestinal damage. In: Marsh MN, ed. *Immunopathology of the Small Intestine*. Chichester: Wiley, 1987:225–52.

32 Mowat A, Ferguson A. Intraepithelial lymphocyte count and crypt hyperplasia measure the mucosal component of the graft-versus-host reaction in mouse small intestine. *Gastroenterology* 1982;83: 417–23.

33 Guy-Grand D, Vassalli P. Gut injury in mouse graft-versus-host reaction: study of its occurrence and mechanisms. *J Clin Invest* 1986;77:1584–95.

34 Paulley JR. Observations on aetiology of idiopathic steatorrhoea. *Br Med J* 1954;ii: 1318–21.
35 Watret KC, Ferguson A. Lymphocyte-mediated intestinal damage — animal studies. In: Peters TJ, ed. *The Cell Biology of Inflammation in the Gastrointestinal Tract*. Hull: Corners Publications, 1989: 191–200.
36 Marsh MN. Lymphocyte-mediated intestinal damage — human studies. In: Peters TJ, ed. *The Cell Biology of Inflammation in the Gastrointestinal Tract*. Hull: Corners Publications, 1989:203–29.
37 Mowat A McI, Felstein M. Intestinal graft-versus-host reactions in experimental animals. In: Burakoff SJ, Ferrar H, eds. *Graft-Versus-Host Disease*. New York: Dekker, 1991:205–44.
38 Fry L, Seah P, McMinn R, Hoffbrand A. Lymphocytic infiltration of epithelium in diagnosis of gluten-sensitive enteropathy. *Br Med J* 1972;3:371–4.
39 Fry L, Seah P, Harper P, Hoffbrand A, McMinn RM. The small intestine in dermatitis herpetiformis. *J Clin Pathol* 1974; 27:817–24.
40 Marsh MN. Studies of intestinal lymphoid tissue. XV. Histopathologic features suggestive of cell-mediated reactivity in jejunal mucosae of patients with dermatitis herpetiformis. *Virchows Arch [A]* 1989;416: 125–32.
41 Marsh MN, Bjarnason I, Shaw J, Ellis A, Baker R, Peters TJ. Studies of intestinal lymphoid tissue. XIV. HLA status, mucosal morphology, permeability and epithelial lymphocyte populations in first degree relatives of patients with coeliac disease. *Gut* 1990;31:32–6.
42 Bjarnason I, Peters TJ, Veall N. A persistent defect in intestinal permeability in coeliac disease demonstrated by a ^{51}Cr-labelled EDTA absorption test. *Lancet* 1983;i: 323–25.
43 Dissanayake AS, Jerrome D, Offord RE, Truelove SC, Whitehead R. Identifying toxic patterns of wheat gluten and their effect on the jejunal mucosa in coeliac disease. *Gut* 1974;15:931–46.
44 Leigh RJ, Marsh MN, Crowe PJ, Garner V, Gordon D. Studies of intestinal lymphoid tissue. IX. Dose-dependent gluten-induced lymphoid infiltration of coeliac jejunal epithelium. *Scand J Gastroenterol* 1985;20: 715–19.
45 Doherty M, Barry RE. Gluten-induced mucosal changes in subjects without overt small-bowel disease. *Lancet* 1981;i:517–20.
46 Ferguson A, Blackwell J, Barnetson R. Effects of additional dietary gluten on the small-intestinal mucosa of volunteers and of patients with dermatitis herpetiformis. *Scand J Gastroenterol* 1987;22:543–9.
47 Freedman A, Macartney J, Nelufer J, Ciclitira PJ. Timing of infiltration of T lymphocytes induced by gluten into the small intestine of coeliac disease. *J Clin Pathol* 1987;40:741–5.
48 Frazer AC, Fletcher RF, Ross CA, Shaw B, Sammons HG, Schneider R. Gluten-induced enteropathy. The effect of partially-digested gluten. *Lancet* 1959;ii:252–5.
49 Marsh MN. Triphasic response of coeliac small intestinal mucosa to challenge with Frazer's digest (FF3) of gliadin. In: MacDonald T, Challacombe S, Bland P, Stokes C, Heatley R, Mowat A, eds. *Advances in Mucosal Immunology*. Dordrecht: Kluwer Academic, 1990:734–7.
50 Marsh MN. Studies of intestinal lymphoid tissue. XI. The immunopathology of cell-mediated reactions in gluten-sensitivity and other enteropathies. *Scanning Microsc* 1988;2:1663–84.
51 MacDonald TT, Ferguson A. Hypersensitivity reactions in the small intestine. II. Effects of allograft rejection on mucosal architecture and lymphoid cell infiltrate. *Gut* 1976;17:81–91.
52 MacDonald TT, Ferguson A. Hypersensitivity reactions in the small intestine. III. The effects of allograft rejection and of graft-versus-host disease on epithelial cell kinetics. *Cell Tissue Kinet* 1977;10:301–12.
53 Mowat A, Ferguson A. Hypersensitivity reactions in the small intestine. VI. Pathogenesis of the graft-versus-host reaction in the small intestinal mucosa. *Transplantation* 1981;32:238–43.
54 Ross IN. Primary immunodeficiency and the small intestine. In: Marsh MN, ed. *Immunopathology of the Small Intestine*. Chichester: Wiley, 1987:283–32.
55 Khojasteh A. Immunoproliferative small intestinal disease (IPSID) in third world countries. In: Marsh MN, ed. *Immunopathology of the Small Intestine*. Chichester: Wiley, 1987:121–50.
56 Katz SI, Hall RP, Lawley TJ, Strober W. Dermatitis herpetiformis: the skin and the gut. *Ann Intern Med* 1980;93:857–74.
57 Gawkrodger DJ, McDonald C, O'Mahony S, Ferguson A. Small bowel function in der-

matitis herpetiformis. *Br J Dermatol* 1989; 121 (Suppl. 34):49.
58 O'Mahony S, Vesley JP, Ferguson A. Similarities in intestinal humoral immunity in dermatitis herpetiformis without enteropathy and in coeliac disease. *Lancet* 1990; 335:1487–90.
59 Fry L. Dermatitis herpetiformis. In: Marsh MN, ed. *Coeliac Disease*. Oxford: Blackwell Scientific Publications, 1992: 81–104.
60 Berg PA, Klein R. Clinical and prognostic relevance of different mitochondrial antibody profiles in primary biliary cirrhosis (PBC). In: Epstein O, ed. Molecular Aspects of Primary Biliary Cirrhosis. *Mol Aspects Med* 1985;8:235–47.
61 Baekkeskov S, Landin M, Kristensen J *et al.* Antibodies to a 64 000 Mr human islet cell antigen precede the clinical onset of insulin-dependent diabetes. *J Clin Invest* 1987;79: 926–34.
62 Kaldany A, Hill T, Wentworth S, Brink S, D'Elia J, Clouse M. Trapping of lymphocytes in the pancreas of patients with acute-onset insulin-dependent diabetes. *Diabetologia* 1982;31:463–6.
63 Signore A, Pozzilli P, Gale E, Andreani D, Beverley P. The natural history of lymphocytes subsets infiltrating the pancreas of NOD mice. *Diabetologia* 1989;32:282–9.
64 Johnston C, Millward B, Hoskins P, Leslie R, Bottazzo G, Pyke D. Islet-cell antibodies as predictors of the later development of Type 1 (insulin-dependent) diabetes. *Diabetologia* 1989;32:382–6.
65 Lampeter E, Signore A, Gale E, Pozzilli P. Lessons from the NOD mouse for the pathogenesis and immunotherapy of human Type 1 (insulin-dependent) diabetes mellitus. *Diabetes* 1989;32:703–8.
66 Nyman E. Ulcerous jejuno-ileitis with symptomatic sprue. *Acta Med Scand* 1949; 134:275–83.
67 Goulston KJ, Skyring AP, McGovern VJ. Ulcerative jejunitis associated with malabsorption. *Am J Med* 1965;14:57–64.
68 Jeffries GH, Steinberg H, Sleisenger MH. Chronic ulcerative (non-granulomatous) jejunitis. *Am J Med* 1968;44:47–59.
69 Baer AN, Bayless TM, Yardley JH. Intestinal ulceration and malabsorption syndromes. *Gastroenterology* 1980;79:754–65.
70 O'Farrelly C, Feighery C, O'Briain D *et al.* Humoral response to wheat protein in patients with coeliac disease and enteropathy associated T cell lymphoma. *Br Med J* 1986;293:908–10.
71 Cooke WT, Holmes GKT. *Coeliac Disease*. Edinburgh: Churchill Livingstone, 1984.
72 Barry RE, Read AE. Coeliac disease and malignancy. *Q J Med* 1973;42:665–73.
73 Cooper BT, Holmes GKT, Ferguson R, Cooke WT. Coeliac disease and malignancy. *Medicine* 1980;59:249–61.
74 Freeman H, Weinstein WM, Shnitka T, Piercey J, Wensel R. Primary abdominal lymphoma. Presenting manifestation of celiac sprue or complicating dermatitis herpetiformis. *Am J Med* 1977;63:585–94.
75 Isaacson PG, Wright DH. Malignant histiocytosis of the intestine. Its relationship to malabsorption and ulcerative jejunitis. *Hum Pathol* 1978;9:661–77.
76 O'Hourihane D, Weir DG. Malignant coeliac syndrome. Report of two cases with malabsorption and microscopic foci of intestinal lymphoma. *Gastroenterology* 1970; 59:130–9.
77 Austad WI, Cornes JS, Gough KR, McCarthy CF, Read AE. Steatorrhea and malignant lymphoma: The relationship of malignant tumors of lymphoid tissue and celiac disease. *Am J Dig Dis* 1967;12:475–90.
78 Swinson CM, Hall P, Bedford P, Booth C. HLA antigens in coeliac disease associated with malignancy. *Gut* 1983;24:925–8.
79 Freeman HJ, Chin BK. Small bowel malignant lymphoma complicating celiac sprue and the mesenteric lymph node cavitation syndrome. *Gastroenterology* 1986;90: 2008–12.
80 O'Driscoll B, Stevens F, O'Gorman T. HLA type of patients with coeliac disease and malignancy in the west of Ireland. *Gut* 1982;23:662–5.
81 Holmes GKT, Prior P, Lane M, Pope D, Allen R. Malignancy in coeliac disease — effect of a gluten free diet. *Gut* 1989;30: 333–8.
82 Freeman HJ, Chin BK. Multifocal small bowel lymphoma and latent celiac sprue. *Gastroenterology* 1986;90:1992–7.
83 Ferguson R, Asquith P, Cooke WT. The jejunal cellular infiltrate in coeliac disease complicated by lymphoma. *Gut* 1974;15: 458–61.
84 Leonard JN, Tucker WF, Fry JS *et al.* Increased incidence of malignancy in dermatitis herpetiformis. *Br Med J* 1983;286: 16–18.
85 Gough KR, Read AE, Naish JM. Intestinal reticulosis as a complication of idiopathic steatorrhoea. *Gut* 1962;3:232–9.
86 Matuchansky C, Colin R, Hemet J,

Touchard J, Babin P, Eugene C. Cavitation of mesenteric lymph nodes, splenic atrophy, and a flat small intestinal mucosa. *Gastroenterology* 1984;87:606–14.

87 Wardrop C, Lee FD, Dyet J, Dagg J, Singh H, Moffat A. Immunological abnormalities in splenic atrophy. *Lancet* 1975;ii:4–7.

88 Foster P, Losowsky MS. Hyposplenism — a review. *J R Coll Physicians Lond* 1987;21: 188–91.

89 O'Grady J, Stevens F, Harding B, O'Gorman T, McNicholl B, McCarthy C. Hyposplenism and gluten-sensitive enteropathy. *Gastroenterology* 1984;87:1326–31.

90 Carvelho E, Bacellar O, Barral A, Badaro R, Johnson WD. Antigen-specific immunosuppression in visceral leishmaniasis is cell mediated. *J Clin Invest* 1989;83:860–4.

91 Hirayama K, Matsushita S, Kikuchi I, Iuchi M, Ohta N, Sasazuki T. HLA-DQ is epistatic to HLA-DR in controlling the immune response to schistosomal antigen in humans. *Nature* 1987;327:426–30.

92 Matsushita S, Muto M, Suemura M, Saito Y, Sasazuki T. HLA-linked non-responsiveness to cryptomeria japonica pollen antigen. I. Non-responsiveness is mediated by antigen-specific suppressor T cell. *J Immunol* 1987;138:109–15.

93 Ellerman K, Powers JM, Brostoff SW. A suppressor T-lymphocyte cell line for autoimmune encephalomyelitis. *Nature* 1988; 331:265–7.

94 Klimpel GR, Annable C, Cleveland M, Jerrells T, Patterson J. Immunosuppression and lymphoid hypoplasia associated with chronic graft versus host disease is dependent upon IFN-γ production. *J Immunol* 1990;144:84–93.

95 Spencer J, MacDonald T, Diss T, Walker-Smith J, Ciclitira P, Isaacson P. Changes in intraepithelial lymphocyte subpopulations in coeliac disease and enteropathy associated T cell lymphoma. *Gut* 1989;30: 339–46.

96 Tongeren JHM, Cluysender OJJ, Schillings PHM. Refractory sprue. In: McNicholl B, McCarthy CF, Fottrell PF, eds. *Perspectives in Coeliac Disease*. Lancaster: MTP Press, 1978:323–9.

97 Egan-Mitchell B, Fottrell, PF, McNichol BF. Early or pre-coeliac mucosa: development of gluten enteropathy. *Gut* 1981;22:65–9.

98 Marsh MN. Studies of intestinal lymphoid tissue. XIII. Immunopathology of the evolving celiac sprue lesion. *Pathol Res Pract* 1989;185:774–7.

99 Watson AJ, Wright NA. Morphology and cell kinetics of the jejunal mucosa in untreated patients. In: Cooke WT, Asquith P, eds. *Coeliac Disease. Clinics in Gastroenterology*. London: WB Saunders, 1974: 11–31.

100 Trier JS, Browning TH. Epithelial-cell renewal in cultured duodenal biopsies in celiac sprue. *N Engl J Med* 1970;283: 1245–50.

101 Creamer B. The dynamics of the small intestinal mucosa. In: Badenoch J, Brooke BN, eds. *Recent Advances in Gastroenterology*. London: Churchill Livingstone 1965: 148–61.

102 Booth CC. Enteropoiesis: structural and functional relationships of the enterocyte. *Postgrad Med J* 1968;44:12–16.

103 Marsh MN, Loft DE, Garner V, Gordon D. The temporal/dose response of coeliac mucosa to graded oral challenges with Frazer's fraction III. *Europ J Gastroenterol Hepatol* 1992;4:667–673.

104 Marsh MN, Leigh RJ, Loft DE, Garner V, Gordon D. Studies of intestinal lymphoid tissue. X. Observations on granular epithelial lymphocytes (gIEL) in normal and diseased human jejunum. *Virchows Archiv [A]* 1988;412:365–70.

105 Marsh MN. Grains of truth. Evolutionary changes in small intestinal mucosa in response to environmental antigen challenge. *Gut* 1990;31:111–14.

106 Weinstein WM. Latent celiac sprue. *Gastroenterology* 1974;66:489–93.

107 Mäki M, Holm, Koskimies S, Hällström O, Visakorpi JK. Normal small bowel biopsy followed by coeliac disease. *Arch Dis Child* 1990;65:1137–41.

108 Challacombe DN, Dawkins PD, Baylis JM, Robertson K. Small-intestinal histology in coeliac disease (Letter). *Lancet* 1975;i: 1345–6.

109 McConnell RB, Whitwell F. Small intestinal histology in coeliac disease (Letter). *Lancet* 1975;ii:418.

110 Scott BB, Losowsky MS. Coeliac disease with mild mucosal abnormalities: a report of four patients. *Postgrad Med J* 1977;53: 134–8.

111 Polanco I, Larrauri J, Prieto G, Guerraro J, Pena AS, Vazquez C. Severe villous atrophy appearing on different ages in two coeliac siblings with identical HLA haplotypes. (Abstract) *Acta Paediatr Belg* 1980;33:276.

112 Auricchio S, Greco L, Troncone R. What is the true prevalence of coeliac disease?

Gastroenterol International 1990;3:140–2.
113 Kamath KR, Dorney SFA. Is discordance for coeliac disease in monozygotic twins permanent? (Abstract) *Paediatr Res* 1983; 17:422.
114 Salazar de Sousa J, Ramos de Almeida JM, Monteiro MV, Magalhaes Ramalho P. Late onset coeliac disease in the monozygotic twin of a coeliac child. *Acta Paediatr Scand* 1987;76:172–4.
115 Loft DE, Marsh MN, Crowe PT, Sandle GI, Garner V, Gordon D. Studies of intestinal lymphoid tissue. XII. Epithelial lymphocyte and mucosal response to rectal gluten challenge in celiac sprue. *Gastroenterology* 1989;97:29–37.
116 Mowat A McI, Borland A, Parrott DMV. Hypersensitivity reactions in the small intestine. VII. Induction of the intestinal phase of murine graft-versus-host reaction by $Lyt2^-$ T cells activated by I-A alloantigens. *Transplantation* 1986;41:192–8.
117 Guy-Grand D, Vassalli P. Gut injury in graft-versus-host reaction. *J Clin Invest* 1986;77:1584–95.
118 MacDonald TT, Spencer J. Evidence that activated mucosal T cells play a role in the pathogenesis of enteropathy in human small intestine. *J Exp Med* 1988;167:1341–9.
119 Monk T, Spencer J, Cerf-Bensussan N, MacDonald TT. Stimulation of mucosal T cells *in situ* with anti-CD3 antibody: location of the activated T cells and their distribution within the mucosal microenvironment. *Clin Exp Immunol* 1988;74: 216–22.
120 Crabbe PA, Heremans JF. Selective IgA deficiency with steatorrhoea. A new syndrome. *Am J Med* 1967;42:319–26.
121 Webster ADB, Slavin G, Shiner M. Coeliac disease with severe hypogammaglobulinaemia. *Gut* 1981;22:153–7.
122 Kieffer M, Frazier PJ, Daniels NWR, Coombs RRA. Wheat gliadin fractions and other cereal antigens reactive with antibodies in the sera of coeliac patients. *Clin Exp Immunol* 1982;50:651–60.
123 Devery JM, LaBrooy JT, Krilis S, Davidson G, Skerritt JH. Anti-gliadin specificity for gluten-derived peptides toxic to coeliac patients. *Clin Exp Immunol* 1989;76: 384–90.
124 Ashkenazi A, Levin S, Idar D, Rosenberg J, Fiandzei TZ. Immunological assay for the diagnosis of coeliac disease: interaction between purified gluten fractions. *Pediatr Res* 1980;14:776–8.
125 Simpson FG, Bullen A, Robertson DAF, Losowsky MS. Leucocyte migration inhibition (LMI) test in coeliac disease: a reappraisal. *Gut* 1981;22:A896.
126 Corazza GR, Rawcliffe P, Frisoni M *et al.* Specificity of leucocyte migration inhibition test in coeliac disease. A reassessment using different gluten sub-fractions. *Clin Exp Immunol* 1985;60:117–22.
127 Corazza GR, Frisoni M, Mule P *et al.* Cytophilic antibodies cause leucocyte migration inhibition in coeliac disease. *J Lab Clin Med* 1989;28:79–83.
128 Guan R, Rawcliffe P, Priddle J, Jewell DP. Cellular hypersensitivity to gluten derived peptides in coeliac disease. *Gut* 1987;28: 426–34.
129 Devery JM, Geczy CL, DeCarle DJ, Skerritt JH, Krilis SA. Macrophage procoagulant activity as an assay of cellular hypersensitivity to gluten peptides in coeliac disease. *Clin Exp Immunol* 1990;82:333–7.
130 Devery JM, Bender V, Penttilla I, Skerritt JH. Identification of reactive synthetic gliadin peptides specific for coeliac disease. *Int Arch Allergy Appl Immunol* 1991;95:356–62.
131 Hopper KE, Geczy CL, Davis WA. A mechanism of migration inhibition in delayed-type hypersensitivity reactions. I. Fibrin deposition on the surface of elicited peritoneal macrophages *in vitro*. *J Immunol* 1981; 126:1052–8.
132 Geczy CL, Hopper KE. A mechanism of migration inhibition in delayed-type hypersensitivity reactions. II. Lymphokines promote procoagulant activity of macrophages *in vivo*. *J Immunol* 1981;126:1059–65.
133 Hogg N. Human monocytes are associated with the formation of fibrin. *J Exp Med* 1983;157:473–85.
134 Dvorak HF, Gulli SJ, Dvorak AM. Expression of cell-mediated hypersensitivity *in vivo*: recent advances. *Int Rev Pathol* 1980;21: 119–94.
135 Penttilla IA, Gibson CE, Forrest BD, Cummins AG, LaBrooy JT. Lymphocyte activation as measured by interleukin 2 receptor expression to gluten fraction III in coeliac disease. *Clin Exp Immunol* 1990;68: 155–60.
136 Crabtree JE, Heatley RV, Juby LD, Howdle PD, Losowsky MS. Serum interleukin-2 receptor in coeliac disease: response to treatment and gluten challenge. *Clin Exp Immunol* 1989;77:345–8.
137 Griffiths C, Barrison I, Leonard J, Cann K, Valdimarrson M, Fry L. Preferential acti-

vation of CD4 T lymphocytes within the lamina propria of gluten-sensitive enteropathy. *Clin Exp Immunol* 1988;72:280–3.
138 Cher DJ, Mosmann TR. Two types of murine helper T cell clone. 2. Delayed-type hypersensitivity is mediated by Th1 clones. *J Immunol* 1987;138:3688–94.
139 Marsh MN, Hinde J. Inflammatory component of celiac sprue mucosa. I. Mast cells, basophils and eosinophils. *Gastroenterology* 1985;89:92–101.
140 Dhesi I, Marsh MN, Kelly C, Crowe P. Morphometric analysis of small intestinal mucosa. II. Determination of lamina propria volumes; plasma cell and neutrophil populations within control and coeliac disease mucosae. *Virchows Arch [A]* 1984;403: 173–80.
141 Hallgren H, Colombel J, Dahl R *et al.* Neutrophil and eosinophil involvement of the small bowel in patients with coeliac disease and Crohn's disease. *Am J Med* 1989;86:56–64.
142 Horvath K, Nagy L, Horn G, Simon K, Csiszar K, Bodensky H. Intestinal mast cells and neutrophil chemotactic activity of serum following a single challenge with gluten in celiac children on a gluten-free diet. *J Paediatr Gastroenterol* 1989;9: 276–80.
143 Wingren U, Hallert C, Norby K, Enerbäck L. Histamine and mucosal mast cells in gluten enteropathy. *Agents Actions* 1986; 18:266–8.
144 Krilis S, Macpherson J, DeCarle DJ, Daggard G, Talley N, Chesterman C. Small bowel mucosa from celiac patients generates 15-hydroxyeicosatetraenoic acid (15-HETE) after *in vitro* challenge with gluten. *J Immunol* 1986;137:3768–71.
145 Lavö B, Knutson L, Lööf L, Hällgren R. Gliadin challenge-induced jejunal prostaglandin E_2 secretion in coeliac disease. *Gastroenterology* 1990;99:703–7.
146 Scott H, Kett K, Halstensen T, Hvatum M, Rognum TO, Brandtzaeg P. The humoral immune system in coeliac disease. In: Marsh MN, ed. *Coeliac Disease.* Oxford: Blackwell Scientific Publications, 1992:239–82.
147 Cummins AG, LaBrooy JT, Stanley DP, Rowland R, Shearman DJC. Quantitative histological study of enteropathy associated with HIV infection. *Gut* 1990;31:317–21.
148 Marsh MN, Mathan M, Mathan VI. Studies of intestinal lymphoid tissue. VII. The secondary nature of lymphoid cell 'activation' in the jejunal lesion of tropical sprue. *Am J Pathol* 1983;89:91–101.
149 Ben Ze'ev A. Cell shape and cell contacts: molecular approaches to cytoskeleton expression. In: Stein WD, Bronner F, eds. *Cell Shape: Determinants, Regulation and Regulatory Role* New York: Academic Press, 1989:95–119.
150 Rodriguez-Boulan E, Nelson WJ. Morphogenesis of the polarized epithelial cell phenotype. *Science* 1989;245:718–25.
151 Kedinger M, Simon-Assmann P, Bouziges F, Haffen K. Epithelial-mesenchymal interactions in intestinal epithelial differentiation. *Scand J Gastroenterol* 1988;23 (Suppl. 151):62–9.
152 Simon-Assmann P, Bouziges F, Arnold C, Haffan K, Kedinger M. Epithelial-mesenchymal interactions in the production of basement membrane components in the gut. *Development* 1988;102:339–47.
153 Gallagher RB, Kelly CP, Neville S, Sheils O, Weir DG. Complement activation within the coeliac small intestine is localised to Brunner's glands. *Gut* 1989;30:1568–73.
154 Janoff A, Zeligs D. Vascular injury and lysis of basement membrane *in vitro* by neutral proteinase of human leukocytes. *Science* 1968;161:702–4.
155 Trier JS, Allan CH, Abrahamson DR, Hagen SJ. Epithelial basement membrane of mouse jejunum. Evidence of laminin turnover along the entire crypt-villus axis. *J Clin Invest* 1990;86:87–95,
156 Marsh MN, Trier JS. The subepithelial fibroblast sheath in mouse jejunum. I. Structural features. *Gastroenterology* 1974;67:622–35.
157 Marsh MN, Trier JS. The subepithelial fibroblast sheath in mouse jejunum. II. Radioautographic studies. *Gastroenterology* 1974; 67:636–45.
158 Granger DN. Role of xanthine oxidase and granulocytes in ischemia-reperfusion injury. *Am J Physiol* 1988;255:H1269–75.
159 Parks DA. Oxygen radicals: mediators of gastrointestinal pathophysiology. *Gut* 1989; 30:293–98.
160 Dvorak AM, Mihm MC, Dvorak HF. Morphology of delayed-type hypersensitivity in man. II. Ultrastructural alterations affecting the microvasculature and tissue mast cells. *Lab Invest* 1976;34:179–91.
161 Marsh MN. Morphologic expression of immunologically-mediated change and injury within the human small intestinal mucosa. In: Batt R, Lawrence TLJ, eds. *Function and Dysfunction of the Small Intestine of Animals.* Liverpool: Liverpool University

Press, 1984:167–98.
162 Dvorak HF, Mihm MC, Dvorak AM, Johnson RA, Manseau J. Morphology of delayed-type hypersensitivity reactions in man. I. Quantitative description of the inflammatory response. *Lab Invest* 1974;31:111–30.
163 Curran RC, Creamer B. Ultrastructural changes in some disorders of the small intestine associated with malabsorption. *J Pathol Bact* 1963;86:1–8.
164 Rubin W, Ross L, Sleisenger MH, Weser E. An electron microscopic study of adult celiac disease. *Lab Invest* 1966;15:1720–47.
165 Shiner M. Ultrastructure of the jejunal surface epithelium in untreated idiopathic steatorrhoea. *Br Med Bull* 1967;23:223–5.
166 Aho AJ, Arstila AU, Ahonen J, Inberg MV, Scheinin T. Ultrastructural alterations in ischaemia lesions of the small intestinal mucosa in experimental superior mesenteric arterial occlusion. *Scand J Gastroenterol* 1973;8:439–47.
167 Marsh MN, Hinde J. Morphometric analysis of small intestinal mucosa. III. The quantitation of crypt epithelial volumes and lymphoid cell infiltrates with reference to celiac sprue mucosae. *Virchows Archiv [A]* 1986;409:11–22.
168 Marsh MN. Studies of intestinal lymphoid tissue. III. Quantitative analyses of epithelial lymphocytes in the small intestine of control subjects and of patients with celiac sprue. *Gastroenterology* 1980;79:481–92.
169 Niazi NM, Leigh R, Crowe P, Marsh MN. Morphometric analysis of small intestinal mucosa. I. Methodology, epithelial volume compartments and enumeration of interepithelial space lymphocytes. *Virchows Archiv [A]* 1984;404:49–60.
170 Marsh MN. Studies of intestinal lymphoid tissue. V. Functional and structural aspects of the epithelial lymphocyte, with implications for coeliac disease and tropical sprue. *Scand J Gastroenterol* 1985;20 (Suppl. 114):55–75.
171 Marsh MN. Studies of intestinal lymphoid tissue. IV. The predictive value of raised mitotic indices among jejunal epithelial lymphocytes in the diagnosis of gluten-sensitive enteropathy. *J Clin Pathol* 1982;35:517–25.
172 Marsh MN, Haeney MR. Studies of intestinal lymphoid tissue. VI. Proliferative response of small intestinal lymphocytes distinguishes gluten-from non-gluten-induced enteropathy. *J Clin Pathol* 1983;76:159–60.
173 Marsh MN, Miller V. Studies of intestinal lymphoid tissue. VIII. The use of epithelial lymphocyte mitotic indices in differentiating untreated celiac sprue mucosae from other childhood enteropathies. *J Pediatr Gastroenterol Nutr* 1985;4:931–5.
174 Selby WS, Janossy G, Bofill M, Jewell D. Lymphocyte populations in the human small intestine. The findings in normal mucosa and in the mucosa of patients with adult coeliac disease. *Clin Exp Immunol* 1983;53:219–38.
175 Selby WS, Janossy G, Jewell D. Immunohistological characterisation of intraepithelial lymphocytes of the human gastrointestinal tract. *Gut* 1981;22:169–76.
176 Cerf-Bensussan N, Schneeberger EE, Bhan AK. Immunohistologic and immunoelectron microscopic characterisation of the mucosal lymphocytes of human small intestine by the use of monoclonal antibodies. *J Immunol* 1983;130:2615–22.
177 Brandtzaeg P, Bosnes V, Halstensen TS, Scott H, Sollid LM, Valnes K. T lymphocytes in human gut epithelium preferentially express the α/β antigen receptor and are often CD45/UCHL1 positive. *Scand J Immunol* 1989;30:123–8.
178 Halstensen TS, Scott H, Brandtzaeg P. Human $CD8^+$ intraepithelial T lymphocytes are mainly CD45 RA^- RB^+ and show increased co-expression of CD45 RO in celiac disease. *Eur J Immunol* 1990;20:1825–30.
179 Streuli M, Murimoto C, Schreiber M, Schlossman SF, Saito H. Characterisation of CD45 and CD45R monoclonal antibodies using transfected mouse cell lines that express individual human common leukocyte antigens. *J Immunol* 1988;141:3910–4.
180 Akbar AN, Timms A, Janossy G. Cellular events during memory T-cell activation *in vitro*: the UCHL1 (180 000 MW) determinant is newly synthesized after mitosis. *Immunology* 1989;66:213–18.
181 Sanders ME, Makgoba MW, Sharrow SO *et al.* Human memory T lymphocytes express increased levels of three cell adhesion molecules (LFA-3, CD2, and LFA-1) and three other molecules (UCHL1, CDw29 and Pgp-1) and have enhanced IFN-gamma production. *J Immunol* 1988;140:1401–7.
182 Cerf-Bensussan N, Quaroni A, Kurnick JT, Bhan AK. Intraepithelial lymphocytes modulate Ia expression by intestinal epithelial cells. *J Immunol* 1984;132:2244–52.

183 Scott H, Sollid LM, Fausa O, Brandtzaeg P, Thorsby E. Expression of MHC Class II subregion products by jejunal epithelium of patients with coeliac disease. *Scand J Immunol* 1987;26:563–72.
184 Scott H, Sollid LM, Brandtzaeg P. Expression of MHC Class II determinants by jejunal epithelium in coeliac disease. *J Pediatr Gastroenterol Nutr* 1988;7:145–6.
185 Malizia G, Trejdosiewicz LK, Wood G, Howdle PD, Janossy G, Losowsky MS. The microenvironment of coeliac disease: T cell phenotypes and expression of the T_2 'blast' antigen by small bowel lymphocytes. *Clin Exp Immunol* 1985;60:437–46.
186 Jarry A, Cerf-Bensussan N, Brousse N, Selz F, Guy-Grand D. Subsets of $CD3^+$ (T cell receptor α/β or γ/δ) and $CD3^-$ lymphocytes isolated from normal gut epithelium display phenotypical features different from their counterparts in peripheral blood. *Eur J Immunol* 1990;20:1097–103.
187 Viney J, MacDonald TT, Spencer J. Gamma/delta T cells in the gut epithelium. *Gut* 1990;31:841–4.
188 Spencer J, Isaacson PG, Diss TC, MacDonald TT. Expression of disulphide linked and non-disulphide linked forms of the T cell receptor or gamma/delta heterodimer in human intestinal intraepithelial lymphocytes. *Eur J Immunol* 1989;19:1335–8.
189 Savilahti E, Arato A, Verkasalo M. Increased numbers of T cell receptor gamma/delta bearing lymphocytes in the epithelium of coeliac patients. In: MacDonald TT, Challacombe SJ, Bland PW, eds. *Advances in Mucosal Immunology*. Dordrecht: Kluwer Academic Publishers, 1990:61–6.
190 Halstensen TS, Scott H, Brandtzaeg P. Intraepithelial T cells of the TCR γ/δ^+ $CD8^-$ and $V\delta1/J\delta1^+$ phenotypes are increased in coeliac disease. *Scand J Immunol* 1989;30: 665–72.
191 Marsh MN. The gut associated lymphoid tissue and immune system. In: Whitehead R, ed. *Gastrointestinal and Oesophageal Pathology*. Edinburgh: Churchill Livingstone, 1989:161–86.
192 Flick AL, Vaergthin KF, Rubin CE. Clinical experience with suction biopsy of the rectal mucosa. *Gastroenterology* 1962;42: 691–705.
193 Dobbins WO, Rubin CE. Studies of the rectal mucosa in coeliac sprue. *Gastroenterology* 1964;47:471–9.
194 Breen EG, Coughlan G, Connolly EC, Stevens FM, McCarthy CF. Coeliac proctitis. *Scand J Gastroenterol* 1987;22:471–7.
195 Dubois RN, Lazenby AJ, Yardley JH, Hendrix TR, Bayless TM, Giardello FM. Lymphocytic enterocolitis in patients with 'refractory sprue'. *J Am Med Assoc* 1989; 262:935–7.
196 Cooke WT, Brooke BN. Non-specific enterocolitis. *Q J Med* 1955;24:6–22.
197 Salem SN, Truelove SC. Small intestine and gastric abnormalities in ulcerative colitis. *Br Med J* 1975;1:827–31.
198 Nugen FW, Gonyea RJ. Development of gluten enteropathy after ileostomy for ulcerative colitis. *Am J Dig Dis* 1968;13: 186–9.
199 Jalan KN, Percy-Robb IW, McManus JPA, Sircus W. In: Girdwood RH, Smith AN, eds. *Malabsorption*. Edinburgh: Edinburgh University Press, 1969:292–302.
200 Jankey N, Price LA. Small intestinal histochemical and histological changes in ulcerative colitis. *Gut* 1969;10:267–9.
201 Binder V, Saltoft J, Gudmard-Moyer E. Histological and histochemical changes in the jejunal mucosa in ulcerative colitis. *Scand J Gastroenterol* 1974;9:293–7.
202 Falchuk KR, Falchuk ZM. Selective immunoglobulin A deficiency, ulcerative colitis and gluten-sensitive enteropathy: a unique association. *Gastroenterology* 1975; 69:503–6.
203 Ansaldi N, Santini B, Dell-Olio D, Lewis F. Proctosigmoiditis and coeliac disease. *Arch Dis Child* 1978;53:645–8.
204 Kumar PJ, O'Donoghue D, Gibson J, Stansfield A, Dawson AM. The existence of inflammatory bowel lesions in gluten-sensitive enteropathy. *Postgrad Med J* 1979; 55:753–6.
205 Kitis G, Holmes GKT, Cooper BT, Thompson H, Allan RN. Association of coeliac disease and inflammatory bowel disease. *Gut* 1980;21:636–41.
206 Gillberg R, Dotevall G, Ahren C. Chronic inflammatory bowel disease in patients with coeliac disease. *Scand J Gastroenterol* 1982; 17:491–6.
207 Glasgow J, Pinkerton C, Sloan J, Serosal miliary Crohn's disease in association with probable coeliac disease. *Arch Dis Child* 1983;58:149–51.
208 Breen EG, Cohlan G, Connolly EC, Stevens FM, McCarthy CF. Increased association of ulcerative colitis and coeliac disease. *Ir J Med Sci* 1987;156:120–1.
209 Bulger K, Griffin M, Dervan P, Lennon J, Crowe J. Coeliac disease in association with

inflammatory bowel disease. *Postgrad Med J* 1988;64:336.
210 Mayberry JF, Smart HL, Toghill PJ. Familial association between coeliac disease and ulcerative colitis. *J R Soc Med* 1986;79: 204–5.
211 Shah A, Mayberry JF, Williams G, Holt P, Loft DE, Rhodes J. Epidemiological survey of coeliac disease and inflammatory bowel disease in first degree relatives of coeliac patients. *Q J Med* 1990;275:283–8.
212 Loft DE. *Coeliac disease: the structural and functional response of large intestinal mucosa to local gluten challenge.* MD Thesis. University of Birmingham, 1990.
213 Trejdosiewicz LK, Badr-el-Din S, Smart CJ *et al.* Colonic mucosal T lymphocytes in ulcerative colitis: expression of CD7 antigen in relation to MHC class II (HLA-D) antigens. *Dig Dis Sci* 1989;34:1449–56.
214 Loft DE, Marsh MN, Crowe P. Rectal gluten challenge and diagnosis of coeliac disease. *Lancet* 1990;335:1293–5.
215 Sandle GI, Hayslett JP, Binder HJ. Effects of glucocorticoids on rectal transport in normal subjects and patients with ulcerative colitis. *Gut* 1986;27:309–16.
216 Hawker PC, McKay JS, Turnberg LA. Electrolyte transport across colonic mucosa from patients with inflammatory bowel disease. *Gastroenterology* 1980;79:508–11.
217 Sandle GI, McGlone F, Crowe P, Marsh MN. Cellular basis for defective electrolyte transport in inflamed human colon. *Gastroenterology* 1990;99:97–106.
218 Doe WF, Henry K, Holt L, Booth CC. An immunological study of adult coeliac disease *Gut* 1972;13:324–5.
219 Shiner M. *Ultrastructure of the Small Intestinal Mucosa.* Berlin: Springer-Verlag, 1983.
220 Askenase PW, Rosenstein RW, Ptak W. T cell production of an antigen binding factor with *in vivo* activity analogous to IgE antibody. *J Exp Med* 1982;157:862–73.
221 van Loveren H, Meade R, Askenase PW. An early component of delayed type hypersensitivity mediated by T cells and mast cells. *J Exp Med* 1983;157:1604–17.
222 Austin LL, Dobbins WO. Studies of the rectal mucosa in coeliac sprue: the intraepithelial lymphocyte. *Gut* 1988;29:200–5.
223 Blumgart HL. Three fatal adult cases of malabsorption of fat. *Arch Int Med* 1923;22: 113–28.
224 Fairley NH, Mackie FP. A progress report on researches in sprue (1924–1925). *Indian J Med Res* 1926;14:105–23.
225 Holmes WH, Starr P. A nutritional disturbance in adults resembling celiac disease and sprue. *J Am Med Assoc* 1929;92:975–80.
226 Hanes FM, McBryde A. Identity of sprue, non-tropical sprue and celiac disease. *Arch Int Med* 1936;58:1–16.
227 Fairley NH. Sprue. Its applied pathology, biochemistry and treatment. *Trans R Soc Trop Med Hyg* 1930;24:131–86.
228 Castle WB, Heath CW, Strauss MB. Observations on the etiologic relationship of achylia gastrica to pernicious anaemia. IV. A biologic assay of the gastric secretion of patients with pernicious anaemia having free hydrochloric acid and that of patients without anaemia having no free hydrochloric acid, and the role of intestinal impermeability to hemopoietic substances in pernicious anaemia. *Am J Med Sci* 1931; 182:741–64.
229 Castle WB, Rhoads CP, Lawson HA, Payne GC. Etiology and treatment of sprue: observations on patients in Puerto Rico and subsequent experiments on animals. *Arch Intern Med* 1935;56:627–99.
230 Badenoch J. Disordered gastro-intestinal function and its relationship to tropical sprue, coeliac disease and idiopathic steatorrhoea. *Trans R Soc Trop Med Hyg* 1952; 46:591.
231 Friedlander PH, Gorvy V. Steatorrhoea. *Br Med J* 1955;2:809–12.
232 Baker SJ. Idiopathic tropical steatorrhoea. *Indian J Med Sci* 1957;11:687–703.
233 Doig A, Girdwood RH. The absorption of folic acid and labelled cyanocobalamin in intestinal malabsorption. *Q J Med* 1960;29: 333–74.
234 Girdwood RH, Delamore IW, Williams AW. Jejunal biopsy in malabsorptive disorders of the adult. *Br Med J* 1961;1:319–23.
235 Floch MH, Thomassen RW, Cox RS, Sheehy TW. The gastric mucosa in tropical sprue. *Gastroenterology* 1963;44:567–77.
236 Hansky J, Shiner M. Gastric studies in idiopathic steatorrhoea. *Gastroenterology* 1963; 45:49–56.
237 Vaish SK, Sampathkumar J, Jacob R, Baker SJ. The stomach in tropical sprue. *Gut* 1965; 6:458–65.
238 Cooke WT. Adult coeliac disease. In: Jerzy Glass GB, ed. *Progress in Gastroenterology.* Vol 1. New York: Grune and Stratton, 1968: 299–338.
239 Moshal MG, Hifg W, Kallichurum S, Pillay K. Endemic tropical sprue in Africa. *J Trop*

Med Hyg 1975;78:2–5.
240 Cream JJ, Scott GL. Anaemia in dermatitis herpetiformis. *Br J Derm* 1970;82:333–42.
241 Andersson H, Dotevall G, Mobacken H. Malignant mesenteric lymphoma in a patient with dermatitis herpetiformis, hypochlorhydria, and small-bowel abnormalities. *Scand J Gastroenterol* 1971a;6: 397–9.
242 Andersson H, Dotevall G, Mobacken H. Gastric secretion of acid and intrinsic factor in dermatitis herpetiformis. *Scand J Gastroenterol* 1971b;6:411–6.
243 Heading RC, Parkin DM, Barnetson R, MacClelland D, Shearman D. Small-intestinal bacterial flora in dermatitis herpetiformis. *Dig Dis* 1974;19:704–8.
244 Fausa O. Vitamin B absorption in intestinal diseases. *Scand J Gastroenterol* 1974;9 (Suppl. 29):75–9.
245 Fausa O, Eeg Larsen T, Husby G, Thune P. Gastrointestinal investigations in dermatitis herpetiformis. *Acta Derm Venereol* 1975; 55:203–6.
246 Stockbrugger R, Andersson H, Gillberg R, Kastrup W, Lundqvist G, Mobacken H. Auto-immune gastritis in patients with dermatitis herpetiformis. *Acta Derm Venereol* 1976;56:111–13.
247 O'Donoghue D, Lancaster-Smith M, Johnson G, Kumar P. Gastric lesion in dermatitis herpetiformis. *Gut* 1976;17:185–8.
248 Thune P, Husby G, Fausa O, Gedde-Dahl D, Baklien K, Solheim B. Immunologic and gastrointestinal abnormalities in dermatitis herpetiformis. *Int J Dermatol* 1979;18: 135–41.
249 Gillberg R, Kastrup W, Mobacken H, Stockbrugger R, Ahren C. Gastric morphology and function in dermatitis herpetiformis and in coeliac disease. *Scand J Gastroenterol* 1985;20:133–40.
250 Witts LJ. *The Stomach and Anaemia*. London: Athlone Press, 1966.
251 Cox AJ. The stomach in pernicious anaemia. *Am J Pathol* 1943;19:491–501.
252 Siurala M, Varis K, Wiljasalo M. Studies of patients with atrophic gastritis: a 10–15 year follow-up. *Scand J Gastroenterol* 1966; 1:40–8.
253 Taylor KB, Fisher JM. Gastritis. In: Jerzy Glass GB, ed. *Progress in Gastroenterology*. Vol 1. New York: Grune and Stratton, 1968: 1–21.
254 Jerzy Glass JB, Spear FD, Nieburgs H, Ishimori A. Gastric atrophy, atrophic gastritis, and gastric secretory failure. *Gastroenterology* 1960;39:429–53.
255 Stockbrugger R, Kastrup W, Lundqvist G, Mobacken H. Development of gastric dysfunction in dermatitis herpetiformis. *Acta Derm Venereol* 1978;58:343–8.
256 Bennett TI, Hunter D, Vaughan JM. Idiopathic steatorrhoea (Gee's disease). A nutritional disturbance associated with tetany, osteomalacia and anaemia. *Q J Med* 1932;1: 603–77.
257 Snell AM. Tropical and non-tropical sprue (chronic idiopathic steatorrhoea): their probable interrelationship. *Ann Intern Med* 1939;12:1632–71.
258 Quigley EMM, Carmichael HA, Watkinson GA. Adult celiac disease (celiac sprue), pernicious anaemia and IgA deficiency. *J Clin Gastroenterol* 1986;8:277–81.
259 Strickland RG, Mackay IR. A reappraisal of the nature and significance of chronic atrophic gastritis. *Dig Dis* 1973;18:426–40.
260 Valnes K, Brandtzaeg P, Elgjo K, Stave R, Baklien K, Fausa O. Local immunoglobulin production is different in gastritis associated with dermatitis herpetiformis and simple gastritis. *Gut* 1987;28:1589–94.
261 Kaye MD, Whorwell PJ, Wright R. Gastric mucosal lymphocyte subpopulations in pernicious anaemia and in normal stomach. *Clin Immunol Immunopathol* 1983;28: 431–40.
262 Hoat J, Jouret-Mourin A, Delos M, Wallez L. Etude anatomoclinique d'une série de gastrites chroniques caractérisées par une infiltration lymphocytaire intra-épithéliale. *Acta Endosc* 1986;16:69–74.
263 Hoat J, Jouret A, Willette M, Gossuin A, Mainguet P. Lymphocytic gastritis — prospective study of its relationship with varioliform gastritis. *Gut* 1990;31:282–5.
264 Dixon M, Wyatt J, Burke D, Rathbone B. Lymphocytic gastritis — relationship to Campylobacter pylori infection. *J Pathol* 1988;154:125–32.
265 Wolber R, Owen D, del Buono L, Appelman H, Freeman H. Lymphocytic gastritis in patients with celiac sprue or spruelike intestinal disease. *Gastroenterology* 1990;98: 310–15.

Chapter 7/Epidemiology of coeliac disease

RICHARD F.A. LOGAN

Epidemiology is concerned with both the study of the distribution of disease within populations, and of the determinants underlying that distribution [1]. This chapter will therefore describe the distribution of coeliac disease (CD) in terms of geography, person and time and then consider the genetic and environmental factors that have been implicated.

Problems of study

In studying CD, the epidemiologist faces three particular problems, namely (1) a low case fatality, (2) its relative rarity and (3) wide variations in its ascertainment.

Low case fatality

By definition, epidemiological studies require some measure of disease occurrence. For diseases in which case fatality rates are high, mortality rates are often an adequate measure, but although the mortality rate of CD is about twice that of the general population, few patients are certified as dying from this disease. For example, in Edinburgh, CD was mentioned on 29% of 115 death certificates but in only 9% was the disease given as the underlying cause of death [2]. As a result, even in those countries where clinical awareness and diagnostic rates are high, it is evident that mortality statistics are unlikely to be a reliable measure of disease occurrence.

Relative rarity

Until recently there had been no test for CD suitable for use in population surveys. Post-mortem autolysis rendered autopsy surveys impossible while blood tests proved unsatisfactory because they were insufficiently specific for use in groups where disease prevalence is low. Even in populations where the prevalence of CD was estimated to be as high as three to four per 1000, a test with a specificity of 95% would identify more than 10 times as many false positives as true cases. However, in a recent study [3] a specificity of greater than 97% for antibodies to gliadin determined by enzyme-linked immunoassay (ELISA) was obtained; in a survey of 1866 adult blood donors, seven out of 43 donors with high gliadin antibody levels had jejunal biopsies which revealed villous flattening. If these results are reproducible then measurement of gliadin antibodies may be sufficiently specific for use in future population surveys.

Variations in case ascertainment

In the absence of population surveys or reliable mortality statistics, most studies on the occurrence of CD have been based on hospital case series collected by clinicians with a particular interest in the disease. These series have usually been relatively small and possibly strongly influenced by the diagnostic acumen of interested clinicians. For example, Swinson and Levi found that the rate of diagnosis of CD at Northwick Park Hospital, London, was three times higher than at two other London hospitals [4]. Of their new coeliacs, only 26% had the classical symptoms of steatorrhoea, osteomalacia or severe anaemia, while 64% had 'trivial, transient or unrelated' symptoms. Similar results have been reported from Edinburgh, where between the periods 1960–64 and 1975–79 there was a three-fold increase in newly diagnosed coeliacs [5]. In the latter period only 27% had classical symptoms compared with 90% previously, while 55% had no gastrointestinal symptoms at all. In both studies, large numbers (44% and 29%, respectively) of coeliacs were only recognized because of unexplained, and often minor abnormalities found on routine blood tests.

If, as these studies suggest, as many as one-half of all adult coeliac patients identified in some populations have few or no symptoms, then much of any apparent difference in prevalence could be accounted for by variations in case ascertainment.

Measures of disease occurrence; prevalence versus incidence

For most chronic diseases their frequency is best assessed by the notion of *incidence*, that is, the number of new cases detected in a given population over a defined time period. For adult coeliac patients, the difficulty in dating the onset of clinical disease and the increasing recognition of mild disease renders calculations of incidence of dubious validity. Most studies derived from hospital case series have therefore assessed frequency in terms of disease *prevalence*, that is, the number of cases identified and alive in a given population irrespective of the date of diagnosis. As mortality rates are low, comparisons of prevalence figures are reasonably valid provided it is recognized that prevalence will tend to be higher in areas where longer established, modern gastroenterological services have been operative for a long time.

In children, disease frequency is usually expressed as the number of cases identified by year of birth with the denominator being the total births in the same year (a birth cohort). Although such figures are, strictly speaking prevalence measures, they can also be viewed as cumulative incidence, and when restricted to the numbers identified by a given age (e.g. cumulative incidence by age 2:1000 births) comparisons can be readily made. However, in some of the studies of children, it is not clear whether comparisons of cumulative incidence have allowed for the longer observation period of earlier (i.e. older) birth cohorts.

Other measures of disease frequency include the use of data on hospital admissions, self- or parent-reported CD, and membership of national coeliac societies (self-help groups) [6–9]. Each of these measures is liable to be influenced by variations in ascertainment, but they do have the advantage of reflecting the diagnostic behaviour of large groups of clinicians. However, the validity of these forms of measurement is not known. Hospital admissions are probably a satisfactory measure of disease frequency in children, particularly those below 5 years of age, since children are virtually always admitted for small intestinal biopsy. The proportion of coeliacs who report membership of self-help groups has varied from 35 to 85%, and in England and Wales the number of Coeliac Society members has been estimated to be no more than half of all known coeliacs [9,10].

Variation by place—geographic distribution

Data on the frequency of CD have predominantly come from countries in western Europe, particularly Scandinavia and the UK (Table 7.1). In most studies of infants and small children, disease frequency has been assessed by counting the numbers diagnosed by paediatric referral services in relation to the number of live births in the population served. Referral practices, the ease of data collection and the effectiveness of the paediatric services are therefore likely to be important influences on both the number of studies and the actual prevalence reported.

As shown in Table 7.1 the childhood prevalence figures show about a four-fold variation across Europe with the highest childhood prevalence being reported from Graz in eastern Austria, and the lowest from Finland. (The figure from Portugal is likely to be an underestimate according to the authors.) The striking feature of the distribution in western Europe is the proximity of high and low prevalence areas such as Graz and northeast Switzerland, and Finland and Sweden. These

Table 7.1 Prevalence of CD* reported from European countries

Region	Number of cases†	Period	Crude prevalence per 100 000 population	Comments
Glasgow [11]	100	1952–62	54	
Edinburgh and Lothian [12]	104	1979	91	Ages 5–14 only, boys — 69, girls — 112
Derby, England [13]	24	1965–72	95	
Western Ireland [14]	97	1960–70	152	168 for County Galway alone
Malmo, Sweden [15]	48	1966–79	111	
Linkoping, central Sweden [16]	167	1970–82	134	
Linkoping, central Sweden [3]	7	1986	370	Result of screening 1866 adult blood donors for antigliadin antibodies
Oulu, northern Finland [17]	35	1970–74	49	Only coeliacs diagnosed before age 2
Tampere, Finland [18]	72	1960–84	55	
Volda, western Norway [19]	35	1980	87	Adults only
Denmark [20]	35	1971–79	71	
Graz, Austria [21]	205	1969–77	203	
Northeast Switzerland [22]	354	1966–75	86	
Naples, Italy [23]	435	1981–86	87	
Portugal [24]	189	1979–83	27	Based on number of referrals to the four specialist paediatric clinics for Portugal

* Childhood CD unless otherwise stated.
† Based on biopsy-confirmed cases.

Table 7.2 Crude prevalence figures* reported outside Europe

Region	Number of cases	Period	Prevalence per 100 000	Comments
Melbourne, Australia [25]	62	1965–68	35	Children only
Otago, New Zealand [9]	20	1975–84	35	Children only
			9	Children and adults
New Zealand [26]	295	1983	9	Range 5–12, based on membership of Coeliac Society
Kuwait [27]	20	1980–85	33	Children only, of which 13 were Palestinians
Israel, west coast [28]	111	1968–81	103	171 per 100 000 if all children with an abnormal biopsy are assumed to be coeliacs
Sudan [29]	7	1974–77	–	No denominator given – all Sudanese
Cuba [30]	50	1972–78	–	No denominator given

* Unless stated, figures are based on biopsy-confirmed cases.

differences have been found consistently and seem to be too large to be due to differing diagnostic criteria and methods.

Outside western Europe there have been few systematic studies (Table 7.2). It is particularly remarkable that none have been reported from the USA or Canada. Nevertheless, there are a large number of reports of small case series which indicate that in Australasia, South Africa and North America CD is not rare. However, the low prevalence of disease in Dunedin and the Otago province of New Zealand is striking when it is considered that this is an area heavily populated by immigrants from Scotland and from the rest of the UK [9,26]. A particularly high prevalence has been found in Israel, where depending on the diagnostic criteria used, between 103 and 171 per 100 000 children have the disease [28]. Prevalence was highest in children whose mothers were of Asian or Middle Eastern origin, and lowest in those with Israeli-born mothers. It is not clear whether the absence of reports of CD from other areas such as the Far East, eastern Europe, much of Africa and South America indicate the rarity of disease or lack of ascertainment.

Variation with age and sex

'Incidence'

For the reasons given earlier, in few studies have estimates of disease incidence been attempted and none have analysed incidence by age. An alternative is to examine age at diagnosis, recognizing that this is affected by the awareness of clinicians and other factors associated with the delivery of health care.

Age at diagnosis shows a similar pattern in several recent series, and is mirrored in Coeliac Society membership data [12,30–33]. The peak age for diagnosis is between age 1 and 2 years (Fig. 7.1) and it can be inferred that the annual incidence of CD at this age, and over the whole period from birth to age 5, is at least two- to three-fold greater than at any later age. The incidence then appears to fall in both sexes reaching a nadir during the teenage years. In most series the frequency of diagnosis in women then rises to a plateau during the later reproductive years which is maintained until old age, except for a slight dip around the menopause.

In men the frequency increases more gradually with age to reach a peak in the fifth decade.

Prevalence

Three recent studies have reported age-specific prevalences of CD in adults (Table 7.3) [12,34,35]. How much the differences in prevalence

Table 7.3 Prevalence of CD by age and sex in surveys of adults (per 100 000 population)

	Lothian, Scotland* 1979 [12]		Linkoping, Sweden 1981 [34]	Orebro, Sweden† 1986 [35]	
Age group	Men (n = 178)	Women (n = 291)	Combined (n = 75)	Men (n = 51) and women (n = 85)	
15–24	57	71	15	39	
25–34	25	72	24	47	
35–44	46	126	58	111	
45–54	49	28	105	107	
55–64	46	84	77	98	
65–74	58	58	37	178	
>75	69	36	24	116	
Sex-specific prevalence	50	74	‡	72§	117§
Crude prevalence	61		56	96	

* Includes 51 (seven per 100 000) with dermatitis herpetiformis.
† Includes 19 (14 per 100 000) with dermatitis herpetiformis.
‡ Figures available for sexes combined only.
§ Figures by age only available for males and females overall.

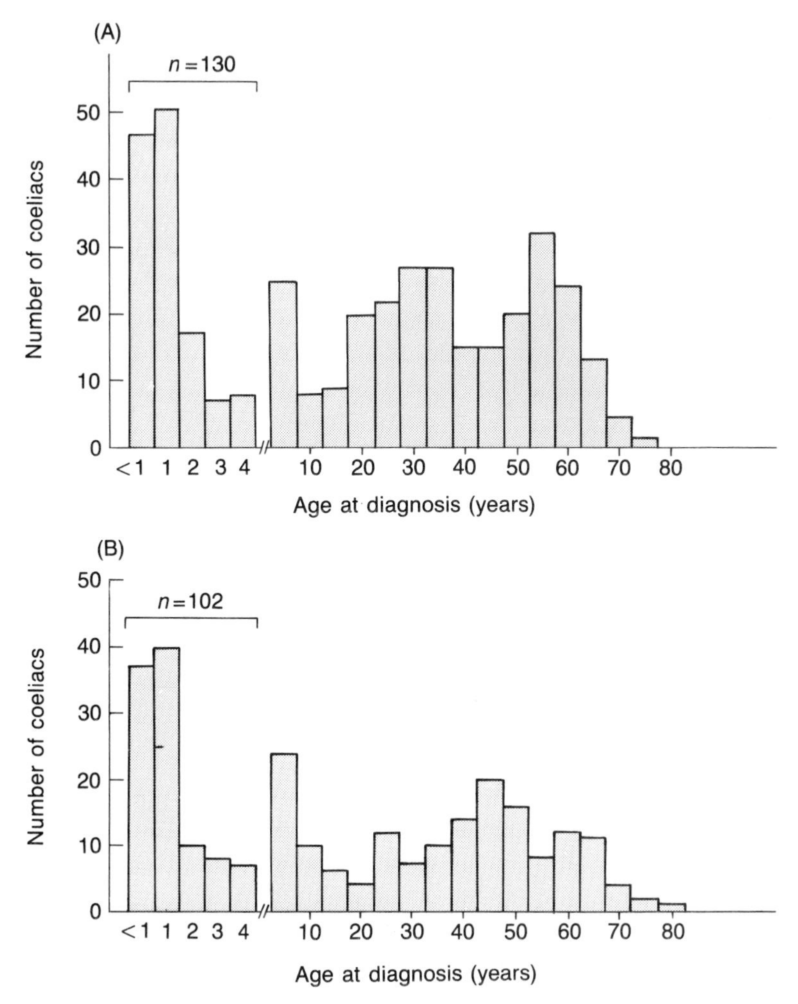

Fig. 7.1 Age at diagnosis for all (A) female and (B) male coeliacs included on coeliac register in Edinburgh (1940–1979). At (A) 130 patients and at (B) 102 patients were diagnosed up to age 4. (From Logan *et al.* [12].)

demonstrated are accounted for by earlier variations in incidence, or by the greater case ascertainment of recent times, is not clear. The timing of the three surveys was such that the many childhood coeliacs diagnosed since 1970 were not old enough to have been included. Prevalence in the younger age groups will therefore be predictably higher in future studies from these areas.

Sex

As few studies have reported disease frequency by gender it is necessary to revert to inferences from published case series. In most series of

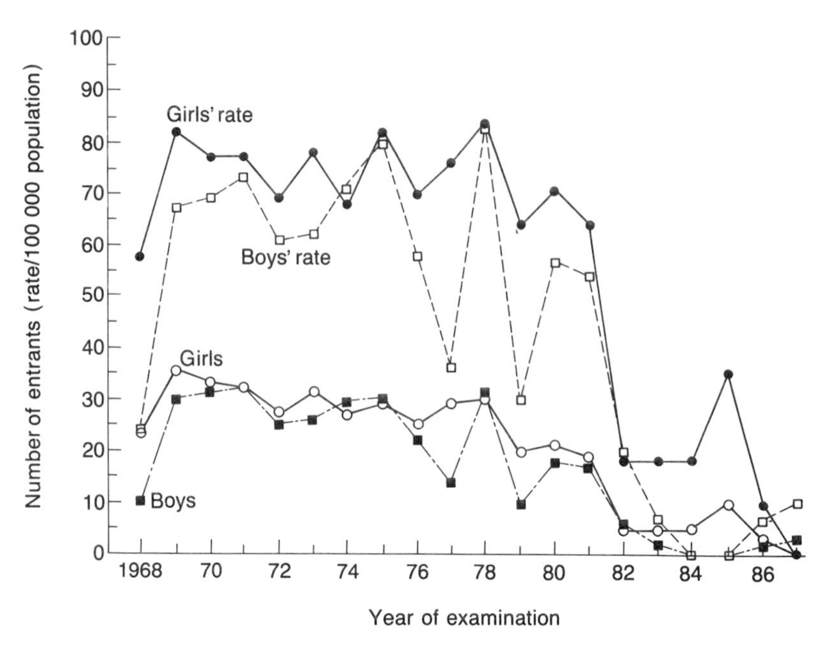

Fig. 7.2 Prevalence and numbers of children with CD reported at school entry medical examinations in Scotland (1968–1987).

childhood cases, girls have slightly outnumbered boys suggesting that the prevalence in girls is marginally higher than in boys. This difference is also evident in the prevalence of CD reported in Scottish school children attending for their first school medical examination (Fig. 7.2) [7]. In contrast, in recent series of adult cases the women have generally outnumbered the men often by as much as 2 : 1 [4,5,32,36]. In the absence of population surveys it is impossible to tell whether this difference simply reflects the greater case ascertainment in women, particularly during their fourth and fifth decades, or whether it indicates a real difference in disease incidence. It is notable that in series of patients with dermatitis herpetiformis (DH) the sex ratio is often reversed [36]. For example, among 76 patients with DH in Edinburgh, the male : female ratio was 1.8 : 1 compared with a male : female ratio of 1 : 1.9 for 324 coeliacs [37].

Variation with time — secular trends

Notwithstanding the fragmentary nature of most of the epidemiological data, a decline in the incidence of CD in children has been apparent in the UK since the mid-1970s (Table 7.4).

The timing and suddenness of this decline is striking, with several studies showing that between 1975 and 1977 there was a greater than 50% fall in the cumulative incidence for these, and subsequent birth cohorts. The decline started at a time when levels of clinical awareness were high so that the likelihood of coeliacs remaining undiagnosed was correspondingly low. Other possible explanations are that there were changes in the referral practices of other paediatricians and doctors, or that childhood coeliacs were being diagnosed when they were older. Both possibilities can be discounted, as the decline is evident in population-based data, while in data analysed by birth cohort no evidence of a rise in diagnosis in older children was apparent [8,12,41]. Evidence of the decline can also be seen in hospital activity analysis data for England and Wales (Fig. 7.3) which show a steep fall in hospital admission rates for CD in infants, with a more gradual decline for the whole age group of 0–4 years. A sharp fall is also evident in the prevalence of CD in Scotland, assessed by the numbers of children reported to have the disease at school medical examinations performed during their first year of local authority schooling (Fig. 7.2). Most children undergo the examination at age 5, and the timing of the decline corresponds with children born in 1976.

In several, but not all studies the decline was preceded by a period of rising birth cohort incidence which reached a peak for cohorts born in the years 1970–1972. Although the peak has usually been ascribed to increasing awareness of CD by paediatricians and a greater use of jejunal biopsy in infants, the subsequent decline suggests that a real increase could also be a contributing factor. A decline in childhood disease has also been seen in Finland but not in neighbouring Sweden (Table 7.4). The data from the west coast of Israel suggests that a decline in childhood cases has occurred there since 1980.

The explanation for the decline is not clear, but in the UK it

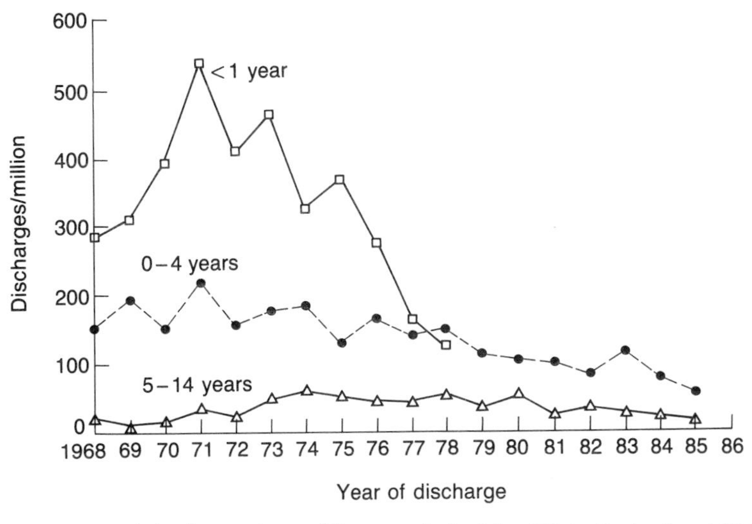

Fig. 7.3 Hospital discharges (per million population) for CD in England and Wales between 1968 and 1985. (From International Classification Disease, Revisions 8 and 9.) ICD8: 269.0; ICD9: 579.0

Table 7.4 Secular trends for incidence of CD in children

Centre	Period of observation 1965–69	1970–74	1975–79	1980–84	Year in which declining incidence became evident
British Isles					
Leeds* [38]	35	42	12	—	1975
Glasgow [39]	55	67	28	—	1976
Edinburgh [12] (male : female)	71/107	81/119	61/64	—	1976
Queen Elizabeth, London* [40]	43	58	27	16	1976
Galway [41]	169	194	73	—	1975
Other countries					
Malmo, Sweden [15]	97	104	135	—	—
Linkoping, Sweden [16]	—	102	157	158	—
Oulu, Finland† [17]	15	49	21	—	n/a
Tampere, Finland‡ [18]	109	61	47	12	—
Rehovot-Ashdod, Israel [28]	59	73	189	90	1980

* Extrapolated from references — no population denominator.
† Number of cases only diagnosis at age <2 years.
‡ Cumulative incidence at all ages — coeliacs diagnosed in teens included in earlier birth cohorts.

followed the publication of a government report on infant feeding practices [42]. The report, published in 1974, recommended that mothers should be encouraged to breast feed and to delay the introduction of cereals and other solids until the child was 4 months of age. The report also suggested that there should be regular surveys of infant feeding practices, and three such surveys have been carried out since 1975 [43–45]. These have shown that the percentage of women still breast feeding 6 weeks after delivery increased from 24 to 42% between 1975 and 1980, falling back slightly to 40% in 1985. Over the same time there was a fall in the number of women introducing solids within 8 weeks of delivery, being 49% in 1975 compared with 24% in 1980 and 1985. Over a longer period there has been a substantial increase in the availability and sales of gluten-free baby foods. However, in Sweden, during a similar time-span, there have been even greater increases in the proportion of mothers breast feeding and in the age when weaning occurs, but without any fall in the incidence of CD in children born [15].

Genetic factors

Familial

Since the 1920s reports were published describing families with two or more affected members [46]. When healthy relatives of coeliacs have been invited to have an intestinal biopsy, about 14% of all biopsies of first degree relatives have been found to be flat, which represents approximately 8% of all such relatives when those not having a biopsy are also included (Table 7.5). Allowing for the greater tendency of those with mild symptoms to have biopsies, the overall figure for affected first degree relatives is about 10%. In general, the disease frequency has been found to be highest in siblings and lowest in parents, with children being intermediate — differences that probably reflect mortality rates and observation times. Most relatives detected in this way are asymptomatic, or have only trivial symptoms that have not required investigation. In some of these studies there was also a small proportion of individuals with less severe mucosal abnormalities that were considered insufficient for a diagnosis of CD [24,50].

Twins

Many examples of monozygotic twin pairs, where one or both twins had CD, have been described. Of 23 pairs reviewed by Polanco *et al.*, 17 were concordant and six were discordant for CD [53]. However, in some of these reports the criteria for monozygosity were inevitably not up to current standards [54]. In one of these discordant pairs, the unaffected twin subsequently developed CD at age 9, and Salazar de Sousa *et al.* have recently reported a second case of an apparently unaffected monozygotic twin who had a normal biopsy at age 2, but 7 years later developed symptoms and was found to have complete mucosal flattening [55]. In four other 'discordant' pairs, CD was diagnosed in infancy and thus it is uncertain whether discordance has been maintained during adulthood. The proportion of monozygotic pairs that show lifetime discordance is therefore likely to be lower than the one in three suggested. Nevertheless, the fact that in childhood, monozygotic twins can be discordant, does underline the aetiological importance of environmental factors acting in addition to dietary gluten.

HLA associations

While a strong familial predisposition could theoretically be due to a shared family environment, associations with genetic markers provide indisputable evidence of a role for such factors in aetiology. An association between CD and the human leucocyte antigen (HLA)-B8 antigen was first reported in 1972 by Falchuk *et al.* and also by Stokes *et al.* [56,57]. In both studies, 88% of coeliacs were HLA-B8 positive compared with 22 and 30% of controls, respectively. In subsequent studies the frequency of B8 positivity has generally been lower and when relative risk is used to assess the strength of the association, the risk of CD in populations where the B8 antigen is common has usually been

Table 7.5 Prevalence of a flat mucosa in first degree relatives in various studies

Reference	Place	Number of families studied	Relationship	Number available	Number biopsied	Number with mucosal flattening	% of those biopsied
MacDonald *et al.* [47]	Washington State, USA	17	Parents	34	12	0	0
			Siblings	63	33	5	15.1
			Children	37	17	2	11.7
Robinson *et al.* [48]	Newcastle, England	22	Parents	41	29	3	10.3
Shipman *et al.* [25]	Melbourne, Australia	32	Parents	64	53	4	7.5
			Siblings	80	78	10	12.8
Mylotte *et al.* [49]	Galway, Ireland	31	Parents	51	28	1	3.6
			Siblings	138	83	12	14.5
			Children	6	6	2	33.3
Rolles *et al.* [50]	Birmingham, England	15	Parents	30	30	2	6.7
			Siblings	42	42	2	4.8
Stokes *et al.* [51]	Birmingham, England	115	Parents	82	41	5	12.2
			Siblings	143	81	18	22.2
			Children	101	60	12	20.0
Ellis *et al.* [52]	Liverpool, England	122	Parents	122	22	4	18.2
			Siblings	177	47	6	12.8
			Children	98	34	1	2.9

about five- to eight-fold greater in HLA-B8 positive, compared with B8 negative, individuals [58]. This can be compared with the apparent 10-fold risk of lung cancer in smokers compared with non-smokers.

It is now clear that the association with HLA-B8 is due to its linkage disequilibrium with the D locus antigen, HLA-DR3 [59]. An association between CD and the DR3 antigen has been found in every population in which it has been sought (Table 7.6). In contrast, an association with another D locus antigen, HLA-DR7, has been found less consistently and has usually been weaker. The relative risks associated with being HLA-DR3 positive have revealed remarkable variability ranging from about four- to six-fold in Israel and southern Europe, to over 20-fold in northern European areas such as Helsinki and Oslo. Why these risks should be so variable is not entirely clear, although it partly reflects the wide variation in prevalence of DR3 alleles across the relevant populations. Nevertheless, the fact that only one-half of coeliacs in Naples, and less than 40% of coeliacs in Israel are HLA-DR3 positive compared with over 85% among northern Europeans suggests that the importance of genetic factors linked to this allele varies from place to place.

With the development of even more detailed methods of genetic analysis, associations with two other HLA loci have recently been described. An association with the DQw2 antigen, first reported from Italy in 1983, has now been confirmed in other countries [71,73]. The DQw2 antigen (previously labelled MB and DC) appears to be more strongly associated with CD than the DR3 antigen, with which the DQw2 antigen is in strong linkage disequilibrium. However, no association with DQw2 has been found in coeliacs who are negative for the DR3 or DR7 antigens [63]. Most recently, several groups have shown associations with a fourth HLA locus, the DP region and CD through the use of restriction fragment length polymorphisms and oligonucleotide probes [74,75]. The association with the DP locus may be independent of linkage to DR3 and DR7 antigens [75]. These studies are discussed in Chapter 8.

Distribution of HLA types and disease prevalence

From the above information it is evident that within populations, or countries, genetic factors are very strong determinants of CD. As the estimated relative risks for being either HLA-B8, or DR3 positive, are reasonably large it might be expected that the prevalence of CD would correlate with the prevalence of these markers of genetic predisposition in different populations.

Across Europe, the prevalence of the B8 antigen shows a greater than three-fold variation with the lowest prevalence occurring in Sardinia (2%) and the highest in the west of Ireland (45%) (Fig. 7.4)

Table 7.6 Frequency of HLA-DR3 and -DR7 in CD

Centre	*n*	-DR3			-DR7		
		Coeliacs (%)	Controls (%)	Relative risk	Coeliacs (%)	Controls (%)	Relative risk
Scandinavia							
Oslo [60]	57 (c)	95	25	54	—	—	—
Helsinki [61]	41 (c)	85	24	18.6	66	11	15.0
Netherlands							
Leiden [62]	23 (a)	96	22	80	21	23	0.9
Britain							
Liverpool [63]	111 (a + c)	87	26	23.3	43	29	1.9
London [64]	42 (c)	93	31	28.9	43	27	2.0
Galway [65]	58 (a + c)	88	41	10.5	27	34	—
France							
St Etienne [66]	—	79	18	17.5	45	17	4.0
Germany							
Munich [67]	91 (c)	64	20	7.0	44	28	2.0
Spain							
Madrid [68]	163 (c)	71	17	12	61	38	2.6
Italy							
Milan [66]	64 (c)	60	13	10.0	42	22	2.7
Turin [69]	100 (c)	68	16	11.2	59	28	3.7
Bologna [70]	51 (a)	69	25	6.6	65	23	6.1
Naples [71]	60 (c)	53	16	6.1	70	24	7.3
Israel							
Jerusalem [28]	43 (c)	39	14	3.9	44	24	2.5
Rehovot-Ashdad	84 (c)	38	14	3.6	46	24	2.7
Australia							
Adelaide [72]	69 (a + c)	83	26	13.1	49	23	3.3

a, adults; c, children.

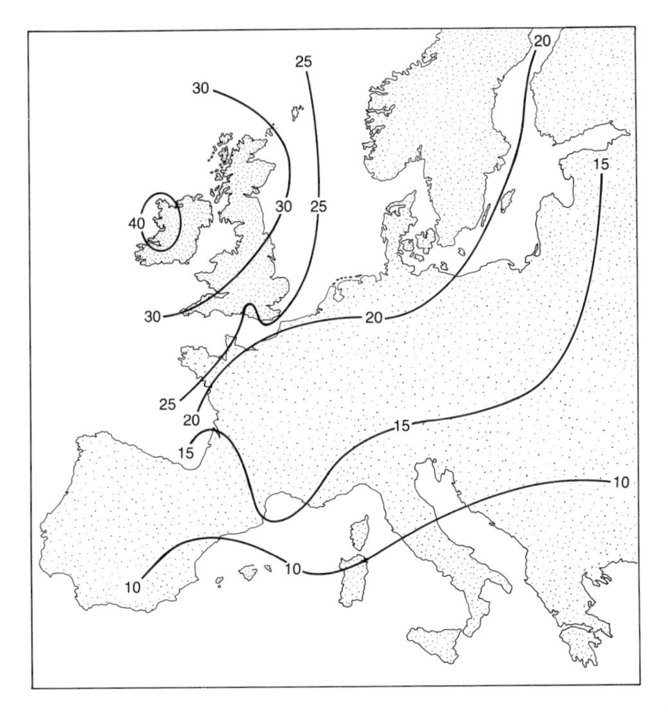

Fig. 7.4 Prevalence (%) of the HLA-B8 antigen across Europe (each line joins areas of equal prevalence). (From Stevens *et al.* [32].)

[76]. The distribution of the D locus antigens is less well characterized, but as shown in Table 7.6 there is a two-fold variation in prevalence of the DR3 antigen. If one assumes that the relative risk of CD in B8 positive individuals is 8, the prevalence of CD could be calculated to be 1.9 times higher in populations where 50% of individuals are B8 antigen positive, compared with those in which only 20% of individuals are B8 antigen positive. Note that such calculations assume that when different populations are compared, case ascertainment (of CD) is similar.

To a limited extent the prevalence of CD does reflect the southeast to northwest gradient in the prevalence of the B8 antigen across Europe. However, there are not many reports of CD prevalence from areas with a low B8 prevalence. It is notable that in Israel, where the prevalence of CD in children is similar to that in the west of Ireland, only 7% of the population carries the B8 antigen [28]. The low prevalence of CD in Otago, New Zealand, is also surprising, given the high proportion of British immigrants. Furthermore, in a recent study of CD in children from the south Tirol area of northern Italy, the prevalence of CD in children from the German population was 105 : 110 000 compared with 33 : 100 000 in children from the Italian population who also had the greater prevalence of the B8 and DR3 haplotype [77].

Thus, the considerable variations in prevalence of the predisposing HLA backgrounds do not relate strongly to the reported prevalence of CD. One reason is that even in the populations where CD is most common, few of the predisposed individuals develop the disease. In Sweden, for example, where one-quarter of the population is known to be positive for the DR3 antigen and the lifetime prevalence of CD may approach four per 1000, it can be quickly calculated that fewer than one in 60 DR3 positive individuals will develop the disease [3].

Environmental factors

Although dietary gluten is a necessary environmental factor in the aetiology of CD, several phenomena indicate that alone it is not sufficient. The discordance of some monozygotic twin pairs, the variable delay in response to gluten challenge and the recent decline in incidence in UK children all point to a role for other important environmental factors. Three factors have received consideration: (1) early weaning on to solid food; (2) breast feeding; and (3) gastrointestinal infection.

Early weaning

Early weaning on to solid foods has been thought to have a particularly adverse effect [78]. Until recently early weaning in many countries implied early introduction of gluten, but since the widespread introduction of gluten-free infant foods, this is no longer always true. Nevertheless, some studies showed that the age at which infants with CD present correlates closely with the age at which gluten-containing foods were first introduced [21,79,80]. To a certain extent such a relationship is predictable, but the period between weaning and presentation with CD has usually been more than 6 months.

In many European countries infant feeding during the post-War decades was characterized by a trend towards the earlier introduction of solid foods. In the UK, Anderson *et al.* found that as cereals were introduced earlier so the age of presentation of CD in Birmingham fell from a mean age of 44 months (1950–1952) to 9 months (1968–1969) [81]. By 1965 in Glasgow, one-quarter of 2-month-old, and 90% of 3-month- old infants had been started on a gluten-containing diet [82]. On the basis of these and other similar observations, the UK report on Present Day Practice in Infant Feeding (1974) recommended that the use of wheat cereal should be discouraged before the age of 4–6 months in the belief that this recommendation would delay presentation, rather than prevent disease [42].

Two large case-control studies carried out by Auricchio *et al.* and

Table 7.7 Relative risk* for CD in Naples by infant feeding practices [84]

		Breast fed†	Bottle fed	Relative risk (bottle vs breast fed)
Early gluten introduction (<2 months)	CD	1	36	14.1
	Controls	54	138	[3.0–67]
Late gluten introduction (>2 months)	CD	37	127	4.4
	Controls	993	764	[3.1–6.3]
Relative risk (early vs late gluten introduction)		0.49 [0.1–3.5]	1.56 [1.0–2.4]	
Adjusted relative risks		1.46 [0.9–2.2] [for differences in bottle vs breast feeding]		4.8 [3.4–6.8] [for differences in early vs late gluten introduction]

* According to Mantel-Haenszel (with 95% confidence limits).
† Breast fed exclusively for ⩾90 days.

Greco *et al.* in Italy examined infant feeding practices in relation to the risk of developing childhood CD [83,84]. In the first study, the feeding practices adopted for 216 coeliac children were compared with those used for their healthy siblings. Siblings eating gluten within the first 2 months of life had a greater risk of developing CD than those who were started on gluten from age 3 months, but the increased risk was not statistically significant. In the second study, the feeding histories of 201 coeliac children (all confirmed by a positive gluten challenge) were compared with those of 1949 healthy children who were accumulated during five community surveys of child health. In 18% of the coeliacs, gluten had been introduced before the end of the second month of life compared with 10% of control children, thus giving a relative risk for early gluten introduction of 2.1 (95% confidence limits; 1.3–3.0). However, as the authors noted, the apparent harmful effect of early gluten introduction could be explained by the additional effect of bottle feeding (Table 7.7).

Breast feeding

Breast feeding has long been thought to be protective [78]. Early studies suggested that the disease predominantly occurred in infants who had not been breast fed [85]. However, Black found that in Glasgow, 37% of 177 children presumed to be coeliacs on clinical and biochemical grounds had been breast fed for 2 months or longer, compared with an expected 33% obtained from an earlier survey of Glasgow children [86]. In a recent study from London, 46% of children with biopsy evidence of CD had been breast fed, although often for only 1 month or less [40].

While these studies demonstrate that breast feeding does not confer absolute protection, the two case-control studies carried out by Auricchio *et al.* and Greco *et al.* produced evidence that breast feeding confers some degree of protection from the disease in childhood [83,84]. In the first study, siblings breast fed for less than 30 days had a relative risk of disease 4.1 times (95% confidence limits; 2.2–7.3) greater than those breast fed for longer periods. The relative risk fell to 2.1 (95% confidence limits; 1.0–4.3) in the subgroup in which the coeliac child was not the first-born sibling. This observation suggests that feeding practices used for younger siblings were influenced by the occurrence of CD in an older sibling. This problem did not arise in their second study, as the feeding histories of the coeliacs were compared with those of unrelated healthy controls. Only 19% of the coeliacs had been breast fed exclusively for 90 days or more compared with 54% of the healthy controls, giving a relative risk of 5 (95% confidence limits; 3.5–6.9) for children breast fed for less than 90 days.

Whether an infant is breast or bottle fed and weaned early or late, are not independent of each other, i.e. they tend to confound one another. One explanation for the apparent adverse effect of early gluten feeding could be that such infants tend to be bottle fed rather than breast fed. When the data from the second case-control study are stratified into early, or late, gluten-weaned categories, the protective effect of breast feeding is unaffected and the adverse effect of early gluten introduction is no longer significant (Table 7.7). This suggests that prolonged breast feeding is considerably more important as a protective factor than delaying the introduction of gluten until the age of 2 months. Whether a longer delay in the introduction of dietary gluten would have a protective effect is still uncertain.

Gastrointestinal infection

Clinical experience suggests that CD is occasionally preceded by gastrointestinal infection, particularly in infants [86,87]. There are anecdotal reports of CD developing after a proven attack of giardiasis [88,89]. The possible role of adenoviral infection, proposed by Kagnoff, is discussed in Chapter 8. At present there are no epidemiological data to support a role for an adenovirus, or any other infection, in the development of CD.

Conclusions

Studies of the epidemiology of CD have been hindered by the lack of a measure of disease occurrence that can be readily applied to populations. Our current understanding is mainly based on studies that have been performed in areas where CD is already thought to be unusually common. This is a particularly difficult problem as in several countries, the reservoir of undiagnosed CD is probably very large.

Recent studies from Israel and Italy have challenged the traditional view that CD is predominantly found in areas where the prevalence of the HLA-B8 antigen is high, like Ireland and northwest Europe. In Israel and Italy, the incidence of CD in children now approaches that reported from Austria and Sweden.

In the UK the incidence in children has fallen by more than 50% since 1976 and this seems to be related to changes in infant feeding practices; the only other country where a similar decline has been demonstrated is Finland. In contrast, the incidence in neighbouring Sweden has not changed despite similar trends in infant feeding. These observations emphasize the aetiological role of environmental factors other than gluten.

One such factor appears to be breast feeding. Two Italian studies have demonstrated that breast feeding for at least 90 days protects against the development of CD even in children given gluten in early life. The importance of gluten-free infant foods, and of delayed introduction of gluten, is not yet clear.

In the future, the measurement of antibodies to α-gliadin looks to be sensitive and specific enough to be used as an effective screening test. If this promise is fulfilled then the next few years should see considerable progress in our understanding of the epidemiology of CD.

References

1 MacMahon B, Pugh TE. *Epidemiology — Principles and Methods*. Boston: Little, Brown & Co, 1970.

2 Logan RFA, Rifkind EA, Turner ID, Ferguson A. Mortality in celiac disease. *Gastroenterology* 1989;97:265–71.

3 Hed J, Lieden G, Ottosson E *et al*. IgA antigliadin antibodies and jejunal mucosal lesions in healthy blood donors (letter). *Lancet* 1986; ii:215.

4 Swinson CM, Levi AJ. Is coeliac disease underdiagnosed? *Br Med J* 1980;281:1258–60.

5 Logan RFA, Tucker G, Rifkind EA, Heading RC, Ferguson A. Changes in clinical features of coeliac disease in adults in Edinburgh and the Lothians 1960–79. *Br Med J* 1981;286: 95–7.

6 O'Reilly D, Murphy J, McLaughlin J, Bradshaw J, Dean G. The prevalence of coeliac disease and cystic fibrosis in Ireland, Scotland, and England and Wales. *Int J Epidemiol* 1974;3:247–51.

7 Logan RFA, Rifkind EA, Ferguson A. The changing clinical picture of coeliac disease in Lothian, Scotland. In: McConnell RB, ed. *The Genetics of Coeliac Disease*. Lancaster: MTP Press, 1981:29–40.

8 Langman MJS, McConnell TH, Spiegelhalter DJ, McConnell RB. Changing patterns of coeliac disease frequency: an analysis of coeliac society membership records. *Gut* 1985;26:175–8.

9 Carrington JM. Coeliac disease: an analysis of Coeliac Society membership records. *NZ Med J* 1986;99:279–81.
10 Barry RE, Henry C, Read AE. The patient's view of a gluten-free diet. In: McNicholl B, McCarthy CF, Fottrell PF, eds. *Perspectives in Coeliac Disease.* Lancaster: MTP Press, 1978:487–93.
11 McCrae WM. Inheritance of coeliac disease. *J Med Genet* 1969;6:129–31.
12 Logan RFA, Rifkind EA, Busuttil A, Gilmour HM, Ferguson A. Prevalence and 'incidence' of celiac disease in Edinburgh and the Lothian region of Scotland. *Gastroenterology* 1986; 90:334–42.
13 Arthur LJH, Langman MJS. Prevalence of coeliac disease in Derby. In: McConnell RB, ed. *The Genetics of Coeliac Disease.* Lancaster: MTP Press, 1981:15–17.
14 Mylotte M, Egan-Mitchell B, McCarthy CF, McNicholl B. Incidence of coeliac disease in the West of Ireland. *Br Med J* 1973;1:703–5.
15 Linberg T. Coeliac disease and infant feeding practices (letter). *Lancet* 1981;i:449.
16 Stenhammar L, Ansved P, Jansson G, Jansson U. The incidence of childhood celiac disease in Sweden. *J Pediatr Gastroenterol Nutr* 1987;6:707–9.
17 Simla S, Kokkonen J, Voulukka P, Kouvalainen K. Childhood coeliac disease (letter). *Lancet* 1981;i:494–5.
18 Mäki M, Kallonen K, Lahdeaho KL, Visakorpi JK. Changing pattern of childhood coeliac disease in Finland. *Acta Paediatr Scand* 1988;77:408–12.
19 Hovdenak N. Prevalence and clinical picture of adult gluten-induced enteropathy in a Norwegian population. *Scand J Gastroenterol* 1980;15:401–4.
20 Tobiasen K. Recent Scandinavian data on the epidemiology of coeliac disease. In: McConnell RB, ed. *The Genetics of Coeliac Disease.* Lancaster: MTP Press, 1981:47–50.
21 Rossipal E. On the incidence of coeliac disease in Austria: a study comprising a nine-year period. In: McConnell RB, ed. *The Genetics of Coeliac Disease.* Lancaster: MTP Press, 1981:23–7.
22 Van Stirum J, Baerlocher K, Fanconi A, Gugler E, Tonz O, Shmerling DH. The incidence of coeliac disease in children in Switzerland. *Helv Paediatr Acta* 1982;37: 421–30.
23 Greco L, Tozzi AE, Mayer M, Grimaldi M, Silano G, Auricchio A. Unchanging clinical picture of coeliac disease presentation in Campania, Italy. *Eur J Pediatr* 1989;148: 610–13.
24 Ramahko PM. *Coeliac disease in Portugal.* MD Thesis. University of Lisbon, 1988.
25 Shipman RT, Williams AL, Kay R, Townley RRW: A family study of coeliac disease. *Aust NZ J Med* 1975;5:250–5.
26 Carrington JM, Hewitt CJ, Dowsett LR, Barbezat GO. The prevalence of coeliac disease in Otago. *NZ Med J* 1987;100:460–2.
27 Khuffash FA, Barakat MH, Shaltout AA, Farwana SS, Adnani MS, Tungekar MF. Coeliac disease among children in Kuwait: difficulties in diagnosis and management. *Gut* 1987;28:1595–9.
28 Dahan S, Slater PE, Cooper M, Brautbar C, Ashknazi A. Coeliac disease in the Rehovot-Ashdod region of Israel: incidence and ethnic distribution. *J Epidemiol Community Health* 1984;38:58–60.
29 Suliman GI. Coeliac disease in Sudanese children. *Gut* 1978;19:121–5.
30 Rabassa EB, Sagaro E, Fragoso T, Castaneda C, Gra B. Coeliac disease in Cuban children. *Arch Dis Child* 1981;56:128–31.
31 Biemond I, Pena AS, Groenland F, Mulder CJJ, Tytgat GNJ. Coeliac disease in The Netherlands: demographic data of a patient survey among the members of the Dutch Coeliac Society. *Neth J Med* 1987;31:263–8.
32 Stevens FM, Egan-Mitchell B, McCarthy CF, McNicholl B. Factors in the epidemiology of coeliac disease in the West of Ireland. In: McConnell RB, ed. *The Genetics of Coeliac Disease.* Lancaster: MTP Press, 1981:7–14.
33 McConnell RB. Membership of the Coeliac Society of the United Kingdom. In: McConnell RB, ed. *The Genetics of Coeliac Disease.* Lancaster: MTP Press, 1981:65–9.
34 Hallert C, Gotthard R, Jansson G, Norrby K, Walan A. Similar prevalence of coeliac disease in children and middle-aged adults in a district of Sweden. *Gut* 1983;24:389–91.
35 Midhagen G, Jarnerot G, Kraaz W. Adult coeliac disease within a defined geographic area in Sweden: A study of prevalence and associated diseases. *Scand J Gastroenterol* 1988;23A:1000–4.
36 Hallert C, Gotthard R, Norrby K, Walan A. On the prevalence of adult coeliac disease in Sweden. *Scand J Gastroenterol* 1981;16: 257–61.
37 Gawkrodger DJ, Blackwell JN, Gilmour HM, Rifkind EA, Heading RC, Barnetson R StC. Dermatitis herpetiformis: diagnosis, diet and demography. *Gut* 1984;25:151–7.

38 Littlewood JM, Crollick AJ, Richards IDG. Childhood coeliac disease is disappearing (letter). *Lancet* 1980;ii:1350.
39 Dossetor JFB, Gibson AAM, McNeish AS. Childhood coeliac disease is disappearing (letter). *Lancet* 1981;i:322–3.
40 Kelly DA, Phillips AD, Elliott EJ, Dias JA, Walker-Smith JA. Rise and fall of coeliac disease 1960–85. *Arch Dis Child* 1989;64: 1157–60.
41 Stevens FM, Egan-Mitchell B, Cryan E, McCarthy CF, McNicholl B. Decreasing incidence of coeliac disease. *Arch Dis Child* 1987;62:465–8.
42 Working Party of the Panel on Child Nutrition. *Present-Day Practice in Infant Feeding*. Report on Health and Social Subjects No 9. London: HMSO, 1974.
43 Martin J. *Infant Feeding 1975: Attitudes and Practice in England and Wales*. London: HMSO, 1978.
44 Martin J, Monk J. *Infant Feeding 1980*. London: Office of Population Censuses and Surveys, 1982.
45 Martin J, White A. *Infant Feeding 1985*. London: Office of Population Censuses and Surveys, 1988.
46 Sauer LW. Coeliac disease (chronic intestinal indigestion) etiology, prognosis and standardisation of treatment. *Am J Dis Child* 1927; 34:934–46.
47 MacDonald WC, Dobbins WO III, Rubin CE. Studies of the familial nature of celiac sprue using biopsy of the small intestine. *N Engl J Med* 1965;272:448–56.
48 Robinson DC, Watson AJ, Wyatt EH, Marks JM, Roberts DF. Incidence of small-intestinal mucosal abnormalities and of clinical coeliac disease in the relatives of children with coeliac disease. *Gut* 1971;12:789–93.
49 Mylotte M, Egan-Mitchell B, Fottrell PF, McNicholl B, McCarthy CF. Family studies in coeliac disease. *Q J Med* 1974;43:359–69.
50 Rolles CJ, Kyaw Mint TO, Sin WK, Anderson CM. A family study of coeliac disease. *Gut* 1974;15:A827.
51 Stokes PL, Ferguson R, Holmes GKT, Cooke WT. Familial aspects of coeliac disease. *Q J Med* 1976;45:567–82.
52 Ellis A, Evans DAP, McConnell RB, Woodrow JC. Liverpool coeliac family study. In: McConnell RB, ed. *Genetics of Coeliac Disease*. Lancaster: MTP Press, 1981: 265–86.
53 Polanco I, Biemond I, van Leeuwen A *et al.* Gluten sensitive enteropathy in Spain: genetic and environmental factors. In: McConnell RB, ed. *Genetics of Coeliac Disease*. Lancaster: MTP Press, 1981: 211–31.
54 Kamath KR, Dorney SFA. Is discordance for coeliac disease in monozygotic twins permanent? (abstract) *Pediatr Res* 1983;17:423.
55 Salazar de Sousa J, Ramos de Almeida JM, Monteiro MV, Magalhaes Ramalho P. Late onset coeliac disease in the monozygotic twin of a coeliac child. *Acta Paediatr Scand* 1987; 76:172–4.
56 Falchuk SM, Rogentine GN, Stober W. Predominance of histocompatibility antigen HL-A8 in patient with gluten-sensitive enteropathy. *J Clin Invest* 1972;51:1602–5.
57 Stokes PL, Asquith P, Holmes GKT, Mackintosh P, Cooke WT. Histocompatibility antigens associated with adult coeliac disease. *Lancet* 1972;ii:162–4.
58 Mackintosh P, Asquith P. HLA and coeliac disease. *Br Med Bull* 1978;34:291–4.
59 Keuning JJ, Pena AS, Van Leeuwen A, Van Hoof JP, van Rood JJ. HLA-Dw3 associated with coeliac disease. *Lancet* 1976;i:506–8.
60 Ek J, Albrechtsen D, Solheim BG, Thorsby E. Strong association between the HLA-Dw3 related B alloantigen DRw3 and coeliac disease. *Scand J Gastroenterol* 1978;13: 229–43.
61 Verkasalo M, Tilikainen A, Kuitunen P, Savilahti E, Backman A. HLA antigens and atopy in children with coeliac disease. *Gut* 1983;24:306–10.
62 Pena AS, Biemond I, Rosekrans PCM, van Leeuwen A, Schreuder I, van Rood JJ. DR locus controlled B-cell alloantigens in coeliac disease in the Netherlands. In: McConnell RB, ed. *Genetics of Coeliac Disease*. Lancaster: MTP Press, 1981:161–71.
63 Ellis A, Taylor CJ, Dillon-Rommy M, Woodrow JC, McConnell RB. HLA-DR typing in coeliac disease: evidence for genetic heterogeneity. *Br Med J* 1984;2:1571–3.
64 Sachs JA, Awad J, McCloskey D *et al.* Different HLA associated gene combinations contribute to susceptibility for coeliac disease and dermatitis herpetiformis. *Gut* 1986;27: 515–20.
65 McKenna R, Stevens FM, Bourke M, McNicholl B, Albert ED, McCarthy CF. B-cell alloantigens associated with coeliac disease. In: McConnell RB, ed. *Genetics of Coeliac Disease*. Lancaster: MTP Press, 1981:153–8.
66 Betuel H, Gebuhrer L, Descos L, Percebois

H, Minaire Y, Bertrand J. Adult coeliac disease associated with HLA-DRw3 and DRw7. *Tissue Antigens* 1980;15:231–8.
67 Scholz S, Rossipal E, Brautbar C *et al.* HLA-DR antigens in coeliac disease. A population and multiple case family study. In: McConnell RB, ed. *Genetics of Coeliac Disease.* Lancaster: MTP Press, 1981:143–9.
68 Mearin ML, Biemond I, Pena AS *et al.* HLA-DR phenotypes in Spanish coeliac children: their contribution to the understanding of the genetics of the disease. *Gut* 1983;24: 532–7.
69 De Marchi M, Carbonara A, Ansaldi N *et al.* HLA-DR3 in coeliac disease: immunogenetic and clinical aspects. *Gut* 1983;24:706–13.
70 Corazza GR, Tabacchi P, Frisoni M, Prati C, Gasbarrini G. DR and non-DR Ia allotypes are associated with susceptibility to coeliac disease. *Gut* 1965;26:1210–13.
71 Tosi R, Vismara D, Tanigaki N *et al.* Evidence that coeliac disease is primarily associated with a DC locus allelic specificity. *Clin Immunol Immunopathol* 1983;28:395–404.
72 Hetzel PAS, Bennett GD, Sheldon AB *et al.* Genetic markers in Australian Caucasian subjects with coeliac disease. *Tissue Antigens* 1987;30:18–22.
73 Hitman GA, Niven MJ, Festenstein H *et al.* HLA class II alpha chain gene polymorphisms in patients with insulin-dependent diabetes mellitus, dermatitis herpetiformis and coeliac disease. *J Clin Invest* 1987;79:609–15.
74 Niven MJ, Caffrey C, Sachs JA *et al.* Susceptibility to coeliac disease involves genes in HLA-DP region (letter). *Lancet* 1987;ii:805.
75 Bugawan TL, Angelini G, Larrick J, Auricchio S, Ferrara GB, Erich HA. A combination of a particular HLA-DP beta allele and an HLA-DQ heterodimer confers susceptibility to coeliac disease. *Nature* 1989;339:470–3.
76 Ryder LP, Andersen E, Svejgaard A. An HLA map of Europe. *Hum Hered* 1978;28: 171–200.
77 Pittschieler K, Reissigl H, Mengarda G. Celiac disease in two different population groups of South Tirol. *J Pediatr Gastroenterol Nutr* 1988;7:400–2.
78 Cooke WT, Holmes GKT. Clinical presentation. In: *Coeliac Disease.* Edinburgh: Churchill Livingstone, 1984:82–105.
79 McNeish AS, Anderson CM. Coeliac disease. The disorder in childhood. *Clin Gastroenterol* 1974;3:127–44.
80 Anderson CM, Burkey V. *Paediatric Gastroenterology.* Oxford: Blackwell Scientific Publications, 1975.
81 Anderson CM, Gracey M, Burke V. Coeliac disease. Some still controversial aspects. *Arch Dis Child* 1972;47:292–8.
82 Arneil GC. *Dietary Study of 4365 Scottish Infants.* Scottish Health Service Studies No 6. Edinburgh: Scottish Home Health Department, 1965.
83 Auricchio S, Follo D, de Ritis G *et al.* Does breast feeding protect against the development of clinical symptoms of celiac disease in children? *J Pediatr Gastroenterol Nutr* 1983;2:428–33.
84 Greco L, Auricchio S, Mayer M, Grimaldi M. Case control study on nutritional risk factors in celiac disease. *J Pediatr Gastroenterol Nutr* 1988;7:395–9.
85 Hardwick C. Prognosis in coeliac disease: a review of seventy-three cases. *Arch Dis Child* 1939;14:279–94.
86 Black JA. Possible factors in the incidence of coeliac disease. *Acta Paediatr* 1964;53: 109–16.
87 Walker-Smith JA. Coeliac disease. In: *Diseases of the Small Intestine in Childhood,* 3rd edn. London: Butterworth, 1988:88–114.
88 Carswell F, Gibson AAM, McAlister TA. Giardiasis and coeliac disease. *Arch Dis Child* 1983;48:414–18.
89 Mendelson RM, Wright SG, Tomkins AM. Coeliac disease presenting as malabsorption from the tropics. *Gut* 1978;19:A992.

Chapter 8/Genetic basis of coeliac disease: role of HLA genes

MARTIN F. KAGNOFF

Major histocompatibility complex and the HLA genes

Coeliac disease (CD) is strongly associated with human leucocyte antigen (HLA) molecules coded for by genes in the major histocompatibility complex (MHC) [1–8]. HLA molecules have been known to exist for several decades and were initially recognized as the major target antigens in transplantation rejection. Experiments in the middle of the twentieth century demonstrated that rejection of skin grafted between different strains of mice was due to an immune reaction to foreign antigens on the surface of the cells present in the grafted skin. Subsequently, it was recognized that such reactions were directed against histocompatibility molecules and that the major molecules involved were coded for by genes located in the MHC which is on chromosome 17 in mice and on the short arm of chromosome 6 in humans. The target molecules of these responses were termed HLA antigens in humans, reflecting their initial demonstration on leucocytes, and H2 antigens in mice.

The role of MHC molecules in normal immune function, and particularly their importance in disease, has been recognized only more recently. Nonetheless, CD was reported to be associated with certain HLA antigens almost two decades ago [9,10].

Genes of the MHC on chromosome 6 are grouped into three major classes [11] (Fig. 8.1). Class 1 genes code for the major transplantation antigens, HLA-A, HLA-B and HLA-C. These class 1 antigens are glycoproteins with a molecular weight of 44 kDa and, together with a second protein (β_2-microglobulin — an invariant protein of molecular weight 12 000), are present on all cells of the body. In addition, and not shown in Fig. 8.1, genes at loci designated HLA-E, HLA-F and HLA-G have been identified in the class 1 region; the HLA-E and HLA-G genes being expressed by extraembryonic tissues (e.g. HLA-G is expressed within placenta and extravillous membranes at various times during pregnancy) [12–16]. In contrast, the class 2 genes present in the HLA-D region, code for HLA glycoproteins found primarily on the surface of cells of the immune system. Both the HLA class 1 and class 2 glycoproteins play a major role in binding peptides and in presenting antigenic peptides to T cells. Class 3 genes code for components of

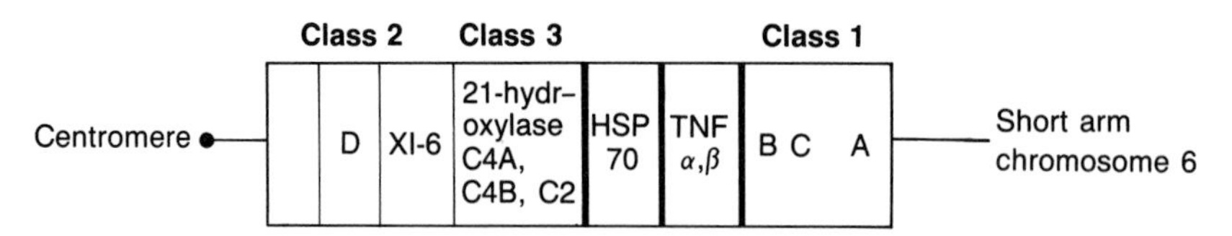

Fig. 8.1 The human MHC on the short arm of chromosome 6 is divided into several regions termed the class 1, class 2 and class 3 regions. The class 2 (also known as the D) region contains genes that code for the HLA class 2 molecules. Other genes which code for molecules involved in intracellular peptide processing and transport are also found in that region. The class 3 region contains genes for components of the complement system (C4A, C4B, C2) and the gene for steroid 21-hydroxylase. Additional genes whose function is less well known are located between the HLA-D region and the gene for steroid 21-hydroxylase. The class 1 region contains genes that code for the classic HLA-A, -B and -C transplantation antigens, as well as other non-classical HLA class 1 genes (HLA-E, -F and -G) (not shown). Genes for the major HSP 70 and tumour necrosis factor (TNF) α and β are found in the region between the class 1 HLA-B locus and the class 3 C2 locus. In addition, many other genes including those termed BAT genes (HLA-B-associated transcripts) are found in that region (not shown).

the complement system and the enzyme steroid 21-hydroxylase. In addition, the MHC contains a number of additional genes as indicated in Fig. 8.1. These include the genes for TNFα and β and the major heat shock protein (HSP) 70. Recent studies have indicated that there are at least 19 or more genes, located between C2 and HLA-B (i.e. in the region that also contains the TNF and HSP 70 genes) [17,18]. The major focus of this chapter will be on the HLA class 2 genes and the association of specific HLA class 2 genes with CD. The class 1 and other MHC genes are mentioned only briefly.

The MHC is a large gene complex that, as indicated above, contains many genes, and additional genes in this region of DNA are still being discovered [17,19–21]. Individual genes within the MHC are located at varying sites, or loci, throughout the complex. The genes encoded at many of the loci in the MHC are extremely polymorphic. This means that within a species, there are many different alleles (i.e. alternative forms of the same gene) at each gene locus. As a result, proteins coded by a polymorphic locus are also highly polymorphic in the species (i.e. between individuals, there are amino acid differences in the proteins that are coded for by a single genetic locus). Such polymorphism is striking in the case of the genes which code the HLA class 1 A, B and C molecules and the HLA class 2 molecules. The combination of extensive polymorphism at individual HLA class 1 and 2 loci, and the presence of multiple polymorphic loci that encode the spectrum of HLA molecules, allows the host immune system to interact with a broad array of peptides.

A further feature of MHC genes which is important for understanding their association with CD is that many of the gene loci along the

MHC exhibit a high degree of linkage disequilibrium. That is, there is less genetic recombination between alleles at different loci than one would expect by chance alone, given the physical distances between the genes. This results in certain groups of MHC alleles being inherited as a group, commonly referred to as an HLA haplotype. In this context, an HLA haplotype contains several alleles that are present at linked loci and are inherited on a single chromosome (genes on a single chromosome are also said to be present in *cis*). This concept will become important in later discussions as we refer to individuals having a particular HLA-DR or HLA-DR/DQ haplotype in CD. Moreover, as also discussed later, a relatively limited number of HLA haplotypes generally make up a large proportion of the population within a geographical region.

HLA class 2 glycoproteins are heterodimers and comprise two polypeptides, the α- and β-chains (Fig. 8.2). The former is encoded by an A gene and the latter by a B gene. The α-chain has molecular weight of 33–35 kDa and the β-chain has a molecular weight of 28–30 kDa. The extracellular amino terminal α_1- and β_1-domains of these molecules are quite polymorphic and involved in binding antigenic peptides;

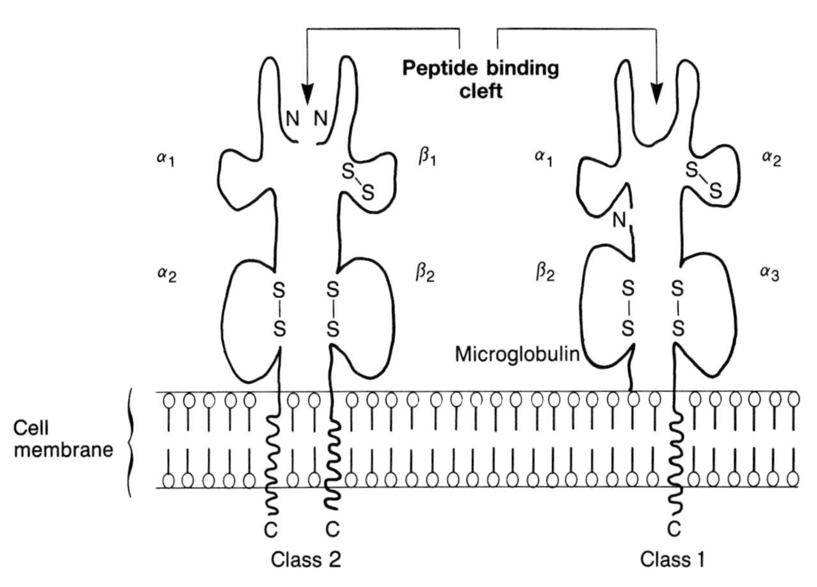

Fig. 8.2 Schematic view of an HLA class 2 and class 1 molecule. HLA class 2 glycoproteins (left side) are present on the cell surface as heterodimers containing two polypeptides, an α-chain and a β-chain. The extracellular part of the α- and β-chains contains a distal polymorphic α_1- and β_1-domain and a more membrane proximal α_2- and β_2-domain. The distal α_1- and β_1-domain form a peptide-binding cleft. The class 1 HLA glycoproteins (right side) contain a single α-polypeptide chain with three extracellular domains (α_1-, α_2-, α_3-). The α-chain is present on the cell surface in association with β_2-microglobulin. Peptides bind in the groove formed by the α_1- and α_2-domains.

more proximal parts of the molecule bind CD4. The corresponding polymorphic peptide binding region on class 1 molecules is formed by the α_1- and α_2-domains.

The HLA class 2 genes are encoded in the HLA-D region at the centromeric end of the MHC (Fig. 8.3). The HLA-D region is divided into three major subregions, termed HLA-DP, HLA-DQ and HLA-DR [22]. Each -DR, -DQ or -DP class 2 molecule on the cell surface is a heterodimer of an α-chain encoded by an A gene, and a β-chain which is encoded by a B gene. In addition, the HLA-D region contains multiple other genes. In some cases, these are pseudogenes which are not structurally capable of being expressed. Thus, the DP region contains pseudogenes at loci termed DPB2 and DPA2. In addition, the DR region contains a pseudogene termed DRB2. The DQ subregion also contains genes at two loci, DQB2 and DQA2, that are not expressed, although these genes appear to be structurally normal (DQB2 and DQA2 previously were termed DXB and DXA). Other genes which may be transcribed, but whose product(s) have not been detected on the cell surface, are located between the DQ and DP subregions. These genes include DN A (also known as DZ A; there is no known DN B counterpart) and DO B (there is no known DO A counterpart). Because protein products of these genes are not expressed on the cell surface, they do not appear to have a role in presenting antigenic peptides to T cells. More recent studies have also described additional genes in the region between DO B and DN A and in the interval between the DR A gene and the gene for steroid 21-hydroxylase in the class 3 region [17–21]. At least some of the genes mapping between DO B and DN A have been suggested to code for products that play a role in the intracellular processing of peptides and the transport of peptides across membranes within the cell [20].

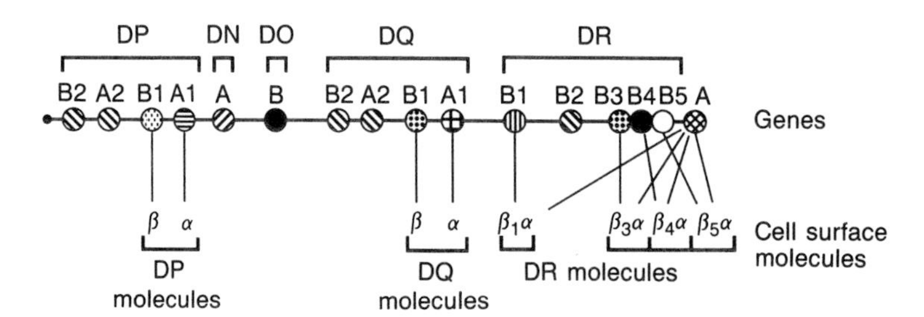

Fig. 8.3 HLA class 2 D region genes. The HLA class 2 D region is subdivided into several subregions. Genes within the HLA-DP, -DQ and -DR subregions code for the -DP, -DQ and -DR glycoproteins that are expressed on the cell surface. Each -DP, -DQ and -DR molecule contains an α-chain encoded by an A gene and a β-chain encoded by a B gene. Genes at the DPB2, A2 and DRB2 loci are pseudogenes. -DQ genes at the B2 and A2 loci are normal structural genes, but are not expressed, perhaps reflecting alterations in their regulatory regions. Of the several expressed -DR loci, the DRB1 locus is the most polymorphic.

Table 8.1 Allelic polymorphism in the HLA class 2 region

Subregion	Locus	No. of alleles
DR	B1	47
	B3	4
	B4	1
	B5	4
DQ	A1	13
	B1	17
DP	A1	4
	B1	21

As shown in Fig. 8.3, the HLA-DR subregion is multigenic. Thus, in addition to the HLA-DRB1 locus, three other HLA-DRB1 loci, known as DRB3, DRB4 and DRB5, code for expressed -DR β-chains [23]. However, genes at each of these other DR loci are not present on all haplotypes. As there is only one DRA allele, as shown, an identical DR α-chain associates with the β-chain encoded by the DRB1, DRB3, DRB4 and DRB5 loci.

Polymorphism is a fundamental characteristic of both the HLA class 1 and class 2 genes and their protein products. For example, there are at least 26 or more different alleles coded for by the class 1 HLA-A locus and 35 or more alleles at the HLA-B locus [23]. As shown in Table 8.1, within the class 2 region, there are 47 or more different alleles at the DRB1 locus. In contrast, the DRB3, DRB4 and DRB5 loci are far less polymorphic. However, the HLA-DQA1, -DQB1 and -DPB1 loci are quite polymorphic. Thus, there are at least 13 different alleles at the DQA1 locus, 17 different alleles at the DQB1 locus and 21 or more different alleles at the DPB1 locus [23–27]. Of note, the DPA1 locus is relatively non-polymorphic and the DRA locus is non-polymorphic with only one allele recognized at that site.

A class 2 bearing cell can express multiple HLA class 2 proteins (Fig. 8.4). Thus, on any class 2 expressing cell, one potentially may find products from the DR, DP and DQ subregions. On most cells studied thus far, DR molecules are expressed at a higher level than DP and DQ molecules [28]. Moreover, not all cells express all of these products [29,30]. However, cells usually express more than one DR molecule (e.g. product of the DRB1 gene together with the DRA1 gene; and product of either the DRB3 or DRB4 or DRB5 gene together with the DRA1 gene). The same cell may also express a DP molecule (e.g. product of the DPA1 gene together with the product of the DPB1 gene) and perhaps a DQ molecule (e.g. product of the DQA1 gene together with the product of the DQB1 gene). In addition, since each individual has two sixth chromosomes, it is possible to form mixed HLA class 2 molecules. For example, the DPB1 gene product from one chromosome

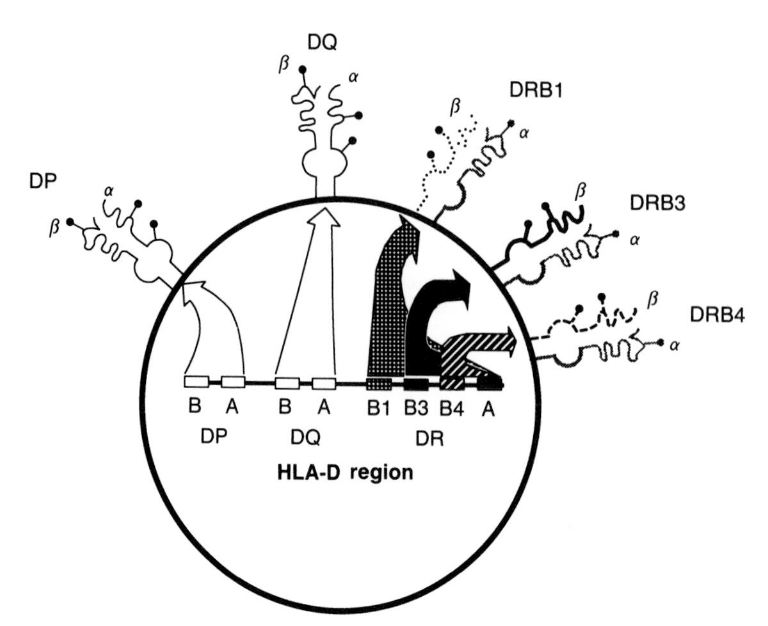

Fig. 8.4 Schematic representation of an antigen presenting cell with HLA-DP, -DR and -DQ genes and the respective cell surface HLA-DP, -DQ and -DR molecules. Each cell surface -DP, -DQ or -DR molecule consists of an α-chain encoded by its respective A gene and a β-chain encoded by its respective B gene. Each cell may express more than one class 2 molecule (i.e. a DP, a DQ and one or more DR molecules). As there is only one non-polymorphic DRA gene, the DR β-chains coded for the B1, B3, B4 or B5 (not shown) loci each combine with the same α-chain.

might combine with the DPA1 product from the second chromosome (i.e. an HLA-DP molecule formed in *trans*). Therefore, in any individual, it is conceivable that a cell may have four different DP molecules (i.e. two encoded on *cis*, two encoded in *trans*) and four different DQ molecules on its surface.

The expression of multiple different HLA class 2 molecules on the cell surface provides the host with the ability to interact with and develop immune responses to an extremely broad array of different antigenic peptides. In addition, extensive polymorphism among alleles at the multiple class 2 loci leads to the hypothetical possibility of an enormous number of different HLA haplotypes within any population. However, this is not the case in that a relatively limited number of different haplotypes is present in most members of a given population. For example, among northern European Caucasians, perhaps 100 major HLA haplotypes comprise the major part of the population.

New understanding of how HLA molecules likely bind peptides for presentation to T cells came with the crystallization and three-dimensional structure analysis of an HLA class 1 molecule [31,32]. Class 2 MHC molecules are thought to have a three-dimensional

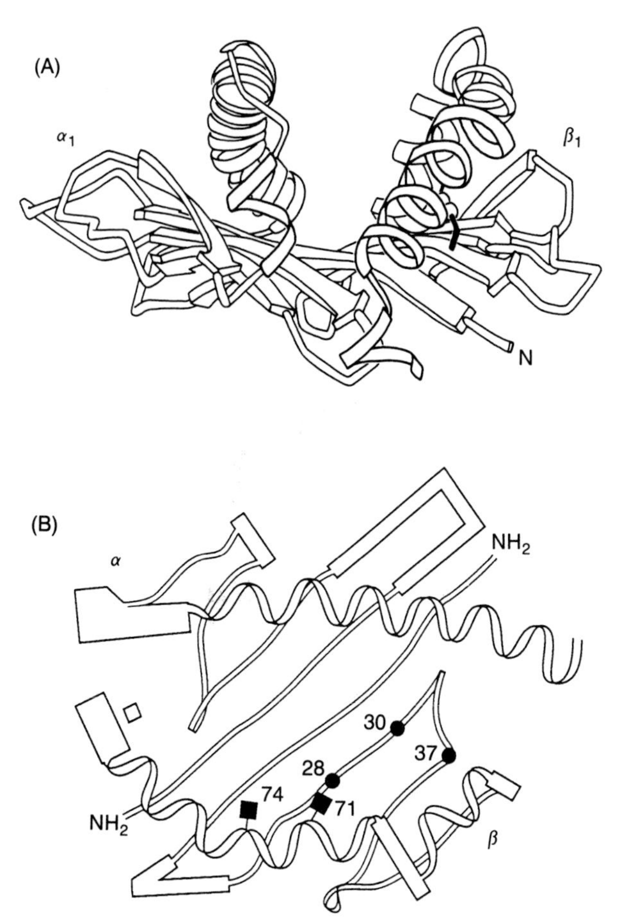

Fig. 8.5 Schematic view of the structure of the binding cleft for peptide on an HLA class 2 molecule. (A) in this side view, the peptide-binding cleft is bounded by two α-helices, one formed by the α_1- and the other by the β_1-domain. The floor of the groove is formed by β-pleated sheets. (B) top view of the peptide-binding cleft with the polymorphic residues that are unique to the DQw2 β-chain shown as solid squares on the α-helix and as solid circles on the β-pleated sheets. These residues are potentially important peptide contact sites. (Adapted with permission from [31] and [33]).

structure analogous to that of class 1 molecules [33]. As shown in Fig. 8.5, HLA proteins contain a peptide-binding groove or cleft located at the amino terminal portion of the molecule. The cleft is formed by two α-helical structures, one α-helix being derived from the α-chain of the class 2 molecule and the second α-helix from the β-chain of the class 2 molecule. The base or floor of the cleft is formed by eight β-strands also derived partially from the α- and partially from the β-chain. The size of the cleft is sufficient to accommodate a peptide of 12–17 amino acids depending on the extent to which the peptide is coiled or bent. Moreover, most of the polymorphic amino acid residues in the class 2 molecules (i.e. those amino acids that vary between the alleles) occur in this part of the molecule and are located inside the groove, either on the sides of the α-helix on the floor (i.e. β-sheets) [33]. These are the locations postulated to interact with and bind peptides. Amino acid polymorphisms also occur on the edges of the α-helices where they are accessible for recognition by the T cell receptor (TCR) [34]. This becomes important later when considering the association of specific HLA class 2 molecules with CD. The extensive polymorphism of the class 2 molecules allows them to bind and present many different foreign peptides. Thus, a relatively limited number of HLA class 2 molecules in an individual can bind an almost unlimited array of peptides.

The proteins coded for by class 1 and class 2 genes have both structural and functional differences. One functional difference between class 1 and class 2 HLA molecules is reflected in their different tissue distribution. Thus, class 1 HLA molecules are present on virtually all nucleated cells, whereas class 2 molecules are largely restricted to cells involved in immune responses, such as macrophages, dendritic cells, B cells and activated T cells. However, class 2 HLA molecules can also be found on several other cell types including intestinal epithelial cells [35–37] and, under certain conditions, the expression of HLA class 2 molecules can be stimulated in cells that normally do not express them.

This is the case in CD in that intestinal crypt cells express HLA class 2 molecules during the course of active disease whereas normal small intestinal crypt epithelial cells do not express HLA class 2 molecules. In the normal small bowel, class 2 expression, especially DR and DP expression, is confined to epithelial cells of the villous tips [38–40]. The cytokines γ-interferon (γ-IFN) and tumour necrosis factor α (TNFα) are important cytokines as regards the induction of class 2 molecules, including their induction on cells that normally do not express class 2 molecules.

Class 1 molecules interact with T cells that have the CD8 molecule on the cell surface. These CD8 T cells functionally mediate cytotoxic and suppressor functions. The presumed reason for the expression of class 1 molecules on all cell types is because class 1 molecules are recognized by CD8 cytotoxic T cells and, in theory, cytotoxic T cells should be able to focus on any cell in the body, especially those infected by viruses or those expressing tumour antigens. Class 2 molecules interact with T cells that have the CD4 molecule on the cell surface. These CD4 T cells function mainly as helper or inducer cells in the immune response. CD4 T cells thus interact with a restricted group of cell types which bear class 2 molecules (i.e. B cells, macrophages, dendritic cells and other cell types including intestinal epithelial cells [41] that constitutively express or can be induced to express class 2 molecules) and, therefore, are potentially capable of presenting antigen to the T cell (Fig. 8.6). Interactions between class 2 expressing antigen presenting cells and CD4 T cells ultimately results in the release of cytokines such as interleukin-2, γ-IFN, IL-4 and IL-5, among others, from the T cell. These cytokines then play a major role in stimulating immune responses among other B and T cells. In addition, these cytokines may interact with and alter the function of a variety of other cells present in the environment in which they are released.

In general, class 1 molecules bind peptides produced within the host cell (i.e. 'endogenous peptides') including viral peptides produced in infected cells [42,43]. In contrast, class 2 molecules bind peptides that result from the degradation of proteins taken up into the cell from the external environment (i.e. 'exogenous peptides'). Those proteins are cleaved to peptides within endosomal and lysosomal compartments of the cell [44,45]. The resulting peptides bind to the class 2 molecules and are reexpressed on the cell surface together with class 2 molecules for presentation to T cells (i.e. class 2 pathway).

As described above, the location of a peptide within the cell and its pathway of intracellular processing largely determine whether or not a given peptide will be presented together with a class 1 or a class 2

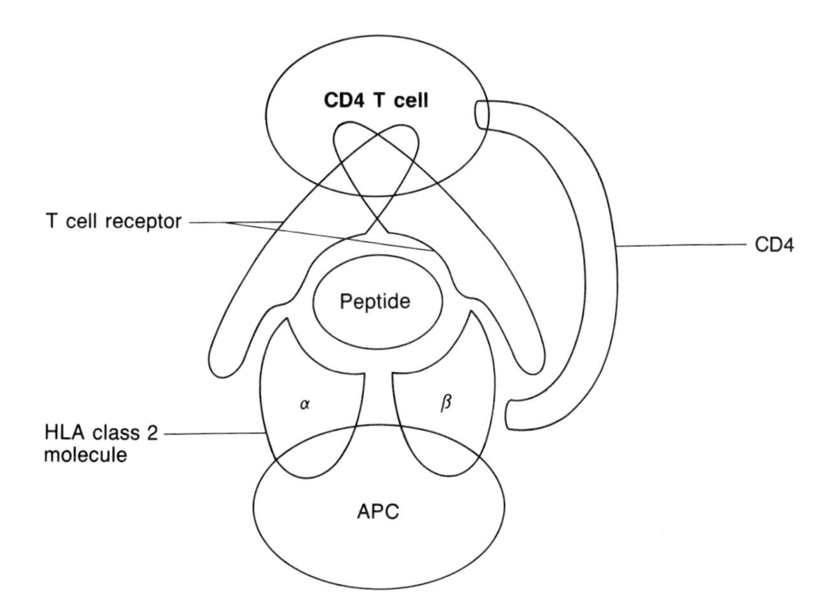

Fig. 8.6 Schematic representation of a CD4 T cell interacting with an HLA class 2 molecule containing a peptide bound in the peptide-binding cleft. The CD4 molecule interacts with the non-polymorphic part of the HLA class 2 molecule. The T cell receptor recognizes determinants on both the HLA class 2 molecule and the peptide. APC, antigen-presenting cell.

molecule [42,43,45]. In general, proteins encoded by viruses in infected cells and tumour antigens behave as 'endogenous' proteins, are processed by the class 1 pathway and are presented in conjunction with class 1 molecules to CD8 T cells. However, there does not seem to be a unique property of the peptides themselves that determines binding to class 1 rather than to class 2 molecules [46]. Rather, whether a given peptide binds to class 1 or class 2 molecules appears to reflect the compartment of the cell in which it is processed. Since class 1 molecules present antigen to T cells which express the CD8 protein, CD8 T cells are said to be HLA class 1 restricted. Similarly, since class 2 molecules present antigen to T cells that have the CD4 molecule, CD4 cells are said to be HLA class 2 restricted.

The above section describes the structure of genes and protein products coded for by the HLA class 2 D region. It is now also recognized that expression of the genes in the HLA-DR, -DQ and -DP subregions may be differentially regulated [47]. Thus, among different cell types and depending on mechanisms controlling regulation, the DR, DP and DQ glycoproteins are variably expressed on any given cell to a greater or lesser extent. Moreover, physiological mediators such as cytokines can play a role in such regulation.

HLA serological markers associated with CD

It has been known for almost two decades that CD is strongly associated with the HLA class 1 B locus marker, HLA-B8. Initial series reported the presence of the HLA-B8, as detected by serology, in approximately 88% of individuals with CD in the USA or the UK compared with 20–30% controls [9,10]. This represented a highly significant difference. In subsequent series [48–54], the frequency of the HLA-B8 marker in coeliac populations has varied markedly. Nonetheless, in series including varying numbers of patients from different geographical locations, such frequencies of HLA-B8 in the CD population have often exceeded 75%.

Later studies, also using serological analysis, revealed that CD had an even stronger association with the HLA class 2 D region serological marker, HLA-DR3 (now known as HLA-DRw17 according to current terminology and hereafter in this chapter referred to as HLA-DRw17). The previously reported association of HLA-B8 with CD was recognized simply to reflect linkage disequilibrium between the allele that codes for HLA-B8 and the allele that codes for HLA-DRw17. The association between CD and HLA-DRw17 has now been confirmed in multiple studies from different geographical areas [55–60]. Nonetheless, the frequency of HLA-DRw17 in CD populations in different geographical areas has varied markedly [56,59–61]. In several studies, the frequency of HLA-DRw17 among the CD population has exceeded 90%. This is particularly the case in populations of CD patients of northern European Caucasian ancestry.

After the recognition of the association of HLA-DRw17 with CD, later studies indicated that the DQw2 serological marker (formerly termed -DC3 or -MB2), was at least and perhaps more strongly associated with CD than was HLA-DRw17 [62–64]. DQw2 is a cell surface HLA class 2 molecule encoded by genes in the DQ subregion. However, in Caucasians, the genes that code for HLA-DQw2 are very strongly linked to DRw17. In fact, virtually all Caucasians having DRw17 also have HLA-DQw2. In some populations, DQw2 is found in 100% of individuals with CD whereas in control populations this marker is present in 25–30% of such individuals, depending on the geographical origin of the population studied.

In populations of southern European origin (Spain and Italy), but also in a study from northern Europe, CD has been associated with increased heterozygosity for certain HLA-DR markers [59–61,64,65]. Thus, there is an increased frequency of patients with HLA-DRw17/7 [60,65,66] and, in some [59,61,64] but not all [60] studies an increased frequency of HLA-DR5/7 heterozygosity among the CD population. How to interpret these observations puzzled investigators for several years. Moreover, the finding that not all individuals with CD had HLA-DRw17 coupled with the finding that there was an increased frequency of non-DRw17 related HLA-DR5/7 heterozygotes in CD, led many to be highly sceptical about the importance of associations between specific HLA alleles and CD as regards disease pathogenesis. The reasoning behind that scepticism was as follows: if not all CD patients had a single HLA marker, the several markers associated with CD must simply represent the presence of an associated gene that is the true 'coeliac' gene. However, it is now recognized from further studies that both individuals with HLA-DR7 and individuals with HLA-DRw17 have DQw2, as determined by serology. This is because the DQB1*0201 allele that codes for the DQw2 β-chain and determines the DQw2 serological typing specificity is tightly linked to both the DRB1*0301 and the DRB1*0701 alleles that determine DRw17 and DR7 serology, respectively [1,26]. Nonetheless, as discussed later (see p. 230), most HLA-DR7 individuals who serologically type as DQw2 do not have the same cell surface DQ α/β glycoprotein as HLA-DRw17 individuals who also type as DQw2 [1]. This is because serological detection of DQw2 depends on the recognition by antibodies of determinants on the β-chain and not on the α-chain of the DQw2 molecule. Thus, although DRw17 and DR7 individuals both type as having DQw2 since they have the same β-chain, they have different α-chains and therefore different cell surface DQ molecules. However, since the DQA1 gene linked to DRw17 and to DR5 are the same, DR5/7 heterozygotes can express the same DQw2 α/β combination as DRw17 individuals by contributing an α-chain from the DQA gene on the chromosome with DR5 and a β-chain from the gene on the chromosome with DR7 [66,67].

It now appears that most, if not all, CD patients have a cell surface molecule detected as DQw2 by serology and that both the DQ A and B genes coding for that HLA-DQw2 molecule are important for CD susceptibility [66–68]. In fact, these genes appear to be necessary, although not sufficient, for disease expression. It should be noted, however, that there is a very small number of patients (5% or less) diagnosed in some series of CD, who lack the DQw2 molecule. They have all expressed DR4 [60,69,70]. In northern European Caucasians, CD is associated with an 'extended haplotype' (also referred to as a DRw17/DQw2 haplotype) (Fig. 8.7). The extended DRw17/DQw2 haplotype is usually associated with a number of other markers [71] including, as discussed above, the class 1 marker HLA-B8. Other markers of this haplotype include HLA-1 (A*0101), HLA-DR52a (DRB3*0101) at the class 2 HLA-B3 locus and the SCO1 complotype [71] (i.e. C2*C, Bf*S, C4A*QO, C4B*1). The same extended haplotype is found also in dermatitis herpetiformis (DH) and at an increased frequency as part of a heterozygous genotype in insulin-dependent diabetes mellitus (IDDM).

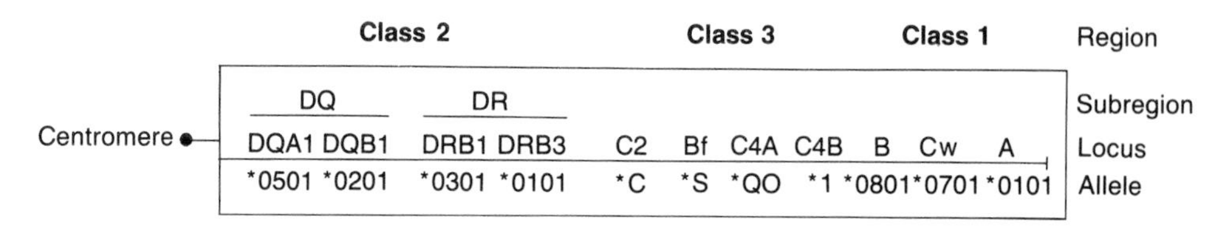

Fig. 8.7 Schematic representation of loci and alleles at those loci on the extended HLA-DRw17 haplotype associated with CD.

The importance of genes in determining susceptibility to CD can be further appreciated from studies of CD concordance among monozygotic twins and studies of HLA haplotype sharing among multiple affected siblings. Among reported identical twins, many of whom are putatively monozygotic, CD is found with a concordance rate of approximately 70% [6]. Since such twins are presumed to ingest similar diets during early life, this suggested that environmental factors, other than dietary grains, may also be involved in the pathogenesis of CD. However, monozygotic twins may not be identical after maturation of the immune system [72]. This is because TCR and immunoglobulin molecules are coded for by groups of rearranging genes that determine the antigen recognition repertoire. In addition, immunoglobulin genes, during maturation, undergo extensive somatic mutation. Thus, although monozygotic twins are genetically identical in the germ line, during maturation they may develop different repertoires in terms of their expressed T cell and immunoglobulin receptors [72].

The concordance rate for CD among siblings who share one or both HLA haplotypes with a CD affected sibling varies from approximately 25–40% [7]. However, in families where more than one sibling has CD, the CD affected siblings almost always (in greater than 95% of cases) share one or both HLA haplotypes [73]. The difference in concordance rates for CD between monozygotic twins (i.e. ~70%) and HLA identical siblings (i.e. ~40%) strongly suggests involvement of additional, as yet undefined, genetic loci in the pathogenesis of CD.

Molecular analysis of the HLA genes associated with CD

The finding that ~25% of a healthy northern European Caucasian population also have the DQw2 serological marker but do not develop CD, despite ingesting similar grain proteins suggests that: (1) the phenotypic expression of CD requires exposure to an enviromental factor in addition to dietary grains; or (2) there are genetic loci in addition to the DRB1 and DQ locus required for the expression of CD; or (3) the DQw2 molecule in CD may be coded for by a variant or a mutant allele of the gene that is not detectable by conventional serological analysis. Such a variant or mutation could be missed by antibody studies since HLA typing antibodies react with only a small region of amino acid sequence on the HLA class 2 α- and β-chains.

Initial molecular biological approaches, designed to examine more precisely the HLA-D region in CD used restriction fragment length polymorphism (RFLP) analysis [74,75]. These studies were designed to determine whether genes coding for the DQw2 molecule in CD differed in any way from the genes coding for the DQw2 molecule in healthy individuals or, alternatively, whether a gene at another HLA-D locus was overrepresented in DRw17/DQw2 CD patients, compared with a control DRw17/DQw2 population.

The technique of RFLP analysis is based on the fact that DNA cutting enzymes, known as restriction endonucleases, cleave DNA at specific sites determined by the nucleotide sequence. If there are differences in gene structure, either within the coding regions (exons) or the flanking regions (introns) of a gene (e.g. differences between the genes that code for DQw2 in CD patients and DQw2 in controls) one might be able to detect such differences by cutting the genomic DNA of these two population groups with a series of several restriction endonucleases. The products of that enzyme digestion are electrophoresed on agarose gels to separate DNA fragments of different sizes. After transfer of the cut DNA from the gel to a solid matrix (e.g. nitrocellulose or nylon) by Southern blotting, the transferred DNA is probed with specific cDNA probes (e.g. -DQ A or B gene probes) to detect the fragments from the relevant HLA class 2 genes. If there are nucleotide substitutions or variations in the particular HLA gene being probed between patients compared to controls, one expects to find different sizes of DNA fragments in the two different populations. This approach has been used successfully in a number of different diseases to detect mutant genes or genes that contain insertions and deletions of DNA that are associated with disease.

Initial studies applied RFLP analysis to compare genomic DNA from the HLA class 2 region of DRw17/DQw2 CD patients to DRw17/DQw2 controls. These studies indicated that the individuals with CD had an increased frequency of a 4.0 kb DPB1 gene fragment detected when genomic DNA was cut with the restriction endonuclease RsaI [74,75]. Ninety-five per cent of DRw17/DQw2 CD patients had the DPB1 gene RFLP whereas <30% of healthy DRw17/DQw2 matched controls had that RFLP [75]. Thus, the presence of this 4.0 kb DNA fragment provided a more accurate means of identifying DRw17/DQw2 individuals at risk for the development of CD than the serological marker HLA-DQw2 alone. The relevance of this 4.0 kb DPB1 gene RFLP as an independent risk factor for CD was further strengthened by the finding that the RFLP was not simply linked to the DQw2 genes. Thus, the frequency of the 4.0 kb DPB gene RFLP in random individuals was as great or greater than in control healthy individuals with DQw2 [75]. Studies have also reported a DPA gene RFLP associated with CD [75]. Taken together, these findings suggested that susceptibility genes for CD, independent of DQ genes, may be found as far centromeric on chromosome 6 as the HLA-DP subregion. Further, this finding lead to the notion that the HLA-associated susceptibility to CD may be multigenic with genes both in the DQ/DR subregion and possibly genes linked to or within the DP subregion determining CD susceptibility. Subsequent studies using different sets of restriction endonucleases detected additional DPA and DPB gene RFLPs and similarly concluded that a DP subregion gene predisposes to CD, independent of DQ genes [76].

The above studies raised several questions. First, what are the specific HLA-DP alleles associated with CD? Further, do the DP alleles associated with CD simply represent one more marker on a disease associated DRw17/DQw2 extended haplotype? Can one detect unique DR, DQ or DP allelic variants (i.e. mutant or variant alleles) in CD but not control individuals on this haplotype? Such questions have been approached using polymerase chain reaction (PCR) technology [77] to amplify the polymorphic alleles on the DRw17/DQw2 haplotype associated with CD and to compare the structure of the polymorphic second exon sequences of the DQ, DR and DP alleles in CD patients and controls (i.e. these are the sequences that form the polymorphic peptide-binding cleft of these molecules and interact with the receptor for the HLA/antigen complex on CD4 T cells). PCR technology enables one to amplify specific segments of DNA from the host genome starting with very small amounts of genomic DNA. This powerful technology now is known to have many applications [78]. In our CD studies, PCR technology was used to amplify polymorphic regions of the HLA-DR, -DQ and -DP genes from CD and control patients [66]. Once amplified (i.e. in order to obtain multiple copies of the gene), the amplified DNA was sequenced [66]. Sequencing of the relevant class 2 alleles from the HLA-DR, -DP and -DQ loci revealed that these alleles are identical in CD patients and controls [66].

Once the sequence of an allele is known, its presence or absence in a patient or control population can be assessed in a more rapid fashion by probing PCR amplified genomic DNA with synthetic oligonucleotides (i.e. short regions of DNA that are synthesized in the laboratory) which are unique in their recognition of DNA sequences that are specific for a particular HLA allele. Such oligonucleotides, known as sequence specific oligonucleotides (SSO) are used to probe host PCR amplified genomic DNA by simple conventional 'dot blot' techniques [66]. This method offers a convenient means for molecular genotyping of the HLA class 2 D region genes in patients or controls.

To analyse the HLA class 2 DP genes associated with CD, SSO were used to probe the PCR amplified second exon regions of -DP genes from our CD patients [66]. Those studies revealed a significant overrepresentation in CD of the relatively rare DP alleles, DPB1*0301 and DPB1*0101 [66]. Moreover, the increased frequency of those alleles in CD accounted for the increased frequency of the 4.0 kb RsaI RFLP in that disease [66]. Subsequent studies showed that DPB1*0301 was also increased in two different Italian CD populations [60,79]. Moreover, the DP allele HLA-DPB1*0301 was associated with CD in northern European Caucasians and Italian CD populations independent of any linkage to DQw2. As in the population of the USA, DPB1*0101 (DPw1) was also increased in CD patients in later studies from the UK [80,81] and Norway [82] (i.e. also northern European Caucasians). However, in those studies, unlike in the USA population, the increased frequency of that allele in CD appeared predominantly to reflect linkage disequilibrium with the DRw17 haplotype. Among southern Italians, but not in a study of northern Italians, HLA-DPB1*0402 was increased in CD [60,79]. Southern Italian CD patients [61,79] differ from northern European Caucasian CD patients and a northern Italian CD population [60] in their distribution of DR markers as determined by serology, in that DRw17 was less common, and DR5/7 heterozygosity more common, among the southern Italians.

The molecular studies of the HLA class 2 D region genes associated with CD are compatible with a disease model in which specific HLA class 2 genes, particularly those that encode a DQw2 molecule, are necessary, although not sufficient, for the phenotypic expression of CD. Nonetheless, the HLA genes associated with CD appear to be structurally normal alleles that simply are overrepresented in CD compared with the control population. In this respect, the findings in CD parallel those in other HLA class 2 associated diseases. Thus, specific alleles of HLA-DR and -DQ on various HLA-DR4 haplotypes are overrepresented in patients with IDDM, rheumatoid arthritis and pemphigus vulgaris, compared with controls [83–86]. Further, the class 2 allelic sequences in those patients are not unique to disease and also are found, although at a lesser frequency, in the control population. Although the peptide-binding regions of the HLA alleles associated with CD are the same in CD patients and controls, such findings do not exclude a possibility that regulatory regions of the alleles present in the CD population differ from the regulatory regions of the same alleles in controls. Such regions affect the level of expression of HLA class 2 molecules on cells.

Considerable evidence supports the importance of a particular DQw2 molecule in disease susceptibility. First, the DQw2 serological specificity is present in virtually all (i.e. 95% or more) coeliacs regardless of their geographical origin. Second, the same DQw2 α/β heterodimer molecule can be present on the cells of CD patients regardless of whether the patient has DRw17 or is heterozygous for -DR5/7 [1,66, 82,87]. Thus, if CD patients are DRw17/DQw2, they have the DQB1*0201 allele and the DQA1*0501 allele that code for the DQ β- and α-chains respectively of a specific DQ molecule (Fig. 8.8). If CD patients are heterozygous for DR5 and DR7, they can form the same DQw2 molecule. This is because DQB1*0201 is present in the DQ subregion linked to DR7, and DQA1*0501 is present in the DQ subregion linked to DR5. Thus, the same DQw2 α/β heterodimer is coded for in *cis*, that is by a single chromosome in DRw17 individuals and in *trans* on DR5/DR7 individuals, in whom the DQA1*0501 allele derives from one chromosome (i.e. DR5 chromosome) and the DQB1*0201 allele derives from the second chromosome (i.e. DR7 chromosome). Further support for this notion is the observation that CD is unusual among African American populations in the USA and the DRw17 haplotype in many African Americans (known as DRw18) has undergone recombination between the DQ and DR loci such that DR3 (DRw18) African Americans lack DQw2 [88]. The rarity of CD in Asian populations also is paralleled by the marked rarity of DQw2 in those populations.

The studies described herein also suggest that more than one gene within the MHC appears to determine, or be linked to, CD susceptibility. Thus, CD is increased among individuals with DQw2 who also have specific DPB1 alleles, that is the DPB1*0301 or DPB1*0101 alleles in

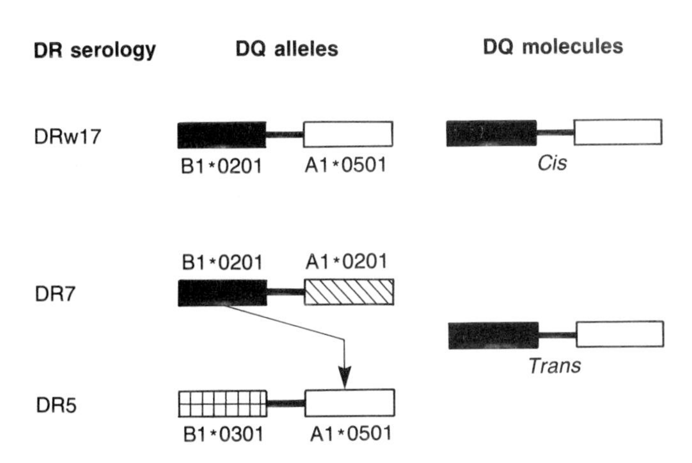

Fig. 8.8 The same DQw2 molecule formed in *cis* on DRw17 haplotypes can be formed in *trans* on DR5/7 haplotypes. As shown, DRw17 is encoded by the alleles B1*0201 and A1*0501. Although the DQB1 allele linked to DR7 (i.e. DQB1*0201) is the same as the DQB1 allele linked to DRw17, the A1 alleles differ. However, the DQA1 allele associated with DR5 (i.e. DQA1*0501) is the same as that of DRw17, although the DQB1 alleles associated with DR5 and DRw17 differ. As indicated, DR7/5 heterozygotes can form the same cell surface DQw2 molecule as DRw17 individuals. This is because a DQ β-chain from the DR7 chromosome can combine with a DQ α-chain from the DR5 chromosome. Since the alleles encoding the cell surface molecule are on opposite chromosomes, the molecule is said to be encoded in *trans*.

northern European Caucasians or alternatively the DPB1*0301 or DPB1*0402 alleles in southern Italians. The association of DPB1 alleles with CD may reflect their direct contribution to disease susceptibility or alternatively an effect of genes linked to the DPB1 locus.

Are there any unique features of the HLA -DQ, -DR or -DP class 2 alleles that are associated with susceptibility to CD? To address this question, one can compare the DQ, DP and DR alleles associated with CD susceptibility with alleles not associated with the disease. The goal of such an approach is to define regions or sequences on the susceptibility alleles that differ from those on non-susceptibility alleles. As described before, the DQ, DP or DR molecules expressed on the cell surface bind antigenic peptides in a cleft-like structure and variations in the amino acid sequences in the cleft are thought to determine which peptides bind in the groove. When one examines variations among the alleles associated with CD, such an analysis reveals distinct, and in some cases, unique amino acid residues on the class 2 alleles associated with CD compared with other non-disease associated alleles. Such residues lie at position 71 of the DQB1*0201 allele and the DRB1*0301 allele or the corresponding position 69 of the DPB1 alleles associated with disease. Most striking is the presence of a positively charged amino acid residue, or the lack of a negatively charged amino acid residue at those sites which are putatively involved in peptide binding [66]. DQA1*0501 has a unique amino acid sequence at position 75 relative to other DQA1 alleles. The latter is also a putative peptide contact site.

Analysis of HLA-DP and -DQ genes associated with DH provides further clues for the importance of HLA class 2 genes in CD

DH is characterized by intensely pruritic papulovesicular cutaneous lesions usually distributed in a symmetrical pattern over the extensor surfaces of the elbows and knees, and on the scalp and buttocks. DH is most prevalent among individuals of Scandinavian or Anglosaxon descent, and is rare in non-Caucasians [89,90]. DH patients also have a small intestinal lesion which is similar to that seen in CD and which responds to a gluten-free diet [91]. However, the intestinal lesion in DH usually is less severe than that in CD. Although most DH patients have a CD-like intestinal lesion, 5% or less of CD patients have skin lesions of DH.

DH and CD share several HLA-D region markers as detected by serology. As in CD, HLA-DRw17 and HLA-DQw2 are found in 95–100% of DH patients of northern European ancestry [92–96]. In addition, cellular typing studies have reported a negative association between DH and HLA-DPw2 [95]. Studies using cellular typing and studies using sensitive molecular techniques, including studies from our laboratory, also have noted an association between DH and specific alleles in the HLA-DP subregion [26,95,96].

PCR technology and SSO probes were used to characterize alleles at the DPB1, DQB1 and DQA1 locus of DH patients. Such studies revealed that the same DQB1 and DQA1 alleles which encode the DQw2 molecule in CD also are overrepresented in DH [26]. In addition, as in CD, DH appears to be associated with the HLA-DP subregion allele DPB1*0301 [26]. Moreover DH, like CD, is negatively associated with a constellation of DPB1 alleles which include DPB1*0202, *0901 or *1301 [26].

Analysis of the DPB1 alleles negatively associated with DH and CD reveals that each of these alleles encodes a negatively charged glutamic acid residue at position 69. In contrast, the -DPB1 alleles positively associated with DH or CD encode a positively charged lysine residue at the same position. Since this is the only consistent difference that distinguishes those alleles, it is tempting to postulate that when present on DRw17, DQw2 haplotypes, DP β-chains lacking a negative charge at position 69 are permissive for the expression of an intestinal lesion such as that seen in DH and CD [26]. Other genes, however, may be necessary for the expression of the more extensive gut involvement in CD and the expression of the cutaneous disease in DH. In addition, analysis of DR and DQ alleles associated with DH and CD indicated that the other expressed HLA-D region β-chains over-represented in these diseases also have a positively charged residue (or lack a negative or neutral residue) at the corresponding position [26,66]. The same amino acid position has been proposed before to be related to susceptibility to pauciarticular juvenile rheumatoid arthritis [97] and is a putative peptide-binding site on the HLA class 2 molecule. Unlike CD, there was no significant increase among DH patients in the frequency of the DPB1*0101 allele [66]. As in CD, the data in DH suggests that disease susceptibility and expression involve an interplay between molecules encoded by HLA alleles at several loci. The requirement for a specific mix of HLA class 2 region susceptibility genes, and perhaps other HLA linked and non-linked genes, also may explain the spectrum of clinical and subclinical disease phenotypes associated with DRw17, DQw2 haplotypes (i.e. DH alone, CD and DH or CD alone) [66].

Unanswered questions and potential approaches to treatment

Several questions have not been answered. For example, little is currently known about the specific mechanism by which the HLA class 2 D region alleles result in CD susceptibility. Further, which other genes, in or outside the MHC, interact with the class 2 D region genes to increase disease susceptibility is not known. In addition, it is not known whether CD is associated with specific HLA class 2 alleles because of events that take place during development of the T cell repertoire in the thymus, because of events that take place during T cell development within the gut epithelium [98,99], or because of events that take place in the periphery following T cell development and differentiation. In addition, the specific antigens and determinants on those antigens that interact with HLA class 2 molecules and T cells as a key element in the pathogenesis of CD are poorly understood. In this regard, the importance of certain dietary grains in disease activation is clearly recognized. Some studies also suggest that a viral protein, perhaps by virtue of having cross-reactive determinants with dietary grains, also may play a role in the pathogenesis of CD [100,101].

Finally, it should be mentioned that knowledge of the role of HLA class 2 D region genes and the role, if any, of TCR genes in the pathogenesis of CD is of interest in terms of potential disease therapies. For example, when the specific peptides known to activate disease and their interactions with specific HLA class 2 D region molecules are better understood, novel therapeutic strategies can be derived to block such interactions. If such reactions are important within the intestinal tract, it may be possible to create 'designer'

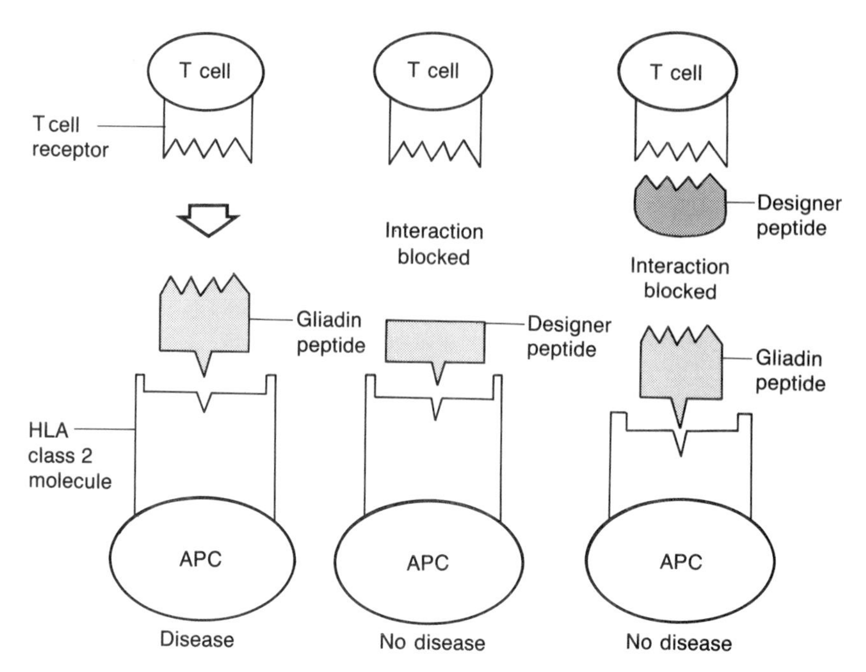

Fig. 8.9 Schematic representation of possible alternative ways for the treatment of CD based on knowledge of the specific HLA class 2 D region genes and T cell receptors important in disease pathogenesis. On the left is shown a T cell interacting with a gliadin peptide bound to an HLA class 2 molecule. In the centre, this interaction has been blocked by administering a 'designer' peptide which binds the HLA class 2 molecule with a higher affinity than the gliadin peptide. As a result, the class 2 molecule is blocked and is no longer available for gliadin peptide binding. On the right, a T cell receptor that recognizes the gliadin peptide bound to the APC is blocked from interacting with the gliadin peptide by administration of a 'designer' peptide which binds to T cell receptor.

peptides that bind, for example, to HLA-DQw2 molecules and prevent binding of the disease-activating peptides (Fig. 8.9). Alternatively, when interaction between specific TCR and the HLA molecules associated with disease and their bound peptides are understood, it may be possible to develop novel strategies to block TCR interactions with those HLA–peptide complexes. Thus, molecular approaches to understanding the genetic basis of CD will provide not only fundamental genetic and immunological information, but the potential for better diagnostic tests of disease and development of new therapeutic strategies as alternatives to the gluten-free diet.

Acknowledgements

Supported by NIH Grant DK35108. The author thanks Miss Colleen Feldpausch for preparation of the manuscript.

References

1 Kagnoff MF. Understanding the molecular basis of coeliac disease. *Gut* 1990;31: 497–9.
2 Kagnoff MF. HLA system and restriction fragment length polymorphisms and coeliac disease. In: Kumar PJ, Walker-Smith JA, eds. *Coeliac Disease: 100 Years*. London: Proceedings for the International Coeliac Symposium, 1991:21–32.
3 Kagnoff MF. Celiac disease. In: Yamada T, ed. *Textbook of Gastroenterology*. Philadelphia: J.B. Lippincott, 1991:1503–20.
4 Kagnoff MF. Celiac disease. In: Targan SR, Shanahan F, eds. *Immunology and Immunopathology of the Liver and Gastrointestinal Tract*. New York: Igaku-Shoin Medical Publishers, 1990:487–505.
5 Kagnoff MF. Celiac disease: Pathogenesis and clinical features. In: Shaffer E, Thomas ABR, eds. *Modern Concepts in Gastroenterology*. New York: Plenum Press, 1989: 277–50.
6 Kagnoff MF. Immunogenetic basis of celiac disease. In: Strober W, Lamm M, McGhee J. eds. *Mucosal Immunity and Infections at Mucosal Surfaces*. Oxford: Oxford University Press, 1988:180–92.
7 Kagnoff MF. A model of an immunologically-mediated intestinal disease. In: Kagnoff MF, ed. *Immunology and Allergy Clinics of North America*. Philadelphia: WB Saunders, 1988:505–20.
8 Cole SG, Kagnoff MF. Celiac disease. In: Olson RE, ed. *Annual Review of Nutrition*. Palo Alto: Annual Reviews, 1985:241–66.
9 Falchuk ZM, Rogentine GN, Strober W. Predominance of histocompatibility antigen HL-A8 in patients with gluten-sensitive enteropathy. *J Clin Invest* 1972;51:1602–5.
10 Stokes PL, Asquith P, Holmes GKT, Mackintosh P, Cooke WT. Histocompatibility antigens associated with adult coeliac disease. *Lancet* 1972;i:162–4.
11 Kappes D, Strominger JL. Human class II major histocompatibility complex genes and proteins. *Ann Rev Biochem* 1988;57: 991–1028.
12 Srivastava R, Chorney MJ, Lawrence SK *et al*. Structure, expression, and molecular mapping of a divergent member of the class I HLA gene family. *Proc Natl Acad Sci USA* 1987;84:4224–8.
13 Koller BH, Geraghty DE, Shimizu Y, DeMars R, Orr HT. HLA-E: A novel HLA class I gene expressed in resting T lymphocytes. *J Immunol* 1987;141:897–904.
14 Geraghty DE, Koller BH, Orr HT. A human major histocompatibility complex class I gene that encodes a protein with a shortened cytoplasmic segment. *Proc Natl Acad Sci USA* 1987;84:9145–9.
15 Geraghty DE, Wei X, Orr HT, Koller BH. Human leukocyte antigen F (HLA-F): An expressed HLA gene composed of class I coding sequences linked to a novel transcribed repetitive element. *J Exp Med* 1990; 171:1–18.
16 Wei X, Orr HT. Differential expression of HLA-E, HLA-F, and HLA-G transcripts in human tissue. *Hum Immunol* 1990;29: 131–42.
17 Spies T, Bresnahan M, Strominger JL. Human major histocompatibility complex contains a minimum of 19 genes between the complement cluster and HLA-B. *Proc Natl Acad Sci USA* 1989;86:8955–8.
18 Kendall E, Sargent CA, Campbell RD. Human major histocompatibility complex contains a new cluster of genes between the HLA-D and complement C4 loci. *Nucleic Acids Res* 1990;18:7251–7.
19 Spies T, Blanck G, Bresnahan M, Sands J, Strominger JL. A new cluster of genes within the human major histocompatibility complex. *Science* 1989;243:214–17.
20 Spies T, Bresnahan M, Bahram S *et al*. A gene in the human major histocompatibility complex class II region controlling the class I antigen presentation pathway. *Nature* 1990;348:744–7.
21 Banerji J, Sands J, Strominger JL, Spies T. A gene pair from the human major histocompatibility complex encodes large proline-rich proteins with multiple repeated motifs and a single ubiquitin-like domain. *Proc Natl Acad Sci USA* 1990;87:2374–8.
22 Gregersen PK. HLA class II polymorphism: Implications for genetic susceptibility to autoimmune disease. *Lab Invest* 1989;61: 5–19.
23 The WHO Nomenclature Committee for factors of the HLA system. Nomenclature for factors of the HLA system, 1989. *Immunogenetics* 1990;31:131–40.
24 Bell JI, Todd JA, McDevitt HO. The molecular basis of HLA-disease association. *Adv Hum Genet* 1989;18:1–41.
25 Bugawan TL, Horn GT, Long CM *et al*.

Analysis of HLA-DP allelic sequence polymorphism using the *in vitro* enzymatic DNA amplification of DPα and DPβ loci. *J Immunol* 1988;141:4024–30.

26 Fronek Z, Cheung MM, Hanbury AM, Kagnoff MF. Molecular analysis of HLA DP and DQ genes associated with dermatitis herpetiformis. *J Invest Derm* 1991;97: 799–802.

27 Fernandez-Vina M, Moraes ME, Stastny P. DNA typing for class II HLA antigens with allele-specific or group-specific amplification. *Hum Immunol* 1991;30:60–8.

28 Volk BA, Brenner DA, Kagnoff MF. Analysis of RNA transcripts for HLA class II genes in human small intestinal biopsies. *Gut* 1989;30:1220–4.

29 Ono SJ, Bazil V, Sugawara M, Strominger JL. An isotype-specific trans-acting factor is defective in a mutant B cell line that expresses HLA-DQ, but not -DR or -DP. *J Exp Med* 1991;173:629–37.

30 Mayer L, Eisenhardt D, Salomon P, Bauer W, Plous R, Piccinini L. Expression of class II molecules on intestinal epithelial cells in humans. Differences between normal and inflammatory bowel disease. *Gastroenterology* 1991;100:3–12.

31 Bjorkman PJ, Saper MA, Samraoui B, Bennett WS, Strominger JL, Wiley DC. Structure of the human class I histocompatibility antigen, HLA-A2. *Nature* 1987; 329:506–12.

32 Bjorkman PJ, Saper MA, Samraoui B, Bennett WS, Strominger JL, Wiley DC. The foreign antigen binding site and T cell recognition regions of class I histocompatibility antigens. *Nature* 1987;329:512–18.

33 Brown JH, Jardetzky T, Saper MA, Samraoui B, Bjorkman PJ, Wiley DC. A hypothetical model of the foreign antigen binding site of class II histocompatibility molecules. *Nature* 1988;332:845–50.

34 Davis MM, Bjorkman PJ. T-cell antigen receptor genes and T-cell recognition. *Nature* 1988;334:395–402.

35 Daar AS, Fuggle SV, Fabre JW, Ting A, Morris PJ. The detailed distribution of MHC class II antigens in normal human organs. *Transplantation* 1984;38:293–8.

36 Gorvel J, Sarles J, Maroux S, Olive D, Mawas C. Cellular localization of class I (HLA-A, B, C) and class II (HLA-DR and DQ) MHC antigens on epithelial cells of normal human jejunum. *Biol Cell* 1984;52:249–52.

37 Scott H, Solheim BG, Brandtzaeg P, Thorsby E. HLA-DR-like antigens in the epithelium of the human small intestine. *Scand J Immunol* 1980;12:77–82.

38 Kelly J, Weir DG, Feighery C. Differential expression of HLA-D gene products in the normal and coeliac small bowel. *Tissue Antigens* 1988;31:151–60.

39 Scott H, Sollid LM, Fausa O, Brandtzaeg P, Thorsby E. Expression of major histocompatibility complex class II subregion products by jejunal epithelium in patients with coeliac disease. *Scand J Immunol* 1987;26: 563–71.

40 Marley NJE, Macartney JC, Ciclitira PJ. HLA-DR, DP and DQ expression in the small intestine of patients with coeliac disease. *Clin Exp Immunol* 1987;70:386–93.

41 Mayer L, Shlien R. Evidence for function of Ia molecules on gut epithelial cells in man. *J Exp Med* 1987;166:1471–83.

42 Bevan MJ. Class discrimination in the world of immunology. *Nature* 1987;325:192–3.

43 Braciale TJ, Morrison LA, Sweetser MT, Sambrook J, Gething MJ, Braciale VL. Antigen presentation pathways to class I and class II MHC-restricted T lymphocytes. *Immunol Rev* 1987;98:95–114.

44 Cresswell P, Blum JS, Davis JE, Marks MS. Transport and expression of HLA class-II glycoproteins. *Immunol Res* 1990;9:190–9.

45 Germain RN. The ins and outs of antigen processing and presentation. *Nature* 1986; 322:687–9.

46 Hickling JK, Fenton CM, Howland K, Marsh SGE, Rothbard JB. Peptides recognized by class I restricted T cells also bind to MHC class II molecules. *Int Immunol* 1990;2: 435–41.

47 Peterlin BM, Andersson G, Lötscher E, Tsang S. Transcriptional regulation of HLA class-II genes. *Immunol Res* 1990;9:164–77.

48 Albert ED, Harms K, Wank R, Steinbauer-Rosenthal I, Scholz S. Segregation analysis of HL-A antigens and haplotypes in 50 families of patients with coeliac disease. *Transplant Proc* 1973;5:1785–9.

49 Evans DAP. Coeliac disease and HL-A8. *Lancet* 1973;ii:1096.

50 McNeish AS, Nelson R, Mackintosh P. HLA 1 and 8 in childhood coeliac disease. *Lancet* 1973;i:668.

51 Dausset J, Hors J. Some contributions of the HL-A complex to the genetics of human diseases. *Transplant Rev* 1975;22:44–74.

52 van Rood JJ, van Hooff JP, Keuning JJ. Disease predisposition, immune responsiveness and the fine structure of the HL-A supergene: A need for a reappraisal. *Transplant Rev*

1975;22:75–104.
53 Seah PP, Fry L, Kearney JW *et al.* A comparison of histocompatibility antigens in dermatitis herpetiformis and adult coeliac disease. *Br J Dermatol* 1976;94:131–8.
54 Solheim BG, Ek J, Thune PO *et al.* HLA antigens in dermatitis herpetiformis and coeliac disease. *Tissue Antigens* 1976;7:57–9.
55 Keuning JJ, Peña AS, van Leeuwen A, van Hooff JP, van Rood JJ. HLA-DW3 associated with coeliac disease. *Lancet* 1976;ii:506–8.
56 Polanco I, Biemond I, van Leeuwen A *et al.* Gluten sensitive enteropathy in Spain: genetic and environmental factors. In: McConnell RB, ed. *The Genetics of Coeliac Disease.* Lancaster: MTP Press, 1981: 211–30.
57 Ek J, Albrechtsen D, Solheim BG, Thorsby E. Strong association between the HLA-Dw3-related B cell alloantigen -DRw3* and coeliac disease. *Scand J Gastroenterol* 1978; 13:229–33.
58 Demarchi M, Carbonara AO, Ansaldi N *et al.* HLA-DR3 and DR7 in coeliac disease: Immunogenetic and clinical aspects. *Gut* 1983; 24:706–12.
59 Mearin ML, Biemond I, Peña AS *et al.* HLA-DR phenotypes in Spanish coeliac children: Their contribution to the understanding of the genetics of the disease. *Gut* 1983;24: 532–7.
60 Colonna M, Mantovani W, Corazza GR *et al.* Reassessment of HLA association with celiac disease in special reference to the DP association. *Hum Immunol* 1990;29: 263–74.
61 Morellini M, Trabace S, Mazzilli MC *et al.* A study of HLA class II antigens in an Italian paediatric population with coeliac disease. *Dis Markers* 1988;6:23–8.
62 Tosi R, Vismara D, Tanigaki N *et al.* Evidence that celiac disease is primarily associated with a DC locus allelic specificity. *Clin Immunol Immunopathol* 1983;28: 395–404.
63 Corazza GR, Tabacchi P, Frisoni M, Prati C, Gasbarrini G. DR and non-DR Ia allotypes are associated with susceptibility to coeliac disease. *Gut* 1985;26:1210–13.
64 Palavecino EA, Mota AH, Awad J *et al.* HLA and celiac disease in Argentina: Involvement of the DQ subregion. *Dis Markers* 1990;8:5–10.
65 Brautbar C, Freier S, Ashkenazi A *et al.* Histocompatibility determinants in Israeli Jewish patients with coeliac disease: Population and family study. *Tissue Antigens* 1981;17:313–22.
66 Kagnoff MF, Harwood JI, Bugawan TL, Erlich HA. Structural analysis of the HLA-DR, -DQ, and -DP alleles on the celiac disease-associated HLA-DR3 (DRw17) haplotype. *Proc Natl Acad Sci USA* 1989;86:6274–8.
67 Sollid LM, Markussen G, Ek J, Gjerde H, Vartdal F, Thorsby E. Evidence for a primary association of celiac disease to a particular HLA-DQ α/β heterodimer. *J Exp Med* 1989; 169:345–50.
68 Roep BO, Bontrop RE, Peña AS, van Eggermond MCJA, van Rood JJ, Giphart MJ. An HLA-DQ alpha allele identified at DNA and protein level is strongly associated with celiac disease. *Hum Immunol* 1988;23: 271–9.
69 Demarchi M, Carbonara AO, Ansaldi N *et al.* HLA-DR3 and DR7-negative celiac disease. In: Albert ED, Baur MP, Mayr WR, eds. *Histocompatibility Testing.* New York: Springer-Verlag, 1984:359.
70 Tosi R, Tanigaki N, Polanco I, De Marchi M, Woodrow JC, Hetzel PA. A radioimmunoassay typing study of non-DQw2-associated celiac disease. *Clin Immunopathol* 1986;39:168–72.
71 Alper CA, Fleischnick E, Awdeh Z, Katz AJ, Yunis EJ. Extended major histocompatibility complex haplotypes in patients with gluten-sensitive enteropathy. *J Clin Invest* 1987;79:251–6.
72 Strominger JL. Biology of the human histocompatibility leukocyte antigen (HLA) system and a hypothesis regarding the generation of autoimmune diseases. *J Clin Invest* 1986;77:1411–15.
73 Scholz S, Albert E. HLA and diseases: Involvement of more than one HLA-linked determinant of disease susceptibility. *Immunol Rev* 1983;70:77–88.
74 Howell MD, Austin RK, Kelleher D, Nepom GT, Kagnoff MF. An HLA-D region restriction fragment length polymorphism associated with celiac disease. *J Exp Med* 1986; 164:333–8.
75 Howell MD, Smith JR, Austin RK, Kelleher D, Nepom GT, Volk B, Kagnoff MF. An extended HLA-D region haplotype associated with celiac disease. *Proc Natl Acad Sci USA* 1988;85:222–6.
76 Caffrey C, Hitman GA, Niven MJ *et al.* HLA-DP and coeliac disease: Family and population studies. *Gut* 1990;31:663–7.
77 Scharf SJ, Horn GT, Erlich HA. Direct cloning and sequence analysis of enzy-

matically amplified genomic sequences. *Science* 1986;233:1076–8.

78 Erlich HA. *PCR Technology*. New York: Stockton Press, 1989.

79 Bugawan TL, Angelini G, Larrick H, Auricchio S, Ferrara GB, Erlich HA. A combination of a particular HLA-DPβ allele and an HLA-DQ heterodimer confers susceptibility to coeliac disease. *Nature* 1989;339: 470–3.

80 Rosenberg WM, Wordsworth BP, Jewell DP, Bell JI. A locus telomeric to HLA-DPB encodes susceptibility to coeliac disease. *Immunogenetics* 1989;30:307–10.

81 Hall MA, Lanchbury JSS, Bolsover WJ, Welsh KI, Ciclitira PJ. Celiac disease is associated with an extended HLA-DR3 haplotype which includes HLA-DPw1. *Hum Immunol* 1990;27:220–8.

82 Spurkland A, Sollid LM, Ronningen KS *et al.* Susceptibility to develop celiac disease is primarily associated with HLA-DQ alleles. *Hum Immunol* 1990;29:157–65.

83 Horn GT, Bugawan TL, Long CM, Erlich HA. Allelic sequence variation of the HLA-DQ loci: Relationship to serology and to insulin-dependent diabetes susceptibility. *Proc Natl Acad Sci USA* 1988;85:6012–16.

84 Todd JA, Acha-Orbea H, Bell JI *et al.* A molecular basis for MHC class II-associated autoimmunity. *Science* 1988;240:1003–9.

85 Scharf SJ, Friedmann A, Brautbar C *et al.* HLA class II allelic variation and susceptibility to pemphigus vulgaris. *Proc Natl Acad Sci USA* 1988;85:3504–8.

86 Sinha AA, Brautbar C, Szafer F *et al.* A newly characterized HLA DQ β allele associated with pemphigus vulgaris. *Science* 1988;239:1026–9.

87 Sollid LM, Thorsby E. The primary association of celiac disease to a given HLA-DQ α/β heterodimer explains the divergent HLA-DR associations observed in various Caucasian populations. *Tissue Antigens* 1990;36:136–7.

88 Hurley CK, Gregersen P, Steiner N *et al.* Polymorphism of the HLA-D region in American blacks: A DR3 haplotype generated by recombination. *J Immunol* 1988; 140:885–92.

89 Katz SI, Hall RP III, Lawley TJ, Strober W. Dermatitis herpetiformis: The skin and the gut. *Ann Intern Med* 1980;93:857–74.

90 Zone JJ, Provost TT. Bullous disease. In: Moschella SL, Hurley HJ, eds. *Dermatology*. Philadelphia: WB Saunders, 1985:579–89.

91 Fry L, McMinn RMH, Cowan JD, Hoffbrand AV. Effect of gluten-free diet on dermatological, intestinal and hematological manifestations of dermatitis herpetiformis. *Lancet* 1968;i:557–61.

92 Strober W. Immunogenetic factors in dermatitis herpetiformis. *Ann Intern Med* 1980;93:857–74.

93 Marrari M, Duquesnoy RJ. Antigen report: HLA-DQw2. In: Albert ED, Baur MD, Mayr WR, eds. *Histocompatibility Testing*. New York: Springer-Verlag, 1984:207–9.

94 Sachs JA, Awad J, McCloskey D *et al.* Different HLA associated gene combinations contribute to susceptibility for coeliac disease and dermatitis herpetiformis. *Gut* 1986;27:515–20.

95 Hall RP, Sanders ME, Duquesnoy RJ, Katz SI, Shaw S. Alterations in HLA-DP and HLA-DQ antigen frequency in patients with dermatitis herpetiformis. *J Invest Derm* 1989;93:501–5.

96 Hall MA, Lanchbury JSS, Bolsover WJ, Welsh KI, Ciclitira PJ. HLA association with dermatitis herpetiformis is accounted for by a *cis* or *trans* associated DQ heterodimer. *Gut* 1991;32:487–90.

97 Begovich AB, Bugawan TL, Nepom BS, Klitz W, Nepom GT, Erlich HA. A specific HLA-DPβ allele is associated with pauciarticular juvenile rheumatoid arthritis but not adult rheumatoid arthritis. *Proc Natl Acad Sci USA* 1989;86:9489–93.

98 Guy-Grand D, Cerf-Bensussan N, Malissen B, Malassis-Seris M, Briottet C, Vassalli P. Two gut intraepithelial CD8+ lymphocyte populations with different T cell receptors: A role for the gut epithelium in T cell differentiation. *J Exp Med* 1991;173:471–81.

99 Bandeira A, Itohara S, Bonneville M *et al.* Extrathymic origin of intestinal epithelial lymphocytes bearing T-cell antigen receptor gamma delta. *Proc Natl Acad Sci USA* 1991;88:43–7.

100 Kagnoff MF, Austin RK, Hubert JJ, Kasarda DD. Possible role for a human adenovirus in the pathogenesis of celiac disease. *J Exp Med* 1984;160:1544–57.

101 Kagnoff MF, Paterson YF, Kumar PJ *et al.* Evidence for the role of the human intestinal adenovirus in the pathogenesis of coeliac disease. *Gut* 1987;28:995–1001.

102 Mautzaris G, Jewell DP. *In vitro* toxicity of a synthetic dodecapeptide from A gliadin in patients with coeliac disease. *Scand J Gastroenterol* 1991;26:392–8.

Chapter 9/The humoral immune system in coeliac disease

HELGE SCOTT, KJELL KETT,
TROND S. HALSTENSEN, METTE HVATUM,
TORLEIV O. ROGNUM AND PER BRANDTZAEG

Introduction — the normal state

In 1965, Tomasi and colleagues established that external secretions contain a unique immunoglobulin (Ig) that is now known as secretory immunoglobulin A, or SIgA [1]. SIgA is generated from dimers or larger polymers of IgA that contain a disulphide-linked polypeptide called 'joining' or J chain [2]. Such polymeric IgA (pIgA) can be transported through the intestinal crypt epithelium together with J chain-containing pentameric IgM (pIgM), by a receptor-mediated mechanism [3]. The pIg receptor comprises the transmembrane secretory component (SC), which is a 100 kDa glycoprotein localized on the basolateral membranes of glandular epithelial cells [3,4]. External pIg transport, or secretory immunity, thus depends on an intimate interaction between the B cell system and exocrine epithelia, where the J chain and SC are to be regarded as 'lock and key' factors essential to its success [4]. The formation of SIgA antibodies depends on the remarkable local preponderance (70–90%) of IgA-producing immunocytes (plasma cells and blasts) as first described by Crabbé *et al.* [5]. The daily translocation of pIgA into the intestinal lumen (~40 mg/kg body weight) exceeds the total daily production of IgG (~30 mg/kg body weight) [6].

Recent observations indicate that interactions between activated leucocytes (e.g. T lymphocytes and macrophages) and the secretory epithelium may upregulate the SC-dependent transport of pIg as part of a local immune response [7–9]. Indirect evidence suggests that lymphoepithelial interactions (perhaps involving the numerous intraepithelial lymphocytes in the gut) may also be involved in modulation of mucosal immunity by normal downregulation, or unwanted upregulation of systemic types of immune responses, to harmless luminal antigens (as reviewed in [10]).

Local humoral immunity

IgG-, IgA- and IgM- producing cells

The most prominent immunohistochemical feature of coeliac disease (CD), as first reported in jejunal mucosae of untreated patients [11], is an increase in the number of IgM-producing cells, an observation confirmed in most subsequent studies of adults and children (Table 9.1). Conversely, IgA cells were reported to be decreased, unchanged or increased (Table 9.1). In most of these studies the number of Ig-producing cells was variably expressed either in terms of mucosal tissue unit area, unit volume or per high-power field of lamina propria [11–17]. In many of these studies, measures of cell density were obtained which failed to reflect the actual size of the mucosal immunocyte population. The quantity of mucosal Ig-producing cells should take into account individual alterations in the volume of the mucosal lamina propria; in two studies, the lamina propria area was on average increased by a factor of 1.7–2.0 in untreated adult CD [18,19]. Moreover, all levels of the lamina propria should be evaluated because of variations in the IgA : IgM : IgG cell ratios; the subepithelial zone usually containing most IgA cells [18].

Our immunohistochemical studies (Table 9.1) have therefore been based on individually defined 'tissue units' which are 'blocks' 6 μm thick and 500 μm wide that extend the full height of the mucosa from the muscularis mucosae to the surface [20]. We found a rise in the absolute number of all three major immunocyte classes in both adults and children with untreated CD (Fig. 9.1); our results have been confirmed by others using comparable approaches [19,21]. However, we found a lower percentage of IgG-producing cells compared with studies from some other laboratories and also a lower percentage of IgM-producing cells (Table 9.1).

These discrepancies are, at least, partly explicable on other methodological differences. Our studies were based on tissue specimens extracted for 48 hours in cold phosphate-buffered saline to remove extracellular diffusible Ig components before ethanol fixation. Several authors [13,14,19,21] used formalin fixed material in which the enumeration of IgG cells, in particular, is difficult to perform because of retained extracellular IgG [22]. Thus, according to our results the mucosal IgG cell fraction is most markedly increased, compared with IgA or IgM, in adult CD [18]. Some authors have reported that IgG cells outnumber IgA cells in diseased mucosa [12], but these results are at extreme variance from all other studies (Table 9.1).

In treated adult CD, we found that both the absolute and relative numbers of immunocytes lay between those observed in untreated patients and controls [18]. However, in coeliac children on a gluten-free diet, the mucosal immunocyte populations were completely normal both in terms of absolute numbers and class ratios [23]. Savilahti [24] reported that a 4-month period of treatment was necessary for such normalization to occur, but his patients still had severe mucosal lesions. Our patients had been treated for 1.2–9 years so that their jejunal mucosa was histologically normal, or revealed only minor changes in

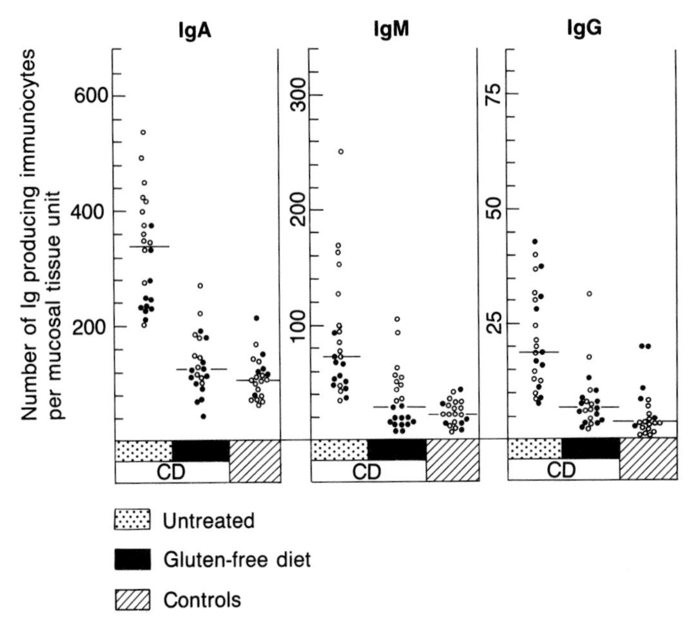

Fig. 9.1 Numbers of IgA-, IgM- and IgG-producing cells in an individually defined mucosal 'tissue unit' (6 μm thick and 500 μm wide) of jejunal mucosa at full height [22]. Results from coeliac patients, untreated or on a gluten-free diet, and controls are indicated by • for children and ○ for adults. In untreated patients the absolute numerical increase was greatest for IgA cells, but the relative increase was most prominent for IgG cells (3.0-, 3.3- and 4.7-fold median increase for IgA, IgM and IgG, respectively). Note different scales on ordinates. (Data from Baklien *et al.* [18] and Scott *et al.* [23].)

villous architecture. Thus, there may be a lag between morphological normalization and the return to a normal mucosal immunocyte pattern. Nevertheless, long-term treatment on a strict gluten-free diet may finally lead to a normal mucosa, at least in children. Since mucosal immunocyte numbers and class ratios in treated adult CD are intermediate between those of untreated patients and controls, it is possible that the adult mucosa does not have the same potential for normalization. However, a strict gluten-free diet may be much more difficult to achieve in adults than in children.

The increase in number of jejunal immunocytes, shown in our paediatric patients at the time of clinical relapse, occurred after 2–11 months on a gluten-containing diet and was more marked than that seen after a standardized 3-month period of challenge [17]. In agreement with the latter study, however, we found no relationship between the jejunal–immunocyte response and the period of gluten-free diet before challenge. Moreover, we could not find any age difference in the response pattern.

Table 9.1 Different studies of class distribution (%) of Ig-producing cells in the proximal small intestinal mucosa of controls (C) and patients with treated (T) or untreated (U) CD*

Authors	Subject category	IgA %	Increase factor	IgM %	Increase factor	IgG %	Increase factor	Tissue preparation	Staining technique
Adults									
Douglas *et al.* [11]	C	84		12		4		Frozen sections	Immunofluorescence
	T	64	0.7	34	2.2	2.1	0.5		
	U	65	0.7	34	3.4	1.8	0.6		
Gasbarini *et al.* [12]	C	59		23		18		Frozen sections	Immunofluorescence
	T†	26	0.7	39	2.6	35	3.0		
	U	—	—	—	—	—	—		
Baklien *et al.* [18]	C	79		18		2.6		Saline extracted, alcohol fixed	Immunofluorescence
	T	70	(1.6)	25	(2.4)	4.6	(2.9)		
	U	66	(2.4)	28	(4.6)	6	(6.5)		
Scott *et al.* [13]	C	55		23		22		Formalin fixed	Peroxidase
	T	—	—	—	—	—	—		
	U	57	2.0	27	1.1	16	0.7		
Dhesi *et al.* [19]	C	69		28		3.0		Formalin fixed	Peroxidase
	T	—	—	—	—	—	—		
	U	52	1.6	32	3.0	5.0	3.5		
Wood *et al.* [14]	C	54		29		17		Formalin fixed	Peroxidase
	T	60	1.4	29	1.3	11	0.8		
	U	56	2.4	32	2.5	13	1.7		

Jenkins *et al.* [15]	C	68		21		11		Frozen sections	Peroxidase
	T	—	—	—	—	—	—		
	U	63	2.0	28	3.0	9.4	2.0		
Children									
Jos *et al.* [16]	C	87		8	5.2			Frozen sections	Immunofluorescence
	T	88	1.1	7.6	1.0	4.4	0.9		
	U	85	1.4	11.5	2.1	3.7	1.0		
Lancaster-Smith *et al.* [17]	C	80		15		5		Frozen sections	Immunofluorescence
	T	75	1.1	19	1.5	5.5	1.2		
	U‡	73	1.3	21	2.1	5.7	1.6		
Scott *et al.* [23]	C	82		11	7.0			Saline extracted, alcohol fixed	Immunofluorescence
	T	83	(0.9)	13	(0.9)	4.5	(0.6)		
	U	75	(2.1)	19	(3.8)	5.5	(2.9)		
Rosenkrans *et al.* [21]	C	70		19		11		Fixed in Bouin solution	Peroxidase
	T	66	(0.9)	22	(1.1)	12	(1.0)		
	U	61	(1.5)	11	(2.7)	29	(1.7)		

* Data from other laboratories have been recalculated to make comparisons possible. Percentage increase factors refers to density of Ig-producing cells compared with normal or numerical increase in individually defined tissue units including the mucosa at full height (figures in parentheses).
† Gluten-free diet for 2 months.
‡ Gluten challenge for 3 months.

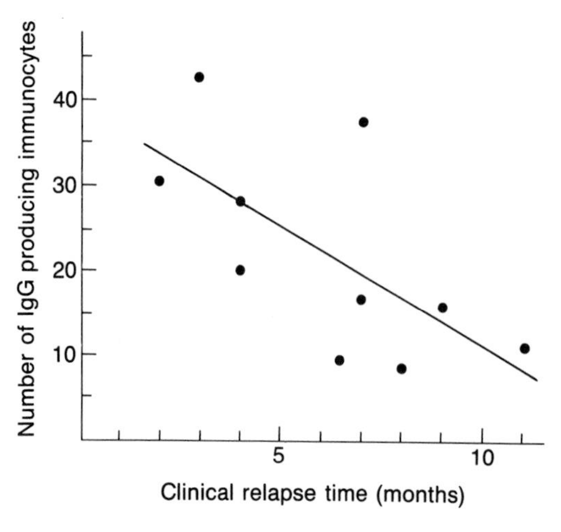

Fig. 9.2 This 'scattergram' illustrates the relationship between time to clinical relapse and the number of IgG-producing cells per 'tissue unit' of jejunal mucosal [22] as revealed by biopsy at the finish of a gluten challenge in 10 children (•) with CD. Relapse time was significantly shorter in those patients with the brisker mucosal IgG response. ($r = -0.645$; $p<0.05$). (Adapted from Scott *et al.* [23].)

There was an inverse relationship between time to clinical relapse, and the number of mucosal IgG cells after challenge in our coeliac children (Fig. 9.2). This limited study should be interpreted with caution, but the striking difference in the mucosal IgG response between children with a short, as opposed to a long time to clinical relapse, suggests that locally produced IgG antibodies to gluten might be of importance in the pathogenesis of CD.

The claim that the epithelial transport of IgA is impaired in CD [25] has not been supported by more recent studies. On the contrary, the hyperplastic crypt epithelium seems to function normally with regard to external transport of both IgA and IgM [18]. The epithelium, in fact, shows increased expression of SC, which agrees with *in vitro* studies suggestive of upregulation of the pIg receptor by various lymphokines (7–9).

The immunocyte pattern in flat jejunal mucosae from other (non-gluten) causes [18] could not be clearly distinguished from that seen in untreated CD. Damage to the mucosal barrier might better explain the intense local IgG cell response as is seen most dramatically in severely inflamed specimens from patients with Crohn's disease and ulcerative colitis [26]. In less pathologically damaged specimens from patients with non-coeliac malabsorption [18], the immunocyte response pattern varied from that seen in CD to one in which a selective rise in the IgA cell population alone was observed.

Gluten specificity of local immune response

According to data from experimental immune responses in animals, only a minor fraction of the stimulated lymphoid cells is engaged in specific antibody production [27]. In a preliminary immunohisto-

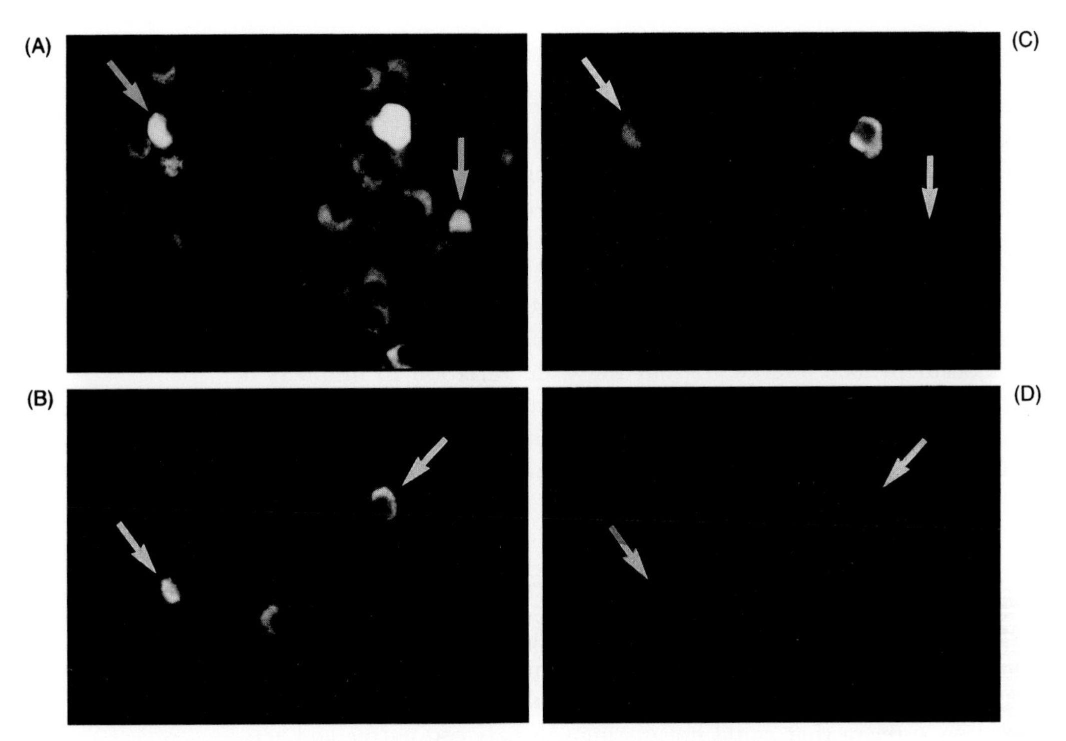

Fig. 9.3 These sections are of duodenal mucosa from an adult coeliac patient. The two left-hand panels are stained by direct immunofluorescence to illustrate IgA cells (A) and IgG cells (B). The same sections, shown in the right-hand panels, are stained indirectly with rhodamine to reveal plasma cells producing specific IgA (C) and IgG (D) antibody to a peptic–tryptic digest of gliadin. Identical positions in each corresponding field of view are indicated by arrows. (Adapted from Brandtzaeg & Baklien [20]; original magnification ×140.)

chemical study of an untreated adult patient with CD, we found a reasonable number of jejunal immunocytes with antibody specificity for gluten (Fig. 9.3) of which, interestingly, a much greater proportion of the IgG than IgA cells (5.7–1.6%) was positive [20]. Very few IgM cells were positive. This suggests that an imbalanced local immune response to gluten, favouring phlogistic antibodies in relative terms, may be involved in the pathogenesis of CD. Another report based on children with CD indicated gluten specificity for 8.4, 8.2 and 5.6% of the jejunal IgG, IgM and IgA cells, respectively [28]. However, in that study an appropriate immunohistochemical 'sandwich' test was not used; the cryostat sections were not treated with a gliadin solution prior to incubation with rhodamine-conjugated rabbit antibody to gliadin. Thus, it cannot be excluded that the results reflected unwanted staining of macrophages or eosinophils rather than of antibody-producing cells.

IgE positive mucosal cells

Mucosal 'IgE positive cells' have been reported to be increased in CD [13,29] but there is controversy as to whether these cells are plasma cells, mast cells, eosinophils or macrophages [4]. IgE positive cells appearing in human intestinal mucosa have recently been identified mainly as mast cells [30]. Increased numbers of mucosal mast cells have been reported in untreated CD [31], but it remains to be established whether mast cell products are of importance in this disorder. A significantly increased number of duodenal IgE positive mast cells does occur in food allergy [32] but the wide variation in numbers of such cells in non-atopic individuals with histologically normal mucosa [32] makes interpretation very difficult. Atopic disease is more frequent in CD than in the normal population [33] but this may be secondary to a 'leaky' mucosa.

Complement factors and immune complexes

Attempts have been made to detect mucosal complement factors and immune complexes in CD but all earlier immunohistochemical reports [34,35] should be interpreted with great caution. Such studies were based on antisera that could not distinguish between native and activated complement factors, while the unwashed tissue sections used contained unpredictable amounts of extracellular plasma proteins [36]. By applying a monoclonal antibody (aE11) to a neoepitope in the C9 part of the terminal complement complex (TCC) which is not expressed in native C9 [37], we recently obtained evidence for subepithelial generation of TCC in untreated coeliac mucosae [38]. Furthermore, in two of five adult patients challenged with gluten for 3 days, trace amounts of C3b were observed within the TCC deposits suggesting recent local complement activation.

IgG and/or IgM containing immune complexes in the epithelial basement membrane zone might thus induce both early- and late-phase complement activation with liberation of the anaphylatoxins C3a and C5a. Such a mechanism could contribute to the increased desquamation of surface epithelial cells seen in untreated CD [39] and attract neutrophils into the lesion [19].

Complement (TCC) deposition around the acini of Brunner's glands was recently described in untreated and treated CD, but also in three of 13 controls [40]. The authors speculated that complement-mediated attack on these glands might be of importance in the pathogenesis of CD. However, such TCC deposition on connective tissue filaments should be interpreted with caution.

Mucosal production of IgG subclasses

IgG1 is the predominant IgG subclass produced locally in CD [41] as is also the case in chronic gastritis [42], ulcerative colitis and Crohn's disease [43]. Our immunohistochemical studies suggest that while the local IgG1 cells mainly reflect systemic immunity, the IgG2 cells may at least partly constitute a response of the mucosal immune system [41–43]. Thus, a raised proportion of IgG2-producing cells (median 35.2%) is observed in patients with untreated compared with treated CD (median 7.3%) or patients with food allergy (median 12.5%) (Fig. 9.4), and IgG2-producing cells are relatively better represented in normal ileal mucosa and Peyer's patches than in peripheral lymph nodes [44]. Moreover, moderate or severe chronic gastritis shows a raised fraction of mucosal IgG2-producing cells compared with mild gastritis [42]. There is likewise a significantly increased fraction of mucosal IgG2 cells in Crohn's colitis compared with active ulcerative colitis [43]. The local immune response of the latter disorder is more systemic in nature also by generating relatively little IgA2 [45] and the preferential IgG1 production may, in addition, have a genetic component [46].

IgG2 shows relatively little complement-activating capacity [47] and poor Fc receptor binding [48]. It is hence unlikely that this subclass contributes to the pathogenesis of CD, although we have previously pointed out the harmful potential of IgG antibodies in relation to the mucosal IgG response [20]. IgG2 may rather be involved in local protective mechanisms in concert with the stimulated secretory IgA and IgM system [49].

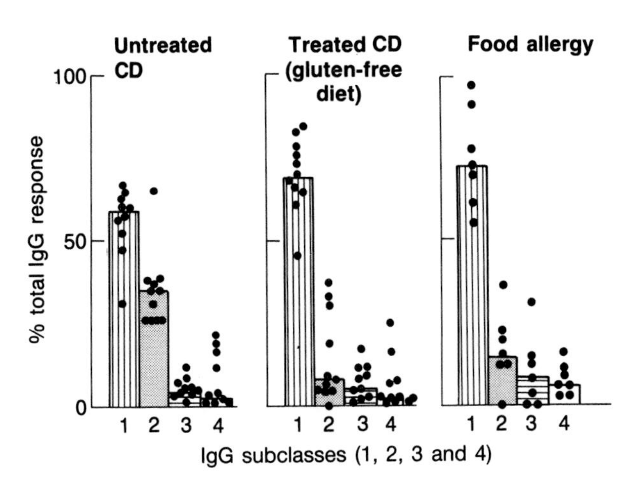

Fig. 9.4 The percentage distribution of IgG1-, IgG2-, IgG3- and IgG4-producing cells in duodenal mucosa in untreated CD, treated CD (gluten-free diet) and in patients with food allergy are shown in this diagram. (Adapted from Rognum *et al.* [41].)

The mechanisms regulating IgG subclass responses are poorly understood, but the nature of the antigen seems to play a decisive role. IgG1 and IgG3 antibodies are thus elicited mainly by protein antigens as, for example, viruses, in contrast to IgG2 which is produced preferentially against bacterial carbohydrates [50]. Such stimulatory differences may explain the disparity between the intestinal mucosa and the nasal mucosa, which tends to show a preference of IgG3 over IgG2 producing cells [51]. Genetic factors will also influence IgG subclass responses [50,52].

Mucosal production of IgA subclasses and associated J chain

A high frequency (about 90%) of J chain expression is preserved in the increased jejunal IgA cell population of CD [53], and the local expansion includes mainly IgA2 cells. Considering the J chain positive IgA immunocyte population, the increase of IgA2 cells averages 3.9- and 1.8-fold in untreated, and treated patients, respectively, compared with 1.7- and 1.4-fold increases for IgA1 cells (Fig. 9.5). The estimated potential for local contribution of IgA2 to SIgA is thus 51% in untreated and 37% for treated patients, compared with 31% in controls. However, there is probably some spillover of IgA2 to the circulation as reflected by the relative increase of this subclass in serum of patients with CD [54].

The determined increase of J chain positive IgA-producing cells in the coeliac lesion [53] agrees with the reported generation of SIgA in organ cultures of untreated jejunal mucosa [14]. These findings, along with the local increase in IgM production [18,20] and the heightened epithelial SC expression [18], clearly reflect an enhanced state of secretory immunity in CD. The preponderance (65–85%) of IgA1-producing cells observed by our laboratory in normal jejunal mucosa [51] has subsequently been confirmed [55] with the same monoclonal antibodies. Conversely, a higher IgA2 cell proportion in jejunal control mucosa was reported in a more recent study which therefore failed to confirm an IgA2 increase in CD [56].

The disease-associated alterations of the mucosal IgA subclasses may be of biological importance [53]. The antimicrobial protective role of IgA2 seems to be superior to that of IgA1. The former subclass has a higher content of mannose-containing oligosaccharides [57] accessible for enterobacterial adhesins [58]; this functional aspect was recently documented by stronger mannose-mediated agglutination of *Escherichia coli* by pIgA2 than pIgA1 [59]. IgA2 is, in addition, resistant to IgA1 specific microbial proteases [60,61].

The effect of the nature of the antigenic or mitogenic stimulus on the immune response within the two IgA subclasses is unresolved [62–65], but antibodies to lipotheichoic acid and bacterial lipopolysac-

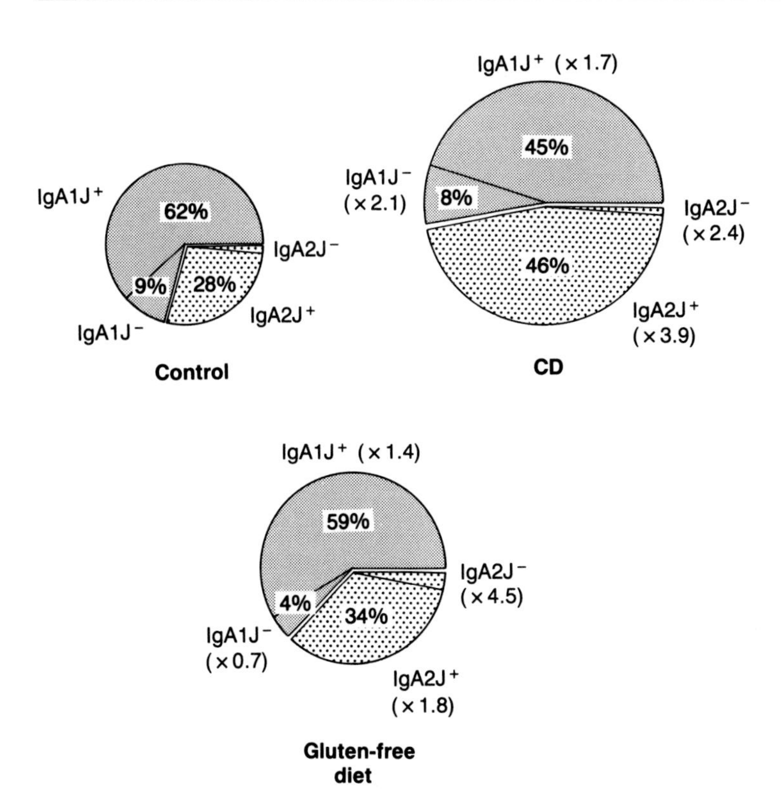

Fig. 9.5 These pie charts illustrate the overall 2.4-fold and 1.5-fold increase in the total jejunal IgA cell populations in untreated CD and in patients on a gluten-free diet. The percentage distributions of various IgA cell subsets are also given for patients in comparison with controls (factors for the absolute increases are given in parentheses). J chain positive (J+) IgA2 immunocytes are increased both in untreated CD ($p<0.01$) and gluten-free diet treated ($p<0.05$) patients, whereas IgA1J+ immunocytes are significantly increased ($p<0.05$) only in untreated CD. (Adapted from Kett *et al.* [53].)

charides have been found preferentially in IgA2 [63]. The increased number of jejunal IgA2-producing cells with preserved J chain expression in CD may therefore, at least in part, reflect an antimicrobial protective mucosal immune response. Enhanced secretory immunity may, in fact be conducive to the relatively well-preserved tissue integrity usually seen in CD and to the reversibility of the mucosal lesion that normally occurs after gluten restriction. Nonetheless, it has been speculated [53] that enhanced local production of mannose rich IgA2 along with carbohydrate-rich SC [66] may render the enterocytes susceptible to damage by lectin-like components in gluten.

Local immunoregulatory events could, in theory, influence IgG and IgA subclass expression. For example, it has recently been suggested from studies of human myeloma cells that IgA1 immunocytes mainly differentiate from IgG1 expressing precursors [67]. Frequent vectorial switching from IgG1 to IgA1 expression may thus explain the striking preponderance of IgA1 immunocytes in respiratory mucosa [51]. Results from stimulated human peripheral blood lymphocytes suggest that most precursors of IgG2-producing cells are relatively immature and express surface IgM, and that switching occurs directly from CHμ to CHγ2 gene activation [68]. As the CHγ2 and CHα2 genes are located on the same chromosomal segment [69] further switching to 3′ genes along this segment could eventually result in IgA2 expression, although a direct switch from CHμ to CHα2 is also possible [70]. Such mechanisms may contribute to the disproportionate increase both in IgG2 and IgA2 immunocytes in CD.

Antibodies to gliadin in duodenal fluid

While numerous studies have focused on aspects of peripheral blood immunity, there is little information about antibodies in the intestinal juice of patients with CD. Precipitins to gliadin and other dietary antigens have been demonstrated in duodenal fluid from untreated patients [71–73] but because the gel precipitation tests used were relatively insensitive, it was not possible to distinguish between Ig isotypes. By means of the enzyme-linked immunoassay (ELISA), high concentrations of IgA and IgM antibody to gliadin have been found in the intestinal fluid of coeliac children [74,75]. IgA antibodies in jejunal fluid were, as expected, mainly of SIgA type, contained a greater proportion of IgA2 compared with serum [76] and were strictly related to the severity of mucosal lesion [75]. Moreover, it was found that the antibodies disappeared more slowly from gut fluid than serum during treatment with a gluten-free diet [74]. Continued intake of minute amounts of gluten in the diet, or enhanced initial priming in mucosa compared with peripheral lymphoid tissues, might be the underlying mechanism here. A similar disparity has been noted in the humoral immune response to enteric bacterial infection; elevated immunity at the gut level persisted 1 year after the decline of serum antibodies [77].

More recently, attempts to study further the local humoral responses have been based on intestinal lavage fluid obtained per rectum in adult patients who had consumed 4 litres of a polyethylenglycol electrolyte solution [78]. Protease inhibitors were added promptly to the samples to prevent proteolysis. Initial serial studies showed that early samples contaminated with faeces contained little IgA whereas once the fluid became clear, a steady state was reached with little variation in IgA content [78]. A positive correlation between gliadin antibody levels in jejunal aspirate and gut lavage fluid was found [79]. Gut lavage IgA was predominantly of SIgA type, comprising 92 and 82% in controls and coeliac patients, respectively [78]. Gut lavage IgM was significantly elevated in untreated adult coeliac patients, and the concentrations were higher in treated patients than controls [79]. Untreated patients had higher levels of IgA and IgM antibodies to gliadin both in jejunal aspirate and in gut lavage fluid than treated patients or controls [79]. Moreover, the IgM antibody activity to gliadin persisted both in jejunal aspirate and gut lavage fluid in treated patients [79]. This might be important in identifying CD patients who have been taking a gluten-free diet for some months before admission to hospital.

Antibodies to gliadin in saliva

Untreated coeliac patients were found to have higher levels of IgA and IgG to gliadin than healthy controls both in stimulated parotid saliva [79] and in unstimulated whole saliva [80]. The salivary antibody levels were generally low, however, and there was considerable overlapping between patients and controls in parotid fluid [79]. No correlation was found between gliadin antibody levels in stimulated parotid saliva and jejunal aspirate [79], and the authors concluded that measurements of such antibodies in saliva did not have diagnostic or screening potential for CD. However, it should be noted that the IgA gliadin antibodies in whole saliva discriminated remarkably well between untreated patients and controls — in fact much better than comparable antibodies in serum [80]. Perhaps the link between gut-associated lymphoid tissue and the parotid gland is poorer than for the remaining salivary glands. Homing studies of IgA precursor cells are not available to support this idea, but further studies of SIgA antibodies to dietary antigens collected from different salivary glands are certainly warranted.

In vitro immunoglobulin production

Cultured biopsy specimens

After organ culture of jejunal biopsy specimens for 24–72 hours, the amounts of IgA and IgM in the medium were found to be higher in untreated patients with CD (both adults and children) than in controls [81–83]; in adult patients the median amounts of total IgA, SIgA and IgM were 6.5, 2.2 and 6.1 times raised, respectively [83]. Earlier studies reported *in vitro* incorporation of ^{14}C-leucine into IgA and IgM in small intestinal biopsy specimens from untreated, and gluten-challenged patients [84,85]. In adults it was found that the changes of *in vitro* Ig production reflected changes in IgA, IgM and IgG immunocyte counts performed on biopsy specimens from the same patients [14]. Treated patients did not differ from the controls [14]. The amounts of IgG released *in vitro* fell rapidly with time [81,82]; the authors therefore concluded that this IgG probably represented extracellular IgG rather than *de novo* synthesis. There was no increase in Ig production after addition of gluten to the culture medium for 24–72 hours [81,82], possibly because the time was too short for putative helper activity to take place.

The Ig class percentages determined in biopsy cultures as specific gliadin antibodies were for controls, treated and untreated coeliac patients, respectively: IgG, 0.7, 0.5 and 2.1%; IgM, 3.2, 10.5 and 12.1%; IgA, 0.7, 0.3 and 4.6% [83]. These figures were in agreement with the small number of cells producing antibodies to gluten demonstrated *in situ* [22]. However, the data contrasted strikingly with a frequently cited early report claiming that approximately half of the net increase of IgA and IgM 2 weeks after gluten challenge could be attributed to synthesis of gliadin antibodies [86].

Isolated cells

Determination of intestinal antibody production *in vitro* is difficult because extracellular Ig components derived from serum are released into the culture medium and various enzymes may degrade the antibodies produced. Although these problems may be avoided by the study of isolated mucosal lymphoid cells, the latter approach yields relatively small cell numbers from biopsy specimens and may introduce an alteration in cell ratios. In small intestinal lymphocyte cultures obtained from untreated patients with CD, *in vitro* Ig secretion was shown by ELISA to be significantly higher for both IgA ($p<0.05$) and IgM ($p<0.001$) compared with controls [87]. Moreover, the secretion of IgM and IgA was increased in a dose-dependent manner by coculture with autologous peripheral blood T lymphocytes, attesting to a T cell-mediated positive immune regulation of intestinal Ig production [87].

Lymphocytes obtained after enzymatic digestion of intestinal biopsy specimens have also been examined for *in vitro* production of gliadin antibodies by the technique known as the enzyme-linked immunospot assay (ELISPOT). This method permits enumeration of antibody secreting cells in relation to Ig class. Patients with untreated CD were found to have relatively high numbers of antigliadin spot-forming cells ($834/10^6$ cultured cells) compared with healthy controls ($49/10^6$ cultured cells) [88]. Specific cells of IgG and IgM class were infrequent while the IgA class predominated in all patients tested (average 68% of total spot-forming cells). Atlhough the number of specific cells was found to be much higher in patients than controls, this study confirmed that only a small fraction of the Ig-producing cells in jejunal mucosa of untreated coeliac patients is engaged in gliadin antibody production [22]. As no patient with a small intestinal disorder other than CD was included for comparison, it remains unknown whether locally produced gliadin antibody is a unique feature of CD.

Peripheral blood mononuclear cells (PBM) producing antibodies to gliadin after culture for only 4 hours were found by ELISPOT in two of six patients with untreated CD and in no controls [88]. After a more prolonged incubation period, PBM obtained from patients with untreated CD did show a higher level of spontaneous antibody production to gliadin (measured by a solid-phase radioimmunoassay) than treated patients [89]. The spontaneous Ig release occurred within the first 3 days of culture; pokeweed mitogen stimulation enhanced the antibody production by cells from treated, but not untreated, patients [89]. In this study the gliadin antibodies were regrettably detected by radio-labelled ^{125}I-Staphylococcal protein A, which binds mainly IgG; circulating Ig-producing cells with specificity for intestinal antigens have in other studies been shown to be mainly of the IgA class [90–92].

Circulating antibodies

Serum immunoglobulins

Abnormal serum Ig levels have been reported in untreated CD, both in children and adults. Eidelman *et al.* [93] found an increase in IgA and several authors have confirmed this finding in adults [18,94–97]. Baklien *et al.* [18] found that this, to some extent, also held true for treated adult patients.

Immonen [97] reported that the raised IgA levels in children with CD fell after gluten withdrawal, and a similar drop has also been noted in most treated adults [18]. Low serum IgM has been found in a varying proportion of untreated coeliac patients [94–96,98], but inconsistently [18,97,99], while serum IgG was deemed to be normal in most patients [18,94–100].

Spillover from the increased mucosal IgA production [10] can, at least in part, explain the increased serum level of IgA in CD; a positive correlation ($r = 0.86$; $p<0.001$) was found between serum levels of IgA gliadin antibodies and the number of jejunal IgA immunocytes per mucosal tissue unit [53]. A reduced serum level of IgM is more difficult to explain. Interestingly, a significant drop in serum IgM was noted in children after gluten challenge for 3 months [17]. Disease-associated mucosal retention of circulating IgM-expressing B cells with specificity for luminal antigens might be one explanation; this would fit with the marked increase in IgM-producing cells in the coeliac lesion (Table 9.1).

About one in 700 normal blood donors shows selective lack of serum IgA. However, the incidence of this deficiency is about 10 times higher among patients with CD [101], a fact that has to be considered in diagnostic tests based on humoral immunity (see pp. 26 and 60).

Table 9.2 Studies of serum IgA and/or IgG activity to gluten (or gliadin) in untreated and gluten-challenged coeliac patients compared with controls

Authors	CD		Controls		Sensitivity* (%)	Specificity* (%)	Antibody class
	Nos	Nos pos.	Nos	Nos pos.			
Signer *et al.* [102]	20 (a)	20	28 (a)	4	100	86	IgG
Unsworth *et al.* [103]	32 (c)	32	152 (c)	22	100	85	IgA
Bürgin-Wolff *et al.* [104]	72 (c)	72	179 (c)	24	100	84	IgG
O'Farrelly *et al.* [105]	44 (NS)	36	46 (a)	6	82	87	IgG
Kilander *et al.* [106]	36 (a) 8 (c)	30 8	62 (NS)	0 0	86 100	100 100	IgA + IgG
Scott *et al.* [107]	20 (a) 18 (c)	16 18	20 (a) 20 (c)	0 0	80 94	100 100	IgA
Stenhammar *et al.* [108]	14 (c)	14	58 (c)	2	100	97	IgA + IgG
Volta *et al.* [109]	15 (a)	14	46 (a)	5	93	89	IgA + IgG

Volta *et al.* [110]	12 (a)	7	166 (a)	0	58	100	IgA + IgG
Kieffer [111]	12 (a)	12	42 (a)	1	100	98	IgG
Juto *et al.* [112]	28 (c)	26	41 (c)	2	93	95	IgA
Ståhlberg *et al.* [113]	31 (c)	29	278 (c)	92	94	66	IgG
		28		39	90	86	IgA
Friis, Gudmand-Høyer [114]	20 (a)	13	205 (a)	0	65	100	IgA + IgG
Montgomery *et al.* [115]	13 (a)	11	10 (a)	1	85	90	IgA
Kelly *et al.* [116]	30 (a)	28	35 (a)	5	93	86	IgA
Bürgin-Wolff *et al.* [117]	331 (a)	331	255 (c)	51	100	80	IgA + IgG
		294		10	89	96	IgA
Scott *et al.* [118]	44 (a)	37	387 (a)	19	84	95	IgA + IgG
Scott *et al.* [119]	43 (c)	43	664 (c)	26	100	96	IgA + IgG

* Nosographic estimates.
a, adults; c, children; NS, not specified.

Serum antibodies to gluten and other dietary antigens

Several early reports [72,120,121] described precipitating antibodies to gluten or its derivatives *in sera* from patients with CD. Wheat grains [122,123], gluten [73], gliadin [104,124,125], α-gliadin [105], or proteolytic fragments of gluten [126] have been used as antigens in various test systems. A significant correlation between the serum IgG titre to gluten and the severity of jejunal damage has been noted [109]. The antibody activity occurs mainly in the IgG class [104,123,127,128]. However, fairly high levels of this antibody class have been detected also in patients with other intestinal disorders and in healthy subjects [74,123]. Moreover, raised IgG antibody activity to dietary antigens other than gluten is present in serum of untreated patients with CD [73,94,107]. Conversely, increased levels of IgA antibodies to gliadin occur regularly in untreated CD but rarely in healthy controls [103, 107,125].

While total serum levels of IgD have been reported to be within the normal range in coeliac patients [129], serum IgD antibody activity to wheat was found to be higher than in normal controls [129]. Short-term sensitizing (STS or anaphylactic IgG) antibody activity to a gluten fraction was detected by passive cutaneous anaphylaxis tests in 33% of patients with CD [130]. It was later suggested that STS IgG is a subfraction of IgG4, as discussed below (see p. 260).

Gluten antibodies in the diagnosis and follow-up of CD

Determination of gluten antibodies in serum has been recommended as a useful adjunct in the diagnosis and follow-up of coeliac patients by several investigators [102–119]. It has been claimed that CD more commonly causes short stature than hypopituitarism. Thus, measurements of gluten antibodies are recommended in children in whom short stature may be the only possible indication of malabsorption [131].

Direct comparisons between the results of various gliadin antibody studies (Table 9.2) are not feasible because of lack of standardization regarding test antigens, and methods of quantitation. Most results have been based on different types of enzyme immunoassay [106–116, 125], while radioimmunosorbent assay [132,133] indirect immunofluorescence performed on wheat grains [134,135], gliadin gel beads [104], gliadin coated red blood cells [136], tissue sections treated with gluten [124] or haemagglutination assays [127,137] have also been used. Moreover, based on ELISA, the results have variably been given as arbitrary optical density units, titres or optical density ratios [103, 107,112,113,125]. In the diffusion-in-gel enzyme-linked immunoassays (DIG-ELISA) the diameter of the reaction zone taken to be indicative of CD has varied [106,114]. To obtain results in mg/litre, it would be necessary in future to isolate gluten specific IgA and IgG antibodies and to establish corresponding reference curves.

Setting the upper reference limit for gliadin antibodies as the highest ELISA reading obtained in healthy controls and patients with other intestinal disorders, we found initially that measurements of IgA afforded virtually 100% diagnostic specificity, detecting 94% of children and 80% of adults with untreated CD [107]. Our results are in agreement with those of others [106,108,114] who characterized their patients with regard both to IgG and IgA activity towards gliadin. The nosographic specificity [138] obtained in our study [107] was better than that reported by Bürgin-Wolff [104] and O'Farrelly [105] who evaluated their patients in terms of IgG activity only.

When we subsequently used the same ELISA setting for the upper reference range in a large prospective study of CD in adults and children [118,119] (Table 9.2), we found that various disorders that could have increased mucosal permeability or affected hepatic IgA catabolism [118,119], were associated with increased serum IgA and/or IgG activities to gliadin. However, the diagnostic specificity for CD increased with increasing IgA activity to gliadin, from 30% in adults (25% in children) with IgA readings between 0.4 and 0.8 optical density units to 90% (100% in children) when readings were above 2.4 optical density units [118,119]. Every child with untreated CD was detected by the ELISA screening in our study (Fig. 9.6). Conversely, the ELISA reading was negative in 16% of untreated adult coeliac patients [118]. It should also be noted that an increased IgA or IgG antibody response to gluten is of less value in the diagnosis of CD in developing countries, as was recently demonstrated in Indian children with protracted diarrhoea [139].

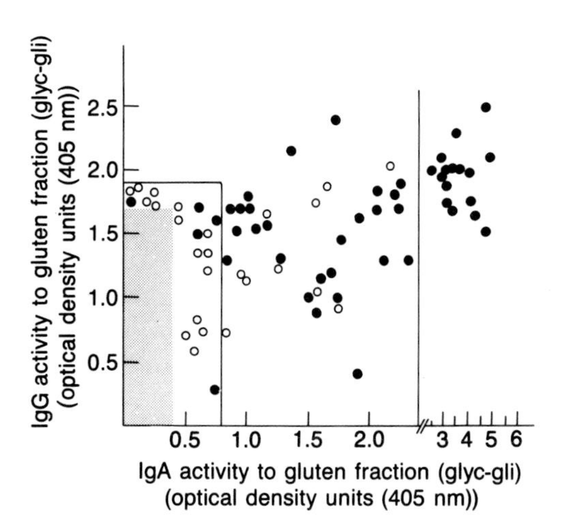

Fig. 9.6 The relationship between serum antibody levels of IgG and IgA (ELISA) to a gluten fraction (glyc-gli) in a group of 72 children with either untreated CD (•) or other disorders (○) is shown in this diagram. The control reference range is indicated by shaded area. Only five of 20 subjects (25%) with IgA activity <0.8 optical density units and an IgG activity <1.9 optical density units had CD (line box). Conversely, 26 of 36 patients (72%) with IgA activities within the range optical density 0.8–2.4 had CD, while all those (28%) remaining with IgA activity >2.4 optical density units (vertical line) had CD. (Adapted from Scott *et al.* [119].)

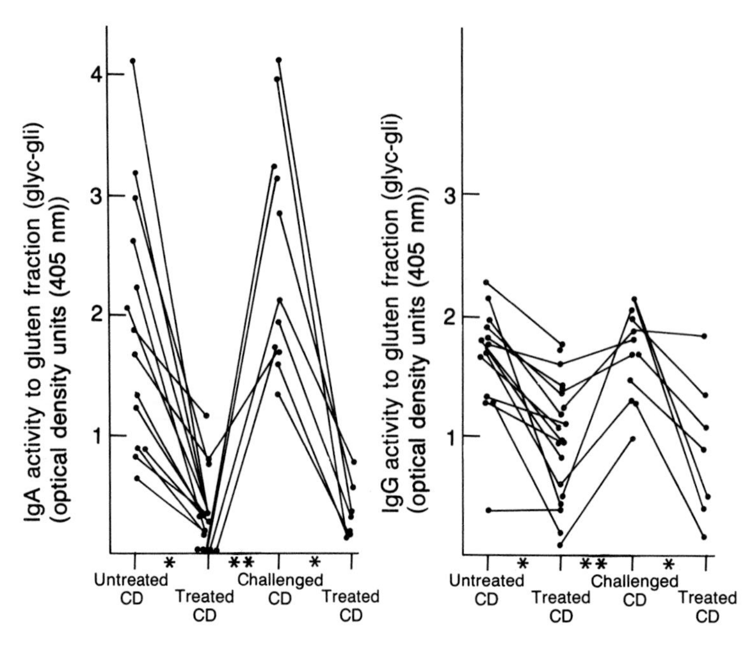

Fig. 9.7 Measurements of IgA and IgG activities (ELISA optical density units at 405 nm) to a gluten fraction (glyc-gli) on duplicate or triplicate serum samples from 24 children with CD are illustrated. The retesting was done after gluten elimination and/or challenge. The time intervals indicated on the horizontal axis represents: * approximately 1 year; ** median 8 months (range 4–19 months). (Adapted from Scott *et al.* [119].)

Treatment with a gluten-free diet results in consistently reduced serum IgA and IgG activities to gluten [117,136,140,141] (Fig. 9.7). We found that IgA activity, in particular, decreased rapidly (Fig. 9.8) being significantly reduced after 3 months gluten restriction [140]. IgA and IgG activities to antigens from egg and cow's milk likewise decreased (Fig. 9.8), although less consistently [140]; nevertheless, the latter variables may also play an important role in the follow-up of CD. Thus, a reduction in serum activity to gliadin after introduction of a gluten-free diet probably reflects both catabolism of existing antibodies and a lack of continued antigenic stimulation, whereas concurrent reduction of activity to other dietary antigens more usefully reflects an improvement in mucosal integrity.

Most challenged coeliac patients showed raised IgG and IgA activities to gluten antigens. When both antibody classes were taken into account in our study [140], relapse was indicated serologically in 15 of 16 children. The antibody activities often reached the diagnostic ELISA level for CD several months before relapse was clinically overt and confirmed by rebiopsy (Fig. 9.9). In addition, raised IgG or IgA activity to one or more of the non-gluten antigens was often found and

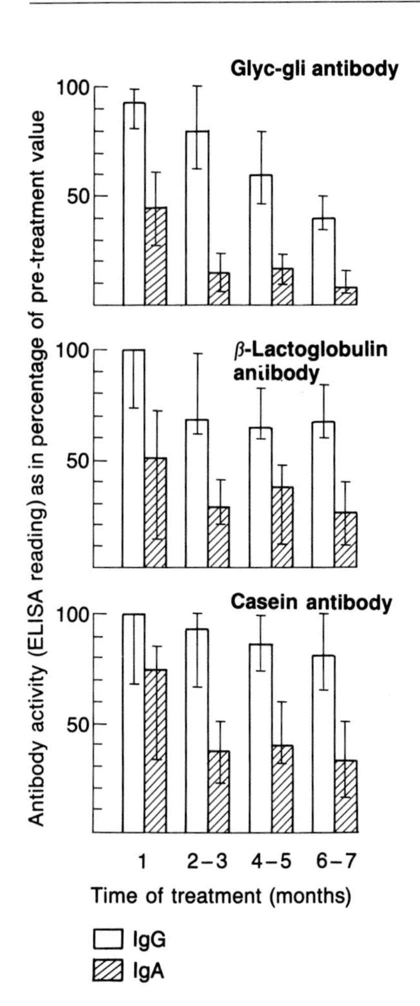

Fig. 9.8 Median ELISA values with 25th and 75th percentile ranges (vertical bars) for serum IgG and IgA activities to a gluten fraction (glyc-gli) and to two bovine milk proteins are shown. Data are from 16 children with CD treated with a gluten-free diet for a variable period as indicated. (Adapted from Scott *et al.* [140].)

strengthened the diagnosis of CD by indicating increased intestinal permeability.

In patients challenged with gluten for 4–15 months we often noted that the highest IgA and IgG activities to gluten and other dietary antigens occurred 1–2 months before gluten intake was discontinued; a decrease in antibody activity, when challenge was prolonged for more than 1 year, was also observed by others [117]. This observation might be explained by enhancement of immunological suppressor mechanisms (induction of 'oral tolerance') or by development of malabsorption resulting in shortage of metabolites necessary for lymphoid cell proliferation and Ig synthesis. We favour the former possibility because intestinal immune responsiveness seems to be intact in patients with CD [142]. However, it remains to be investigated whether such a putative 'oral tolerance' phenomenon is associated with one of the different subsets of T cells [10] that migrate into the jejunal epithelium after gluten challenge [21,143].

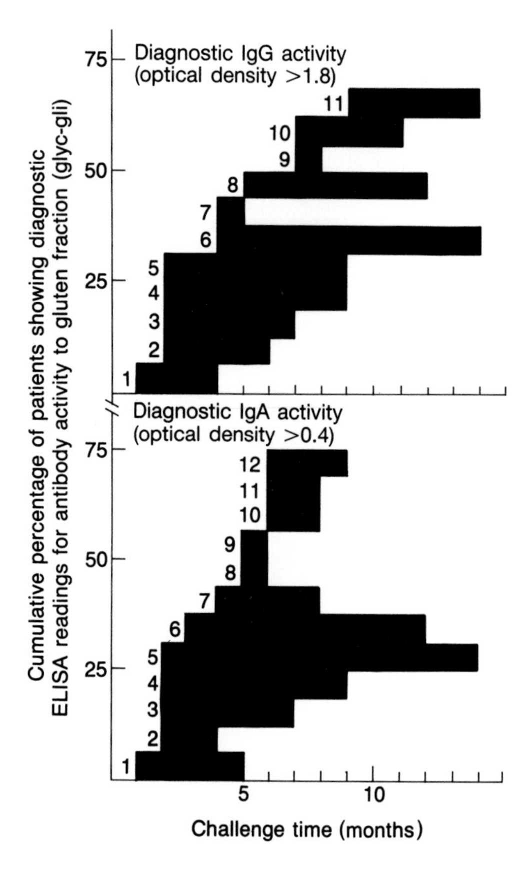

Fig. 9.9 The intervals required to elicit diagnostic levels of serum IgG and IgA activities to a gluten fraction (glyc-gli) in 16 gluten-challenged children with CD are illustrated in this diagram. The diagnostic levels adapted from optical density readings (ELISA) are indicated, the shaded areas representing the time to overt clinical relapse once the first diagnostic reading had been obtained. Diagnostic activity levels were reached for 11 patients (69%) with regard to IgG, and for 12 patients (75%) with regard to IgA. When measurements of both IgG and IgA activities were taken into account, a serological diagnosis of CD could be made in 15 of the 16 patients after challenge. (Adapted from Scott *et al.* [140].)

IgG and IgA subclasses of food antibodies

In healthy individuals serum IgG consists of 60–70% IgG1, 12–18% IgG2, 5–8% IgG3 and 0.7–5% IgG4 [49,144]. Nevertheless, using an ELISA with optimal sensitivity for antibodies to all four IgG subclasses, we found a predominant IgG4 activity to ovalbumin (Fig. 9.10) and β-lactoglobulin both in untreated coeliac patients and in controls with various intestinal disorders [145]. Similar findings have been reported by others [146–148]. The IgG subclass patterns to gliadin (Fig. 9.10) and casein reveal wide individual variations, but the activity seems to occur predominantly in the IgG1 and IgG4 subclasses. There is a significantly lower IgG4 activity to gluten in untreated coeliac patients compared with controls.

Husby *et al.* [146] reported IgG1 and IgG3 antibodies to gliadin in most coeliac patients on a normal diet whereas none of the controls had appreciable IgG1 activity and only one of 22 had IgG3 activity. IgG2 and IgG4 antibodies were found in only a few patients and controls. Conversely, the IgG activity to ovalbumin and β-lactoglobulin

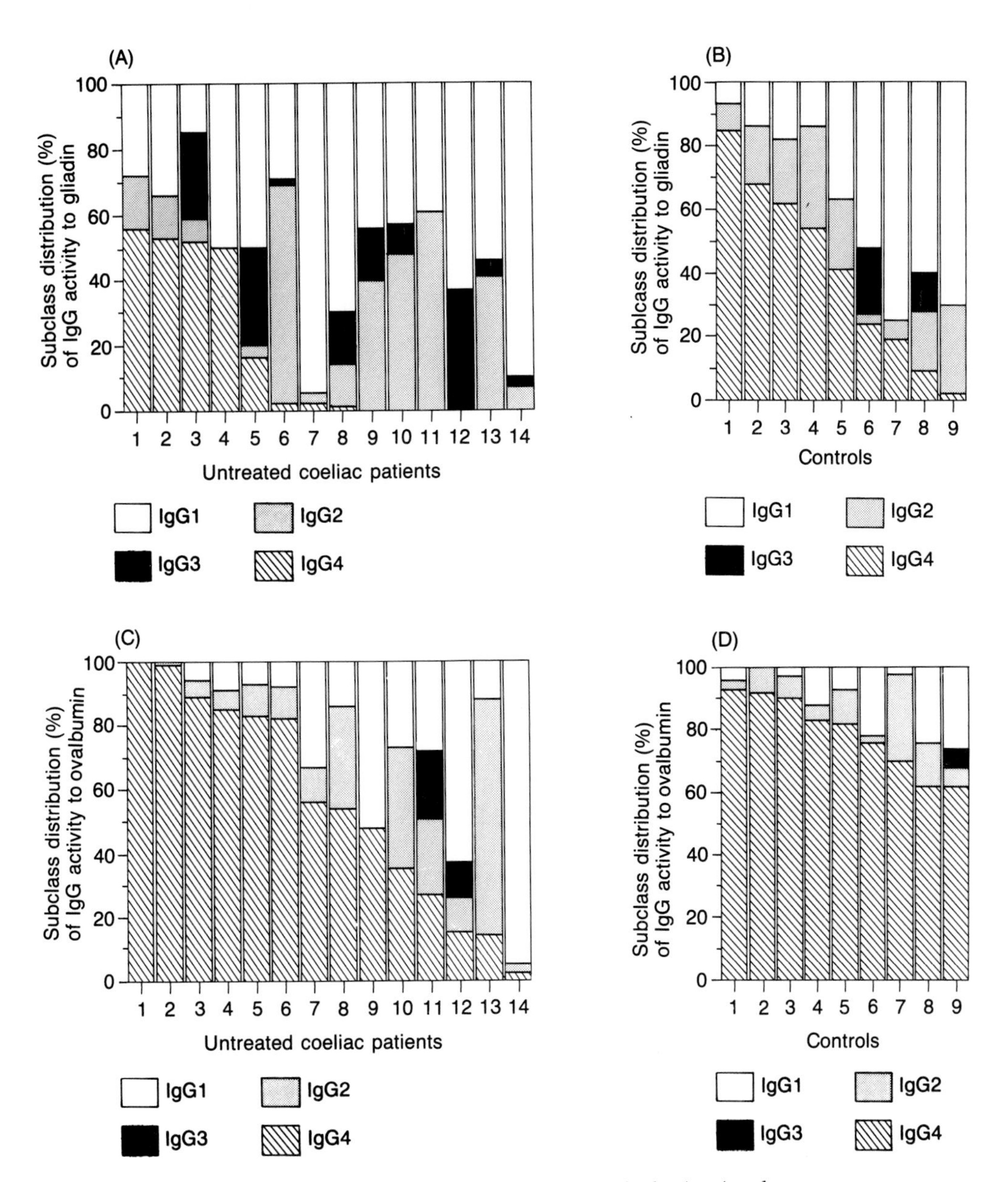

Fig. 9.10 Subclass distributions (%) of IgG ELISA activity to gliadin (A,B) and ovalbumin (C,D) in 14 adults with untreated CD (A,C) and in nine control patients with other intestinal disorders (B,D). There is a significantly ($p<0.02$) lower percentage of IgG4 antibody activity to gliadin in untreated coeliac patients compared with the disease controls.

occurred mainly in IgG1 and IgG4. A predominant increase of IgG1 activity to gluten in untreated CD has also been reported by others [130,147,149]. Conversely, Barnes *et al.* [148] found that IgG antibodies to milk and gluten were often restricted to IgG4 both in adults with CD or dermatitis herpetiformis (DH) and healthy individuals.

Altogether, it seems that the serum IgG subclass activity to dietary antigens exhibits a much higher IgG4 proportion than expected from the subclass distribution of IgG-producing cells in the small intestine [41]. Perhaps most of the IgG antibodies to gluten are produced in mesenteric lymph nodes. It is well-established that the IgG subclass response varies with the antigen [144]. As we and some others [147,148] have found a much higher fraction of IgG4 activity to gluten, casein, β-lactoglobulin and ovalbumin in serum than that expected from the total IgG4 level, it is possible that the production of IgG4 may be part of a normal immune response to dietary proteins [148]. Notably, IgG4 has been reported to increase after prolonged antigen stimulation [150], and the proportion of IgG4-producing cells is relatively higher in Peyer's patches than in lymph nodes [44].

IgG4 antibodies are unable to activate the classical complement pathway [50] and show no significant binding to Fcγ receptors on human monocytes and lymphocytes [50]. The role of this subclass in allergic conditions is still being debated. The existence of subtypes of IgG4 with different biological functions has also been postulated [151]. IgG4 may have a protective role against hypersensitivity by blocking antigen binding to IgE on basophils and mast cells [152]. It has been speculated that IgG4 (or a fraction of this isotype) present in small amounts on mast cells and basophils may act as a sensitizer (STS IgG) whereas large amounts of IgG4 may act as blocking antibodies [151]. The observed shift away from IgG4 towards phlogistic IgG1 antibodies to gluten in CD (Fig. 9.10) may thus be of pathogenic importance.

Kemp *et al.* [153] found elevated serum levels of IgA1 to the gluten fraction glyc-gli in 10 of 11 children with CD challenged with gluten; the patient without elevated IgA1 to glyc-gli had a markedly reduced total serum IgA level. The IgA2 antibody levels to gluten were low in both treated and challenged coeliac patients and of the same magnitude as in healthy individuals. We could likewise detect only trace amounts of IgA2 antibodies to gliadin in untreated coeliac patients (unpublished).

It is controversial as to what extent serum IgA antibodies to gliadin are derived from the intestinal mucosa. A significant relationship between the number of mucosal IgA-producing cells and the serum level of IgA antibodies to gliadin [53] supports a substantial mucosal origin. The finding that almost 80% of the serum IgA antibodies to gliadin comprised IgA1 [76] and that the latter fraction increased upon gluten challenge [153], does not exclude a mucosal origin because presumably more IgA1 than IgA2 cells are engaged in gluten antibody production. Such antibodies produced by J chain negative IgA cells will not be transported externally and may therefore reach serum as monomeric IgA. Eight times more J chain negative IgA1 than IgA2 immunocytes were, in fact, found in the coeliac lesion [53].

Monomeric/polymeric IgA antibodies to gluten

Mascart-Lemone *et al.* [154,155] found that 57% of circulating IgA antibodies to gliadin was pIgA in children with untreated CD compared with 17% in children with other intestinal disorders (acute gastroenteritis, chronic Giardia infections, cow's milk protein intolerance, inflammatory bowel disease) or hospitalized for various other reasons. The pIgA fraction comprised mainly dimers with a small proportion of SIgA. The presence of considerable pIgA activity to gliadin was related to a high level of total serum IgA. After 6 weeks of gluten restriction, the pIgA activity dropped to 15%; during gluten challenge it rose from 20% before, to 59% at the end of the challenge when clinical symptoms reappeared [155]. Circulating pIgA activity to gliadin thus seems to be related to relatively long-lasting gluten exposure and is most likely explained by spillover from mucosal production. A more rapid decrease in pIgA than monomeric IgA (mIgA) antibodies after gluten restriction was probably not caused by the small difference (about 2 days) in plasma half-life of pIgA and mIgA in humans [156] but rather by an efficient external transport of the reduced amounts of pIgA produced in the gut mucosa.

Specificity of gluten antibodies

Gluten consists of four heterogeneous groups: gliadins, glutenins, albumins and globulins [157] of which gliadin and glutenin comprise most of the wheat grain proteins. Each of the gliadin fractions (α, β, γ, ω) separated by electrophoresis [158–160] contains multiple subcomponents [160].

The specificity of gluten antibodies in CD has been investigated in numerous studies [133,161–166]. Gliadins separated by ion-exchange chromatography have often been used as test antigens [133,161,162], but these fractions are not homogeneous with regard to electrophoretically distinct gliadin components [165]. Nevertheless, separation of wheat proteins by sodium dodecyl sulphate (SDS) polyacrylamide gel electrophoresis followed by Western blotting has shown that both normal and CD sera contain antibodies that react with a variety of gliadins [164,165]; only a few coeliac patients and controls react with the high molecular weight glutenin subunits and none with wheat albumin or globulin [165]. It has not been possible to identify any particular gliadin component that binds antibodies only from coeliac patients [164,165]. Skerritt *et al.* [165] reported that the specificites of serum IgG and IgM antibodies were similar in each patient while Vaino [164] found IgA antibodies to be more restricted. This disparity might be explained by different assay sensitivities. When gliadin antibodies in serum and jejunal aspirates were compared, the specificity of the latter showed a broader range [165].

Serum and intestinal antibodies from coeliac patients and healthy individuals have been studied with regard to their activity towards gluten-derived peptides claimed to be 'toxic' in CD [166]: Frazer fraction III (FF3) [167], Cornell fractions [168], glyc-gli [169], A-gliadin fragment B 1342 [170], and adenovirus 12 homologous A-gliadin peptide [171]. Untreated patients were generally found to have higher levels of serum antibodies to some of these peptides, but the specificities did not differ between patients and controls [166]. At present, therefore, a selective humoral immune response to one particular 'toxic' gluten peptide(s) has not been identified.

Antibodies to WGA

It has been postulated that gluten or a component in gluten acts as a lectin and binds to the surface of enterocytes; villous flattening may then follow because of either a direct toxic, or immunological, attack [172]. A lectin-like activity has in fact been demonstrated in gluten [169,173,174], and was recently shown to be present in trace amounts in commercial gluten powder [175]. Patients with untreated CD were found to have significantly higher antibody levels to wheat germ agglutinin (WGA) than patients with other intestinal disorders or healthy controls; the WGA antibodies did not cross-react with gluten antigens [176].

Intraluminal administration of WGA to rats has been reported to produce dose-dependent lesions [177] and permeability alterations [178] characteristic of CD [179,180]. The pathogenetic effect of WGA may be potentiated by its resistance to gastrointestinal degradation [181]. Moreover, low concentrations of WGA are apparently mitogenic to the $CD8^+$ subset of T lymphocytes [182]; it is of interest in this context that the first immunopathological feature observed in coeliac mucosae after gluten challenge is a dose-dependent migration of $CD8^+$ lymphocytes into the jejunal epithelium [21,144].

Antibodies to adenovirus Type 12

Kagnoff *et al.* [171] discovered that A-gliadin (an α-gliadin with known-amino acid sequence) shares a region of striking amino acid sequence homology with the 54 kDa E1b protein of human adenovirus Type 12 (Ad12). This region spans 12 amino acid residues, including eight residue identities and an identical pentapeptide which is hydrophilic in both proteins. A murine monoclonal antibody to E1b was found to cross-react with A-gliadin [171]. It was further reported [183] that 89% of untreated patients with CD had serological evidence of previous Ad12 infection; there was an increased prevalence of neutralizing antibody to Ad12 among treated adult (33%) and paediatric (30.8%) patients compared with controls (0–12.8%) both in western USA and London.

Howdle *et al.* [184] were unable to detect antibodies to E1b in sera from 23 coeliac patients and 10 healthy subjects when tested by radio-immunoprecipitation with metabolically labelled Ad12 transformed rat cells followed by separation on polyacrylamide gels. Devery *et al.* [166], moreover, failed to reveal antibody activity to the crossreacting 12 amino acid A-gliadin peptide in sera from patients with CD or controls, and none of eight monoclonal antibodies to different gliadin proteins showed binding to this peptide [166]. It seems unlikely, therefore, that the 12 amino acid A-gliadin peptide acts as a target for antibody-mediated attack in CD. In addition, DNA of Ad12 could not be detected in small intestinal biopsy specimens from coeliac patients by the Southern blot technique, providing evidence against a persistent Ad12 infection [185]. Thus, the putative role of Ad12 in the pathogenesis of CD remains uncertain although it might possibly be involved in an initial T cell activation.

Antibody activity to other viral antigens and bacteria

The possibility that patients with CD respond abnormally to a variety of enteric antigens has initiated a few studies of immune responses to viral or bacterial antigens. Mawhinney and Love [143] found that serum IgG and/or IgA antibodies to Type II oral polio vaccine were elicited in 50% of treated coeliac patients compared with 18% of controls. Conversely, others reported lower antibody responses in serum of patients with CD than in controls after oral polio vaccination [186]. The same authors found similar serum antibody responses to intramuscular tetanus toxoid injection in coeliac patients and controls whereas Pettingale [187] reported a lower antitoxin response in the patients. Thus, the results are conflicting and have apparently not been followed up by more recent studies. It therefore remains an open question whether patients with CD have an altered immune response to other microbial antigens than Ad12 (see p. 264). Since there is a marked difference in systemic and local humoral activity in CD [79], more effort obviously needs to concentrate in the future on local responses to fed antigens.

Antibodies to reticulin and endomysium

Demonstration of serum antibody to reticulin was proposed as a promising screening test for childhood CD as early as 1971 [188]. Sera from coeliac patients were shown to produce a characteristic staining pattern of reticulin fibres in indirect immunofluorescence tests on frozen tissue sections of rat kidney and liver [189] (Fig. 9.11). However, subsequent studies suggested that the reticulin antibody test was of little diagnostic

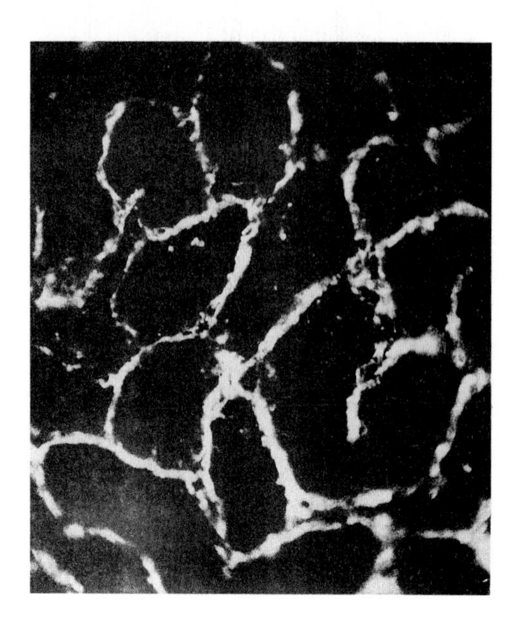

Fig. 9.11 This micrograph illustrates the R1 staining pattern [189] of reticulin fibres in rat kidney demonstrated by indirect immunofluorescence. A cryostat section was first incubated with serum (dilution 1 : 50) from a patient with untreated CD, washed in phosphate-buffered saline and then reincubated with a fluorescein-conjugated rabbit antihuman IgA. Original magnification ×400.

value [123,189–191], being positive in only about one-half of children with untreated CD (Table 9.3). Nevertheless, the test was considered more disease specific (Table 9.3) than antibodies to gliadin, and some studies have claimed that IgA reticulin antibodies are of particular value in screening for CD [190,195,196,198] (Table 9.3). Non-specific reticulin-like reactions should be avoided by starting with a serum dilution of no lower than 1 : 50 [195]. Note that antibodies to reticulin were considered useful for diagnosing CD in India [197] in contrast to gluten antibodies (see p. 256).

Reticulin is not a single entity [199] but is composed of collagen, fibronectin, and at least one additional non-collagenous glycoprotein [200]. Both IgG and IgA reticulin antibodies are unaffected by absorption with gluten, gliadin or a peptic–tryptic digest of gluten [201]. Antibodies to reticulin have also been found in DH [189,194,199], rheumatoid arthritis [189,202], Sjögren's syndrome [189] and chronic heroin addicts [189]. Although different staining patterns have been seen in these disorders compared with CD, it is not known whether the actual antibodies are directed against the same or dissimilar antigens.

Teppo and Maury [203] isolated a 90 kDa pemphigus-like mannose-rich intercellular substance antigen ('reticulin glycoprotein') which was shown to be present in human small intestinal epithelium and normal skin. Interestingly, it was found to share some antigenic properties with gluten and reticulin and had an amino acid composition similar to that of the previously described non-collagenous reticulin antigen [200]. Antibodies to the 90 kDa antigen were found in CD, DH, Sjögren's syndrome and massive cutaneous hyalinosis [204,205]

Table 9.3 Studies of reticulin antibodies in serum of untreated coeliac patients compared with controls

	CD		Controls				
Authors	Nos	Nos pos.	Nos	Nos pos.	Sensitivity* (%)	Specificity* (%)	Test system
Seah *et al.* [188]	10 (c)	9	28	1	90	96	Anti-IgG
Von Essen *et al.* [192]	40 (c)	27	20	0	68	100	Anti-IgG
Seah *et al.* [193]	51 (a) 26 (c)	30 22	479	14	60 85	97	Anti-IgG
Rizzetto *et al.* [189]	50 (not specified)	22	3542	142	44	96	Anti-F(ab)$_2$
Magalhaes *et al.* [190]	92 (a)	36 13	109	6 0	39 14	94 100	Anti-IgG Anti-IgA
Eade *et al.* [194]	28 (a + c)	22	23	3	78	87	Anti-IgA
Etermann, Feltkamp [106]	36 (a) 6 (c)	12 2	95 14	2 0	33 33	98 100	Anti-F(ab)$_2$
Unsworth *et al.* [191]	32 (c)	15	249	3	46	99	Not defined
Mäki *et al.* [195]	29 (c)	28	245	4	97	98	Anti-IgA
Monteiro *et al.* [196]	48 (c)	36	32	4	75	88	Anti-IgG
Khoshoo *et al.* [197]	12 (c)	10	123	0	83	100	Anti-IgG
Hällström [198]	32 (a) 14 (c)	29 14	45 24	0 0	90 100	100 100	Anti-IgA Anti-IgA

* Nosographic estimates.
a, adults; c, children.

but did not completely parallel antibodies to reticulin in appearance; they increased more slowly during gluten challenge and disappeared later after introduction of a gluten-free diet [205]. Moreover, the antibody levels in untreated coeliac patients were positively related to age, perhaps as a reflection of disease duration and extent of tissue damage. The reticulin antibody levels, however, showed no significant change with age [205].

Chorzelski *et al.* [206] reported in 1983 that sera from patients with CD or DH contain antibody activity against the connective tissue filaments (endomysium) surrounding smooth muscle fibres in the gastrointestinal tract. These antibodies are detected by indirect immunofluorescence tests on frozen tissue sections of monkey oesophagus, a substrate of choice also for pemphigus and pemphigoid antibodies [207–209]. The antigen(s) reactive with endomysial antibodies is mainly available in the lower portion of the oesophagus, decreasing towards the uppermost part. Antibodies of the IgA class have been reported to be a valuable adjunct in the diagnosis of CD because they show high specificity for this disorder, and DH with small intestinal villous flattening [210].

The antibodies to endomysium and reticulin are most likely different; absorption with rat liver homogenates removed the rodent specific reticulin antibodies but not the endomysial antibodies reactive with monkey oesophagus [198]. Gliadin binding to endomysial antigenic sites has been reported [211]. However, in these studies, frozen sections were pre-treated with a solution of undigested gliadin in distilled water, so non-specific binding of gliadin to various tissue elements could not be excluded.

Antibodies to reticulin and endomysium in the diagnosis and follow-up of CD

The highest sensitivity for CD determined by the reticulin antibody test (Table 9.3) is comparable to the best results obtained from measurements of IgG and IgA antibodies to gluten antigens (Table 9.2). The reticulin antibody specificity for CD is also high (Table 9.3). IgA antibodies to endomysium have been detected in 90–100% of untreated adults, in all untreated children with CD (Table 9.4) and in about 70% of patients with DH, namely those with a coeliac 'flat' jejunal lesion [215,216]. Only 15% of patients with CD have IgG endomysial antibodies, but high titres of such antibodies have been reported in IgA deficient coeliac patients [198,217]. Interestingly, endomysial antibodies have not as yet been found in other skin or gut diseases, including Crohn's disease [214,216]. It is important to note in this context that antibodies to gluten cannot distinguish Crohn's disease with extensive involvement of the ileum from CD [129,130].

Table 9.4 Studies of IgA endomysium antibodies in serum of untreated coeliac patients compared with controls

Authors	CD		Controls		Sensitivity* (%)	Specificity* (%)
	Nos	Nos pos.	Nos	Nos pos.		
Chorzelski *et al.* [210]	28 NS	19	107	0	68	100
Kapuscinska *et al.* [212]	33 (c)	100	140	0	100	100
Rossi *et al.* [213]	46 (c)	46	160	0	100	100
Kumar *et al.* [214]	38 (c)	38	278	0	100	100
Hällström [198]	14 (c)	14	24	0	100	100
	32 (a)	29	45	0	90	100

* Nosographic estimates.
NS, adults or children not specified; both untreated and treated patients.
a, adults; c, children.

Children with treated CD showed increasing anti-endomysium titres during gluten challenge, whereas the antibody levels decreased in all cases after a gluten-free diet for 6–12 months [212]. Moreover, aggressive gluten challenge made DH patients positive for endomysial antibodies [218].

Circulating immune complexes

Observations suggesting the presence of circulating 'immune' complexes have been obtained in patients with CD on the basis of the C1q precipitin test [219], ^{125}C1q binding assay [220,221], polyethylene glycol precipitation test [221], and inhibition of binding of ^{125}I-labelled human aggregated IgG to guinea pig peritoneal macrophages [221]. Moreover, passage of ovalbumin and β-lactoglobulin into the blood of children with CD after a test meal has been demonstrated; the size distribution of the absorbed antigen suggests formation of immune complexes [222]. In one study, larger amounts of circulating complexes in patients on a normal diet than in those treated with a gluten-free diet were reported [219], but this disparity was not confirmed by others, either in CD [221] or in DH [223].

The circulating immune complexes in CD contain IgG and IgM [221], but it should be emphasized that the assays used could not identify other associated Ig classes. Later studies have shown that DH, which is closely related to CD, gives rise to circulating immune complexes mainly containing IgA [224,225]. Sodium dodecyl sulphate extracts of patients' skin contain monomers, dimers and larger polymers of IgA [226], but gluten antigens have never been detected in dermal deposits [225]. Such antigens have been demonstrated in the sera of DH patients [227], although a distinction between immune complexes and free gluten molecules could not be made with the assay employed. The only antigen unequivocally shown to be associated with immune complexes is the mannose-rich 90 kDa epithelial glycoprotein [228], which is a constituent of both small intestinal mucosa and skin.

It may be concluded that although a role for circulating immune complexes has not been related to pathogenesis, such complexes may be a link between DH and CD, and between CD and IgA mesangial nephropathy, fibrosing alveolitis and rheumatoid arthritis [229]. Increases in serum IgA activity to gluten have, in fact, been found in a fraction of patients with IgA nephropathy [230], while some children with rheumatoid arthritis have flat small intestinal mucosae and reticulin antibodies [231].

Genetic aspects of antibody production

The IgG response to gluten has been claimed to be associated with the IgG heavy chain allotype G2m(n) in American adult Caucasian patients with CD. Persistent IgG activity to gluten after treatment with a gluten-free diet for more than 18 months was found mainly in patients with this genetic marker, regardless of whether they did or did not express the histocompatibility antigens HLA-B8 or HLA-DR3, which are closely associated with CD [232]. However, the G2m(n) association was neither confirmed in an Italian study of adult CD [233] nor in a Finnish study of diseased children [234]; our study was likewise negative in this respect. We found the G2m(n) allotype in 72% of adult Norwegian coeliac patients, in 71% of patients with food allergy and in 70% of healthy blood donors [41].

It has been claimed that all coeliac patients lacking HLA-B8 and -DR3 have the Gm(f;n;b) phenotype of the IgG heavy chain [235]. Moreover, an interplay of HLA- and Gm-linked genes with gender in the pathogenesis of CD was also suggested [233]. Thus, raised gluten antibody levels have been reported to persist mainly in treated HLA-DR3 negative female patients [236]. Furthermore, higher gluten antibody titres occur in HLA-$DR7^{+}DR3^{-}$ compared with HLA-$DR7^{-}DR3^{+}$ coeliac children [237]. In most of these studies the genetic influences have been evaluated in a relatively small number of patients; the results therefore must be interpreted with great caution.

Antibodies and immune complexes in the pathogenesis of CD

CD is most likely initiated by an inappropriate T lymphocyte response [10,143,238,239] leading to a release of different lymphokines which in turn may be responsible for overstimulation of the mucosal B cell system [240,241], induction of crypt hyperplasia [242], increased epithelial permeability [243], and upregulated epithelial MHC class 2 [244–247] and SC expression [7–9,244].

Although mucosal humoral immunity in CD is dominated by a typical pIgA and pIgM response and enhanced SC-mediated transport of SIgA and SIgM, overstimulation of the B cell system leads to a disproportionate local and systemic IgG response both to gluten and other dietary antigens. Serum-derived, and locally produced, IgG antibodies may be considered as a second line of humoral defence against luminal antigens. However, if immune elimination is unsuccessful due to continuous penetration of antigens, persistently altered immunological homostasis in the mucosa may contribute to pathogenesis [10].

A putative pathogenic role for IgG antibodies in CD is suggested both by the disproportionate IgG cell response and by the fact that the serum IgG antibody activity to gluten is much more persistent than the IgA class after treatment of children with a gluten-free diet [140]. The same is true for serum antibodies to β-lactoglobulin, ovalbumin and casein [140]. IgG antibodies may be phlogistic and tissue damaging by forming complement-activating immune complexes, or by arming K cells expressing Fcγ receptors.

The mucosal IgG response in CD comprises more than 50% IgG1-producing cells [41] and there is an isotype shift of circulating gluten antibodies from IgG4 to IgG1 in untreated patients; these features favour the complement-activating potential of the humoral immune response. Complement activation has indeed been demonstrated by immunohistochemistry beneath the epithelium in jejunal mucosa from patients with untreated CD. Complement activation may obviously contribute to epithelial damage and increased mucosal penetrability, not only for gluten but for various other dietary bystander antigens [248]. Thus, a vicious circle may conceivably develop. Lim and Rowley [249] showed in an experimental *in vivo* model that phlogistic immune complexes can cause considerable mucosal damage; they concluded that only IgA antibodies are able to mediate uncomplicated inhibition of antigenic uptake. The dominating local SIgA (and SIgM) response seen in CD is probably able to limit the tissue destructive aspects of the lesion and contribute to successful normalization of the mucosa in patients who adhere strictly to a gluten-free diet.

Despite the emphasis in this chapter on antibodies, and their possible role in the pathogenesis of CD and DH, it should be noted that similar mucosal lesions have also been reported in individuals with common variable immunodeficiency [250]. In these circumstances, it is evident that T cells must play the most important role in pathogenesis, although it may be incorrect to designate such lesions as CD. The pathogenetic role of T cells is considered in greater depth in the next chapter.

Acknowledgements

Studies in the authors' laboratory were supported by The Norwegian Research Council for Science and the Humanities, The Norwegian Cancer Society and Anders Jahre's Foundation.

References

1 Tomasi TB, Tan EM, Solomon A, Prendergast RA. Characteristics of an immune system common to certain external secretions. *J Exp Med* 1965;121:101–24.

2 Mestecky J, McGhee JR. Immunoglobulin A (IgA): Molecular and cellular interactions in IgA biosynthesis and immune response. *Adv Immunol* 1987;40:153–245.

3 Brandtzaeg P. Role of J chain and secretory component in receptor-mediated glandular and hepatic transport of immunoglobulins in man. *Scand J Immunol* 1985;22:111–46.

4 Brandtzaeg P, Baklien K, Bjerke K, Rognum TO, Scott H, Valnes K. Nature and properties of the human gastrointestinal immune system. In: Miller K, Nicklin S, eds. *Immunology of the Gastrointestinal Tract.* Florida: CRC Press, 1987:1–85.

5 Crabbé PA, Carbonara AO, Heremans JF. The normal human intestinal mucosa as a major source of plasma cells containing A-immunoglobulin. *Lab Invest* 1965;14:235–48.

6 Conley ME, Delacroix DL. Intravascular and mucosal immunoglobulin A: Two separate but related systems of immune defence? *Ann Intern Med* 1987;106:892–9.

7 Sollid LM, Kvale D, Brandtzaeg P, Markussen G, Thorsby E. Interferon-γ enhances expression of secretory component, the epithelial receptor for polymeric immunoglobulins. *J Immunol* 1987;138:4303–6.

8 Kvale D, Løvhaug D, Sollid LM, Brandtzaeg P. Tumor necrosis factor-α upregulates expression of secretory component, the epithelial receptor for polymeric Ig. *J Immunol* 1988;140:3086–9.

9 Kvale D, Brandtzaeg P, Løvhaug D. Upregulation of the expression of secretory component and HLA molecules in a human colonic cell line by tumor necrosis factor-α and gamma interferon. *Scand J Immunol* 1988;28:351–7.

10 Brandtzaeg P, Halstensen TS, Kett K *et al.* Immunobiology and immunopathology of human gut mucosa: Humoral immunity and intraepithelial lymphocytes. *Gastroenterology* 1989;97:1562–84.

11 Douglas AP, Crabbe PA, Hobbs JR. Immunochemical studies of the serum, intestinal secretions and intestinal mucosa in patients with adult celiac disease and other forms of the celiac syndrome. *Gastroenterology* 1970;59:414–25.

12 Gasbarini G, Miglio F, Serra MA, Bernardi M. Immunological studies of the jejunal mucosa in normal subjects and adult celiac patients. *Digestion* 1974;10:122–8.

13 Scott BB, Goodall A, Stephenson P, Jenkins D. Small intestinal plasma cells in coeliac disease. *Gut* 1984;25:41–6.

14 Wood GM, Howdle PD, Trejdosiewicz LK, Losowsky MS. Jejunal plasma cells and *in vitro* immunoglobulin production in adult coeliac disease. *Clin Exp Immunol* 1987;69:123–32.

15 Jenkins D, Goodall A, Scott B. T cells and plasma cell populations in coeliac small intestinal mucosa in relation to dermatitis herpetiformis. *Gut* 1989;30:955–8.

16 Jos J, Rey J, Frezal J. Etude immunohistochemique de la muqueuse intestinale chez l'enfant. *Arch Fr Pediatr* 1972;29:681–98.

17 Lancaster-Smith M, Packer S, Kumar PJ, Harries JT. Immunological phenomena in the jejunum and serum after reintroduction of dietary gluten in children with treated coeliac disease. *J Clin Pathol* 1976;29:592–7.

18 Baklien K, Brandtzaeg P, Fausa O. Immunoglobulins in jejunal mucosa and serum from patients with adult coeliac disease. *Scand J Gastroenterol* 1977;12:149–59.

19 Dhesi I, Marsh MN, Kelly C, Crowe P. Morphometric analysis of small intestinal mucosa. II. Determination of lamina propria volumes; plasma cell and neutrophil populations within control and coeliac disease mucosae. *Virchows Arch [A]* 1984;403:173–80.

20 Brandtzaeg P, Baklien K. Immunohistochemical studies of the formation and epithelial transport of immunoglobulins in normal and diseased human intestinal

mucosa. *Scand J Gastroenterol* 1976; 11(Suppl 36):1–45.
21 Rosenkrans PCM, Meijer CJLM, Polanco I, Mearin ML, Van der Wal AM, Lindeman J. Long-term morphological and immunohistochemical observations on biopsy specimens of small intestine from children with gluten-sensitive enteropathy. *J Clin Pathol* 1981;34:138–44.
22 Brandtzaeg P, Rognum TO. Evaluation of tissue preparation methods and paired immunofluorescence staining for immunohistochemistry of lymphomas. *Histochem J* 1983;15:655–89.
23 Scott H, Ek J, Baklien K, Brandtzaeg P. Immunoglobulin-producing cells in jejunal mucosa of children with coeliac disease on a gluten-free diet and after gluten challenge. *Scand J Gastroenterol* 1980;15:81–8.
24 Savilahti E. Intestinal immunoglobulins in children with coeliac disease. *Gut* 1972; 13:958–64.
25 Shiner M, Ballard J. Mucosal secretory IgA and secretory piece in adult coeliac disease. *Gut* 1973;14:778–83.
26 Baklien K, Brandtzaeg P. Comparative mapping of the local distribution of immunoglobulin-containing cells in ulcerative colitis and Crohn's disease of the colon. *Clin Exp Immunol* 1975;22:197–209.
27 Mottica EJ. The non-specific stimulation of immunoglobulin secretion following specific stimulation of the immune system. *Immunology* 1974;27:401–12.
28 Stern M, Dietrich R. Gliadin- and immunoglobulin-containing cells of small intestinal lamina propria in childhood coeliac disease. *Eur J Pediatr* 1982;139:13–7.
29 Savilahti E. Immunoglobulin containing cells in the intestinal mucosa and immunoglobulins in the intestinal juice in children. *Clin Exp Immunol* 1972;11:415–25.
30 Rognum TO, Brandtzaeg P. IgE-positive cells in human intestinal mucosa are mainly mast cells. *Int Arch Allergy Appl Immunol* 1989;89:256–60.
31 Strobel S, Busuttil A, Ferguson A. Human intestinal mast cells: Expanded population in untreated coeliac disease. *Gut* 1983;24: 222–7.
32 Bengtsson U, Rognum TO, Brandtzaeg P, Kilander A, Hanson LÅ, Ahlstedt S. IgE positive duodenal mast cells in patients with food-related diarrhoea. *Int Arch Allergy Appl Immunol* 1991;95:86–91.
33 Verkasalo M, Tilikainen A, Kuitunen P, Savilahti E, Backman A. HLA antigens and atopy in children with coeliac disease. *Gut* 1983;24:306–10.
34 Shiner M, Ballard J. Antigen–antibody reactions in jejunal mucosa in childhood coeliac disease after gluten challenge. *Lancet* 1972;i:1202–5.
35 Scott BB, Scott DG, Losowsky MS. Jejunal mucosal immunoglobulins and complement in untreated coeliac disease. *J Pathol* 1977; 121:219–23.
36 Baklien K, Brandtzaeg P. Immunohistochemical localization of complement in intestinal mucosa. *Lancet* 1974;ii:1087–8.
37 Mollnes TE, Lea T, Harboe M, Tschopp J. Monoclonal antibodies recognizing a neoantigen of poly(C9) detect the human terminal complement complex in tissue and plasma. *Scand J Immunol* 1985;22:183–95.
38 Halstensen TS, Hvatum M, Scott H *et al.* Association of subepithelial deposition of activated complement and immunoglobulin G and M response to gluten in coeliac disease. *Gastroenterology* 1992;102:751–9.
39 Wright N, Watson A, Morley A, Appleton D, Marks J, Douglas A. The cell cycle time in the flat (avillous) mucosa of the human small intestine. *Gut* 1973;14:603–6.
40 Gallagher RB, Kelly CP, Neville S, Sheils O, Weir DG, Feighery CF. Complement activation within the coeliac small intestine is localised to Brunner's glands. *Gut* 1989; 30:1568–73.
41 Rognum TO, Kett K, Fausa O *et al.* Raised number of jejunal IgG2-producing cells in untreated adult coeliac disease compared with food allergy. *Gut* 1989;20:1574–80.
42 Valnes K, Brandtzaeg P. Subclass distribution of mucosal IgG-producing cells in gastritis. *Gut* 1989;30:322–6.
43 Kett K, Rognum TO, Brandtzaeg P. Mucosal subclass distribution of immunoglobulin G producing cells is different in ulcerative colitis and Crohn's disease of the colon. *Gastroenterology* 1987;93:919–24.
44 Bjerke K, Brandtzaeg P. Terminally differentiated human intestinal B cells IgA and IgG subclass-producing immunocytes in the distal ileum, including Peyer's patches, compared with lymph nodes and palatine tonsils. *Scand J Immunol* 1990;32:61–7.
45 Kett K, Brandtzaeg P. Local IgA subclass alterations in ulcerative colitis and Crohn's disease of the colon. *Gut* 1987;28:1013–21.
46 Helgeland L, Kett K, Tysk C, Brandtzaeg P. Evaluation of genetic impact on the mu-

cosal IgG-subclass response in inflammatory bowel disease. In: Tsuchiya M, Nagura H, Hibi T *et al.*, eds. *Frontiers of Mucosal Immunology*. Amsterdam: Excerpta Medica, Elsevier, 1991:807–8.
47 Spigelberg HL. Biological activities of immunoglobulins of different classes and subclasses. *Adv Immunol* 1974;19:259–93.
48 Unkeless JC, Fleit H, Mellman JS. Structural aspects and heterogeneity of immunoglobulin Fc-receptors. *Adv Immunol* 1981;31: 247–70.
49 Brandtzaeg P, Valnes K, Scott H, Rognum TO, Bjerke K, Baklien K. The human gastrointestinal secretory immune system in health and disease. *Scand J Gastroenterol* 1985;20(Suppl 114):17–38.
50 Papeda C, Check IJ. Human immunoglobulin G and immunoglobulin G subclasses: biochemical, genetic and clinical aspects. *Crit Rev Clin Lab Sci* 1989;27:27–58.
51 Brandtzaeg P, Kett K, Rognum TO *et al.* Distribution of mucosal IgA and IgG subclass-producing immunocytes and alterations in various disorders. *Monogr Allergy* 1986;20:179–94.
52 Van Loghem E. The immunoglobulin genes: genetics, biological and clinical significance. *Clin Immunol Allergy* 1984;4: 607–22.
53 Kett K, Scott H, Fausa O, Brandtzaeg P. Secretory immunity in celiac disease: cellular expression of immunoglobulin A subclass and joining chain. *Gastroenterology* 1990;99:386–92.
54 Soppi E, Granfors K, Leino RJ. Serum secretory IgA1 and IgA2 subclasses in inflammatory bowel and chronic liver disease. *Clin Lab Immunol* 1987;23:15–17.
55 Hene RJ, Schurman HJ, Kater L. Immunoglobulin A subclass-containing plasma cells in the jejunum in primary IgA nephropathy and in Henoch-Schönlein purpura. *Nephron* 1988;48:4–7.
56 Mearin F, Mearin ML, Pena AS. Distribution of IgA1 and IgA2 immunocytes in the jejunum of adult coeliac patients and controls. *J Clin Nutr Gastroenterol* 1986;1: 79–82.
57 Tomana M, Niedermeier W, Mestecky J, Skvaril F. The difference in carbohydrate composition between the subclass of IgA immunocytes. *Immunochemistry* 1976; 13:325–9.
58 Duguid JP, Gillies RR. Fimbriae and adhesive properties in dysenteric bacilli. *J Pathol Bact* 1957;74:397–411.
59 Wold AE, Mestecky J, Svanborg Eden C. Agglutination of *E coli* by secretory IgA: a result of interaction between bacterial mannose-specific adhesins and immunoglobulin carbohydrate? *Monogr Allergy* 1988;22:307–9.
60 Plaut AG. The IgA1 protease of pathogenic bacteria. *Ann Rev Microbiol* 1983;37: 603–22.
61 Kilan M, Reinholdt J. Interference with IgA defence mechanisms by extracellular bacterial enzymes. *Med Microbiol* 1986;5: 173–208.
62 Brown TA, Murphy BR, Radl J, Haaijman JJ, Mestecky J. Subclass distribution and molecular form of immunoglobulin A hemagglutinin antibodies in sera and nasal secretions after experimental secondary infections with influenza A virus in humans. *J Clin Microbiol* 1985;22:256–64.
63 Brown TA, Mestecky J. Immunoglobulin A subclass distribution of naturally occuring salivary antibodies to microbial antigens. *Infect Immun* 1985;49:459–62.
64 Conley ME, Briles DE. Lack of IgA subclass restriction in antibody response to phosphorylcholine, lactoglobulin and tetanus toxoid. *Immunology* 1984;53:419–26.
65 Hammarström L, Persson MAA, Smith CIE. Immunoglobulin subclass distribution of human anti-carbohydrate antibodies: Aberrant pattern in IgA-deficient donors. *Immunology* 1985;54:821–6.
66 Mizoguchi A, Mizuochi T, Kobata A. Structures of the carbohydrate moieties of secretory component purified from human milk. *J Biol Chem* 1982;257:9612–21.
67 Hammarström L, Mellstedt H, Persson MAA, Smith CIE, Ahre A. IgA subclass distribution in paraproteinemias: Suggestion of an IgG-IgA subclass switch pattern. *Acta Pathol Microbiol Immunol Scand Sect C* 1984;92:207–11.
68 Conley ME, Brown P, Bartelt MS. IgG subclass potential of surface IgM- negative and surface IgM-positive human peripheral blood B cells. *Clin Immunol Immunopathol* 1987;43:211–22.
69 Flanagan JG, Rabbits TH. Arrangement of human immunoglobulin heavy chain constant region genes implies evolutionary duplication of a segment containing gamma, epsilon and alpha genes. *Nature* 1982;300: 709–13.
70 Conley ME, Bartelt MS. *In vitro* regulation

of IgA subclass synthesis. II. The source of IgA2 plasma cells. *J Immunol* 1984;133: 2312–6.
71 Katz J, Kantor FS, Herskovic T. Intestinal antibodies to wheat fractions in celiac disease. *Ann Intern Med* 1968;69:1149–53.
72 Herscovic T, Katz J, Gryboski JD, Spiro HM. Coproantibodies to gluten in coeliac disease. *J Am Med Assoc* 1968;203:887–8.
73 Ferguson A, Carswell F. Precipitins to dietary proteins in serum and upper intestinal secretions of coeliac children. *Br Med J* 1972;i:75–7.
74 Labrooy JT, Hohmann AW, Davidson GP, Hetzel PAS, Johnson RB, Sherman DJC. Intestinal and serum antibody in coeliac disease: A comparison using ELISA. *Clin Exp Immunol* 1986;66:661–8.
75 Volta U, Bonazzi C, Lazzari R *et al.* Immunoglobulin A antigliadin antibodies in jejunal juice: Markers of severe intestinal damage in coeliac children. *Digestion* 1988; 39:35–9.
76 Mascart-Lemone F, Colombel JF, Rambaud JC *et al.* Jejunal and serum IgA in adult coeliac disease. *Gastroenterology* 1989;96 (Suppl):A324.
77 Labrooy JT, Sherman DJC, Rowley D. Antibodies in serum and secretions one year after Salmonella gastroenteritis. *Clin Exp Immunol* 1982;48:551–4.
78 O'Mahony S, Barton JR, Crichton S, Ferguson A. Appraisal of gut lavage in the study of intestinal humoral immunity. *Gut* 1990;31:1341–4.
79 O'Mahony S, Arranz E, Barton JR, Ferguson A. Dissociation between systemic and mucosal humoral immune responses in coeliac disease. *Gut* 1991;32:29–35.
80 Al-Bayaty HF, Aldred MJ, Walker DM *et al.* Salivary and serum antibodies to gliadin in the diagnosis of celiac disease. *J Oral Pathol Med* 1989;18:578–81.
81 Fluge G, Aksnes L. Quantification of immunoglobulins after organ culture of human duodenal mucosa. *J Pediatr Gastroenterol Nutr* 1983;2:62–70.
82 Wood GM, Shires S, Howdle PD, Losowsky MS. Immunoglobulin production by coeliac biopsies in organ culture. *Gut* 1986;27: 1151–60.
83 Ciclitira PJ, Ellis HJ, Wood GM, Howdle PD, Losowsky MS. Secretion of gliadin antibody by coeliac jejunal mucosal biopsies cultured *in vitro*. *Clin Exp Immunol* 1986; 64:119–24.
84 Loeb PM, Strober W, Falchuk ZM, Laster L. Incorporation of Leucine-^{14}C into immunoglobulins by jejunal biopsies of patients with celiac sprue and other gastrointestinal diseases. *J Clin Invest* 1971;50:559–69.
85 Falchuk ZM, Strober W. Increased jejunal immunoglobulin synthesis in patients with nontropical sprue as measured by a solid phase immunoadsorption technique. *J Lab Clin Med* 1972;79:1004–13.
86 Falchuk ZM, Strober W. Gluten sensitive enteropathy: Synthesis of antigliadin antibodies *in vitro*. *Gut* 1974;15:947–52.
87 Crabtree JE, Heatley RV, Losowsky MS. Immunoglobulin secretion by isolated intestinal lymphocytes: spontaneous production and T-cell regulation in normal small intestine and in patients with coeliac disease. *Gut* 1989;30:347–54.
88 Lycke N, Kilander A, Nilsson L-Å, Tarkowski A, Werner N. Production of antibodies to gliadin in intestinal mucosa of patients with coeliac disease: A study at the single cell level. *Gut* 1989;30:72–7.
89 Troncone R, Farris E, Donatiello A, Auricchio S. *In vitro* gliadin antibody production by peripheral blood mononuclear cells from patients with coeliac disease. *J Clin Lab Immunol* 1987;23:179–83.
90 Kantele A, Arvilommi H, Jokinen I. Specific immunoglobulin-secreting human blood cells after peroral vaccination against *Salmonella typhii*. *J Infect Dis* 1986;153: 1126–31.
91 Czerkinsky C, Prince SJ, Michalek SM *et al.* IgA antibody-producing cells in peripheral blood after antigen ingestion: Evidence for a common mucosal immune system in humans. *Proc Natl Acad Sci USA* 1987;84:2449–53.
92 Forrest BD. Identification of an intestinal immune response using peripheral blood lymphocytes. *Lancet* 1988;i:81–3.
93 Eidelman S, Davis SD, Lagunoff D, Rubin CE. The relationship between intestinal plasma, cells and serum immunoglobulin A (IgA) in man. *J Clin Invest* 1966;45: 1113–14.
94 Kenrick KG, Walker-Smith JA. Immunoglobulins and dietary protein antigens in childhood coeliac disease. *Gut* 1970;11: 635–40.
95 Asquith P, Thompson RA, Cooke WT. Serum-immunoglobulins in adult coeliac disease. *Lancet* 1969;ii:129–31.
96 Blecher TE, Brzechwa-Ajdukiewicz A,

McCarthy CF, Read AE. Serum immunoglobulins and lymphocyte transformation studies in coeliac disease. *Gut* 1969;10:57–62.

97 Immonen P. Levels of serum immunoglobulins IgA, IgG and IgM in the malabsorption syndrome in children. *Ann Paediat Fenn* 1967;13:115–52.

98 Hobbs JR, Hepner GW. Deficiency of M-globulin in coeliac disease. *Lancet* 1968;i:217–20.

99 Brown IL, Ferguson A, Carswell F, Horne CHW, MacSween RNM. Autoantibodies in children with coeliac disease. *Clin Exp Immunol* 1973;13:373–82.

100 Ashkenazi A, Levin S, Miskin A. Immunoglobulin levels in children with celiac disease: variations with age and diet. *Isr J Med Sci* 1980;16:843–6.

101 Thomas HC, Jewell DP. *Clinical Gastrointestinal Immunology*. Oxford: Blackwell Scientific Publications, 1979:100–20.

102 Signer E, Bürgin-Wolff A, Berger R, Birbaumer A, Just M. Antibodies to gliadin as a screening test for coeliac disease. A prospective study. *Helv Paediatr Acta* 1979;34:41–52.

103 Unsworth DJ, Kieffer M, Holborow EJ, Coombs RRA, Walker-Smith JA. IgA antigliadin antibodies in coeliac disease. *Clin Exp Immunol* 1981;46:286–93.

104 Bürgin-Wolff A, Bertele RM, Berger R *et al.* A reliable screening test for childhood coeliac disease: fluorescent immunosorbent test for gliadin antibodies. *J Pediatr* 1983;102:655–60.

105 O'Farrelly CO, Kelly J, Hekkens W *et al.* Gliadin antibody levels: a serological test for coeliac disease. *Br Med J* 1983;286:2007–10.

106 Kilander AF, Dotevall G, Fellström SP, Gillberg RE, Nilsson LÅ, Tarkowski A. Evaluation of gliadin antibodies for detection of coeliac disease. *Scand J Gastroenterol* 1983;18:377–83.

107 Scott H, Fausa O, Ek J, Brandtzaeg P. Immune response patterns in coeliac disease. Serum antibodies to dietary antigens measured by an enzyme linked immunosorbent assay (ELISA). *Clin Exp Immunol* 1984;57:25–32.

108 Stenhammar L, Kilander AF, Nilsson LÅ, Strömberg L, Tarkowski A. Serum gliadin antibodies for detection and control of childhood coeliac disease. *Acta Paediatr Scand* 1984;73:657–63.

109 Volta U, Cassani F, De Franchis R *et al.* Antibodies to gliadin in adult coeliac disease and dermatitis herpetiformis. *Digestion* 1984;30:263–70.

110 Volta U, Lenzi R, Cassani F. Antibodies to gluten detected by immunofluorescence and a micro-ELISA method: Markers of active childhood and adult coeliac disease. *Gut* 1985;26:667–71.

111 Kieffer M. Serum antibodies to gliadin and other cereal proteins in patients with coeliac disease and dermatitis herpetiformis. *Dan Med Bull* 1985;32:251–62.

112 Juto P, Fredrikzon B, Hernell O. Gliadin specific serum immunoglobulins A, E, G, and M in childhood: Relation to small intestine mucosal morphology. *J Pediatr Gastroenterol Nutr* 1985;4:723–9.

113 Ståhlberg MR, Savilahti E, Viander M. Antibodies to gliadin by ELISA as a screening test for childhood coeliac disease. *J Pediatr Gastroenterol Nutr* 1986;5:726–9.

114 Friis SU, Gudmand-Høyer E. Screening for coeliac disease in adults by simultaneous determination of IgA and IgG gliadin antibodies. *Scand J Gastroenterol* 1986;21:1058–62.

115 Montgomery AMP, Goka AKJ, Kumar PJ, Farthing MJG, Clark ML. Low gluten diet in the treatment of adult coeliac disease: Effect on jejunal morphology and serum antigluten antibodies. *Gut* 1988;29:1564–8.

116 Kelly J, Feighery CF, Weir DG. Biotin-streptavidin ELISA: A sensitive, standardised assay for serum antigliadin IgA in coeliac disease. *Gastroenterology* 1988;94:A221.

117 Bürgin-Wolff A, Berger R, Gaze H, Huber H, Lentze MJ, Nussle D. IgG, IgA and IgE gliadin antibody determinations as screening test for untreated coeliac disease in children, a multicentre study. *Eur J Pediatr* 1989;148:496–502.

118 Scott H, Fausa O, Ek J, Valnes K, Blystad L, Brandtzaeg P. Measurements of serum IgA and IgG activities to dietary antigens: A prospective study of their diagnostic usefulness in adult coeliac disease. *Scand J Gastroenterol* 1990;25:287–92.

119 Scott H, Ek J, Havnen J *et al.* Serum antibodies to dietary antigens: A prospective study of the diagnostic usefulness in coeliac disease of children. *J Pediatr Gastroenterol Nutr* 1990;11:215–20.

120 Heiner DC, Lahey ME, Wilson JF, Gerrard JW, Shwachman H, Shaw KT. Precipitins to

antigens of wheat and cow's milk in celiac disease. *J Pediatr* 1962;61:813–30.
121 Kievel RM, Kearns DH, Liebowitz D. Significance of antibodies to dietary proteins in the serums of patients with nontropical sprue. *N Engl J Med* 1964;271:762–72.
122 Eterman KP, Hekkens WThJM, Peña AS, Lems van Kahn PH, Feltkamp TEW. Wheat grains: A substrate for the determination of gluten antibodies in serum of gluten sensitive patients. *J Immunol Methods* 1977; 14:85–92.
123 Eterman KP, Feltkamp TEW. Antibodies to gluten and reticulin in gastrointestinal disease. *Clin Exp Immunol* 1978;31:92–9.
124 Unsworth DJ, Manuel PD, Walker-Smith JA, Campbell CA, Johnson GD, Holborow EJ. New immunofluorescent blood test for gluten sensitivity. *Arch Dis Child* 1981; 56:864–8.
125 Savilahti E, Viander M, Perkkiö M, Vaino E, Kalimo K, Reunala T. IgA antigliadin antibodies: A marker of mucosal damage in childhood coeliac disease. *Lancet* 1983;i: 320–2.
126 Cornell HJ. Circulating antibodies to wheat gliadin fractions in coeliac disease. *Arch Dis Child* 1974;49:454–8.
127 Stern M, Fischer K, Grüttner R. Immunofluorescent serum gliadin antibodies in children with coeliac disease and various malabsorptive disorders. II. Specificity of gliadin antibodies: Immunoglobulin classes, immunogenic properties of wheat protein fractions, and pathogenic significance of food antibodies in coeliac disease. *Eur J Pediatr* 1979;130:165–72.
128 Bürgin-Wolff A, Hernandez R, Just M, Signer E. Immunofluorescent antibodies against gliadin: a screening test for coeliac disease. *Helv Paediatr Acta* 1976;31:375–80.
129 Bahna SL, Tateno K, Heiner D. Elevated IgD antibodies to wheat in celiac disease. *Ann Allergy* 1980;44:146–51.
130 Rawcliffe PM, Jewell DP, Faux JA. Specific IgG subclass antibodies, IgE, and IgG S-TS antibodies to wheat gluten fraction B in patients with coeliac disease. *Clin Allergy* 1985;15:155–62.
131 Cacciari E, Volta U, Lazzari R *et al.* Can antigliadin antibody detect symptomless coeliac disease in children with short stature? *Lancet* 1985;i:1469–71.
132 Troncone R, Pignata C, Farris E, Ciccimarra F. A solid-phase radioimmunoassay for IgG gliadin antibodies using ^{125}I-labelled staphylococcal protein A. *J Immunol Methods* 1983;63:163–70.
133 Ciclitira PJ, Ellis HJ, Evans DJ. A solid-phase radioimmunoassay for measurement of circulating antibody titres to wheat gliadin and its subfractions in patients with adult coeliac disease. *J Immunol Methods* 1983;62:231–9.
134 Kalimo K, Vaino E. Wheat grain immunofluorescent antibodies as an indication of gluten sensitivity? *Br J Dermatol* 1980; 103:657–61.
135 Rosenthal E, Golan DT, Benderly A, Shmuel Z, Levy J. Immunofluorescent antigluten antibody test titer and profile of gluten antibodies in celiac disease. *Am J Dis Child* 1984;138:659–62.
136 Blazer S, Naveh Y, Berant M, Merzbach D, Sperber S. Serum IgG antibodies to gliadin in children with celiac disease as measured by an immunoflourescence method. *J Pediatr Gastroenterol Nutr* 1984;3:205–9.
137 Kieffer M, Frazier PJ, Daniels NWR, Ciclitira PJ, Coombs RRA. Serum antibodies (measured by MRSPAH) to alcohol-soluble gliadins in adult coeliac patients. *J Immunol Methods* 1981;42:129–36.
138 Wulff HR. *Rational Diagnosis and Treatment.* Oxford: Blackwell Scientific Publications, 1976:78–100.
139 Khoshoo V, Bahn MK, Puri S *et al.* Serum anti-gliadin antibody profile in childhood protracted diarrhoea due to coeliac disease and other causes in a developing country. *Scand J Gastroenterol* 1989;24:1212–16.
140 Scott H, Ek J, Brandtzaeg P. Changes of serum antibody activities to various dietary antigens related to gluten withdrawal or challenge in children with coeliac disease. *Int Arch Allergy Appl Immunol* 1985;76: 138–44.
141 Kilander AF, Nilsson LÅ, Gillberg R. Serum antibodies to gliadin in coeliac disease after gluten withdrawal. *Scand J Gastroenterol* 1987;22:29–34.
142 Mawhinney H, Love AHG. The immunoglobulin class response to oral poliovaccine in coeliac disease. *Clin Exp Immunol* 1975; 21:399–406.
143 Leigh RJ, Marsh MN, Crowe P, Kelly C, Garner V, Gordon D. Studies of intestinal lymphoid tissue. IX. Dose-dependent, gluten-induced lymphoid infiltration of coeliac jejunal epithelium. *Scand J Gastroenterol* 1985;20:715–19.
144 Urbanek R. IgG subclasses and subclass

distribution in allergic disorders. *Monogr Allergy* 1988;23:33–40.
145 Hvatum M, Scott H, Brandtzaeg P. Serum subclass antibodies to a variety of food antigens in patients with coeliac disease. *Gut* 1992;33:632–38.
146 Husby S, Foged N, Oxelius VA, Svehag SE. Serum subclass antibodies to gliadin and other dietary antigens in children with coeliac disease. *Clin Exp Immunol* 1986; 64:526–35.
147 Kemeny DM, Urbanek R, Amlot PL, Ciclitira PJ, Richards D, Lessof MH. Subclass of IgG in allergic disease. 1. IgG subclass antibodies in immediate and non-immediate food allergy. *Clin Allergy* 1986; 16:571–81.
148 Barnes RMR, Harvey MM, Blears J, Finn R, Johnson PM. IgG subclass of human serum antibodies reactive with dietary proteins. *Int Arch Allergy Appl Immunol* 1986;81: 141–7.
149 Ciclitira PJ, Ellis HJ, Richards D, Kemeny DM. Gliadin IgG subclass antibodies in patients with coeliac disease. *Int Arch Allergy Appl Immunol* 1986;80:258–61.
150 Aalberse RC, van der Gaag R, Leeuwen J. Serologic aspects of IgG4 antibodies. 1. Prolonged immunization results in an IgG4 restricted response. *J Immunol* 1983;130: 722–6.
151 Halpern GM, Scott JR. Non-IgE antibody mediated mechanisms in food allergy. *Ann Allergy* 1987;58:14–27.
152 Van der Giessen M, Homan WL, Van Kernebeek G, Alberse RC, Dieges PH. Subclass typing of IgG antibodies formed by grass pollen-allergic patients during immune therapy. *Int Arch Allergy Appl Immunol* 1976;50:625–40.
153 Kemp M, Husby S, Larsen ML, Svehag SE. ELISA analysis of IgA subclass antibodies to dietary antigens. Elevated IgA1 antibodies in children with coeliac disease. *Int Arch Allergy Appl Immunol* 1988;87:247–53.
154 Mascart-Lemone F, Cadranel S, Van den Broeck J, Dive C, Vaerman JP, Duchateau J. IgA immune response patterns to gliadin in serum. *Int Arch Allergy Appl Immunol* 1988;86:412–19.
155 Mascart-Lemone F, Cadranel S, Delacroix DL, Duchateau J, Vaerman JP. Changes in molecular size of antigliadin IgA in serum related to presence of antigen in the gut. *Monogr Allergy* 1988;24:310–14.
156 Delacroix DL, Elkon KB, Geubel AP, Hodgson HF, Dive C, Vaerman JP. Changes in size, subclass and metabolic properties of serum immunoglobulin A in liver diseases and in other diseases with high serum immunoglobulin A. *J Clin Invest* 1983;71: 358–67.
157 Patey AL. Gliadin: the protein mixture toxic to coeliac patients. *Lancet* 1974;i:722–3.
158 Woychik JH, Boundy JA, Dimler RJ. Starch gel electrophoresis of wheat gluten proteins with concentrated urea. *Arch Biochem Biophys* 1961;94:477–82.
159 Bietz JA, Wall JS. Wheat gluten subunits: Molecular weight determined by sodium dodecyl sulphate-polyacrylamide gel electrophoresis. *Cereal Chem* 1972;49:416–30.
160 Brown JWS, Flavell RB. Fractionation of wheat gliadin and glutenin subunits by two-dimensional electrophoresis and the role of group 2 and group 6 chromosomes in gliadin synthesis. *Theor Appl Genet* 1981;59: 349–59.
161 Kieffer M, Frazier PJ, Daniels NWR, Coombs RRA. Wheat gliadin fractions and other cereal antigens reactive with antibodies in the sera of coeliac patients. *Clin Exp Immunol* 1982;50:651–60.
162 Levenson SD, Austin RK, Dietler MD, Kasarda DD, Kagnoff MF. Specificity of antigliadin antibody in coeliac disease. *Gastroenterology* 1985;89:1–5.
163 Friis SU, Noren O, Sjöström M, Gudmand-Höyer E. Patients with coeliac disease have a characteristic gliadin antibody pattern. *Clin Chim Acta* 1986;155:133–41.
164 Vaino E. Immunoblotting analysis of anti-gliadin antibodies in the sera of patients with dermatitis herpetiformis and gluten sensitive enteropathy. *Int Arch Allergy Appl Immunol* 1986;80:157–64.
165 Skerritt JH, Johnson RB, Hetzel PA, La Brooy JT, Shearman DJ, Davidson GP. Variation of serum and intestinal gluten antibody specificities in coeliac disease. *Clin Exp Immunol* 1987;68:189–99.
166 Devery JM, La Brooy JT, Krilis S, Davidson G, Skerritt JH. Anti-gliadin antibody specificity for gluten-derived peptides toxic to coeliac patients. *Clin Exp Immunol* 1989; 76:384–90.
167 Frazer AC, Fletcher RF, Ross AC, Shaw B, Sammons MG, Schneider R. Gluten-induced enteropathy, the effect of partially digested gluten. *Lancet* 1959;i:252–5.
168 Cornell HJ, Townley RR. The toxicity of certain cereal proteins in coeliac disease.

Gut 1974;15:862–9.

169 Douglas AP. The binding of a glycopeptide component of wheat gluten to intestinal mucosa of normal and coeliac human subjects. *Clin Chim Acta* 1976;73:357–61.

170 Wieser H, Belitz HD, Ashkenazi A. Amino acid sequence of the coeliac active gluten peptide B3142. *Z Lebensmu Forsch* 1984; 179:371–6.

171 Kagnoff MF, Austin RK, Hubert JJ, Bernardin JE, Kasarda DD. Possible role of a human adenovirus in the pathogenesis of coeliac disease. *J Exp Med* 1984;160:1544–57.

172 Weiser MM, Douglas AP. An alternative mechanism for gluten toxicity in coeliac disease. *Lancet* 1976;i:567–9.

173 Köttgen E, Volk B, Kluge F, Gerok W. Gluten, a lectin with oligomannosyl specificity and the causative agent of gluten-sensitive enteropathy. *Biochem Biophys Res Commun* 1982;109:168–73.

174 Auricchio S, de Ritis G, de Vincenzi M *et al.* Agglutinating activity of gliadin-derived peptides from white bread: Implications for coeliac disease pathogenesis. *Biochem Biophys Res Commun* 1984;121: 428–33.

175 Kolberg J, Sollid L. Lectin activity of gluten identified as wheat germ agglutinin. *Biochem Biophys Res Commun* 1985;130: 867–72.

176 Sollid LM, Kolberg J, Scott H, Ek J, Fausa O, Brandtzaeg P. Antibodies to wheat germ agglutinin in coeliac disease. *Clin Exp Immunol* 1986;63:95–100.

177 Lorenzsonn V, Olsen WA. *In vivo* response of rat intestinal epithelium to intraluminal dietary lectins. *Gastroenterology* 1982;82: 838–48.

178 Sjolander A, Magnusson KE, Latkovic S. The effect of concanavalin A and wheat germ agglutinin on the ultrastructure and permeability of rat intestine. *Int Arch Allergy Appl Immunol* 1984;75:230–6.

179 Hamilton I, Cobden I, Rothwell JR, Axon ATR. Intestinal permeability in coeliac disease: The response to gluten withdrawal and single dose-gluten challenge. *Gut* 1982; 23:202–10.

180 Bjarnason I, Peters TJ, Veall N. A persistent defect in intestinal permeability in coeliac disease demonstrated by a ^{51}Cr-labelled EDTA absorption test. *Lancet* 1983;i: 323–5.

181 Brady PG, Vannier AM, Banwell JG. Identification of the dietary lectin, wheat germ agglutinin, in human intestinal contents. *Gastroenterology* 1978;75:236–42.

182 Boldt DH, Dorsey SA. Interactions of lectins and monoclonal antibodies with human mononuclear cells. 1. Specific inhibition of OKT4 and OKT8 binding by Ricinus communis agglutinin and wheat germ agglutinin. *J Immunol* 1983;130:1645–53.

183 Kagnoff MF, Paterson YJ, Kumar PJ *et al.* Evidence for the role of a human intestinal adenovirus in the pathogenesis of coeliac disease. *Gut* 1987;28:995–1001.

184 Howdle PD, Blair Zaidel ME, Smart CJ, Trejdosiewicz LK, Blair GE, Losowsky MS. Adenovirus 12 infection and coeliac disease. *Scand J Gastroenterol* 1989;24:282–6.

185 Carter MJ, Willcocks MM, Mitchinson HC, Record CO, Madley CR. Is a persistent adenovirus infection involved in coeliac disease? *Gut* 1989;30:1563–7.

186 Beale AJ, Parish WE, Douglas AP, Hobbs JR. Impaired IgA responses in coeliac disease. *Lancet* 1971;i:1198–200.

187 Pettingale KW. Immunoglobulin and specific antibody responses to antigenic stimulation in adult coeliac disease. *Clin Sci* 1970;38:16P.

188 Seah PP, Fry L, Rossiter MA, Hoffbrand AV, Holborow EJ. Anti-reticulin antibodies in childhood coeliac disease. *Lancet* 1971;ii: 681–2.

189 Rizzetto M, Doniach D. Types of reticulin antibodies detected in human sera by immunofluorescence. *J Clin Pathol* 1973;26: 841–51.

190 Magalhaes AFN, Peters TJ, Doe WF. Studies on the nature and significance of connective tissue antibodies in adult coeliac disease and Crohn's disease. *Gut* 1974;15:284–8.

191 Unsworth DJ, Walker-Smith JA, Holborow EJ. Gliadin and reticulin antibodies in childhood coeliac disease. *Lancet* 1983;i: 874–5.

192 Von Essen R, Savilahti E, Pelkonen P. Reticulin antibody in children with malabsorption. *Lancet* 1972;i:1157–9.

193 Seah PP, Fry L, Holborow EJ *et al.* Anti-reticulin antibody: Incidence and diagnostic significance. *Gut* 1973;14:311–15.

194 Eade OE, Lloyd RS, Lang C, Wright R. IgA and IgG reticulin antibodies in coeliac and non-coeliac patients. *Gut* 1977;18:991–3.

195 Mäki M, Hällström O, Vesikari T, Visakorpi K. Evaluation of a serum IgA-class reticulin antibody test for the detection of childhood celiac disease. *J Pediatr* 1984;105:901–5.

196 Monteiro E, Menezes ML, Ramalho P. Antireticulin antibodies: A diagnostic and monitoring test for childhood coeliac disease. *Scand J Gastroenterol* 1986;21:955–7.
197 Khoshoo V, Bhan MK, Unsworth DJ, Kumar PJ, Walker-Smith JA. Anti-reticulin antibodies: Useful adjunct to histopathology in diagnosing celiac disease, especially in a developing country. *J Pediatr Gastroenterol Nutr* 1988;7:864–6.
198 Hällström O. Comparison of IgA class reticulin and endomysium antibodies in coeliac disease and dermatitis herpetiformis. *Gut* 1989;30:1225–32.
199 Unsworth DJ, Scott DL, Almond TJ, Beard HK, Holborow EJ, Walton KW. Studies on reticulin. 1. Serological and immunohistological investigation of the occurrence of collagen type III, fibronectin and the non-collagenous glycoprotein of Pras and Glynn in reticulin. *Br J Exp Pathol* 1982;63: 154–66.
200 Pras M, Johnson GD, Holborow EJ, Glynn LE. Antigenic properties of a non-collageneous reticulin component of normal connective tissue. *Immunology* 1974;27: 469–85.
201 Unsworth DJ, Holborow EJ. Does the reticulin binding property of cereal proteins demonstrable *in vitro* have pathogenetic significance for coeliac disease? *Gut* 1985; 26:1204–9.
202 Williamson N, Housley J, McCormick JN. An antibody to renal glomeruli, synovial membrane and reticulin found in rheumatoid arthritic sera. *Ann Rheum Dis* 1967; 26:348–9.
203 Teppo AM, Maury CPJ. Enzyme immunoassay of antibodies to epithelial glycoprotein: Increased level of antibodies in coeliac disease. *J Immunol Methods* 1984;74: 327–36.
204 Teppo AM, Maury CPJ. Antibodies to gliadin, gluten and reticulin glycoprotein in rheumatic diseases: Elevated levels in Sjøgren's syndrome. *Clin Exp Immunol* 1984;57:73–8.
205 Teppo AM, Mäki M, Hallström O, Maury CP. Antibodies to 90 kilodalton glycoprotein in childhood and adolescent coeliac disease: Relationship to reticulin antibodies. *J Pediatr Gastroenterol Nutr* 1987;6:908–14.
206 Chorzelski TP, Sulej T, Tchorzewska H, Jablonska S, Beutner EH, Kumar V. IgA class endomysium antibodies in dermatitis herpetiformis and celiac disease. In: Beutner EH, Nisengard RJ, Albini B, eds. *Defined Immunofluorescence and Related Cytochemical Methods. Ann N Y Acad Sci* 1983;420:325–34.
207 Chorzelski TP, Beutner EH. Factors contributing to occasional failures in demonstration of pemphigus antibodies by the immunofluorescence test. *J Invest Dermatol* 1969;53:188–91.
208 Fiebelman C, Stolzner G, Provost TT. Superior sensitivity of monkey oesophagus in the determination of pemphigus antibody. *Arch Dermatol* 1981;117:561–2.
209 Judd KP, Lever WJ. Correlation of antibodies in skin and serum with disease severity in phemphigus. *Arch Dermatol* 1979;115: 428–32.
210 Chorzelski TP, Beutner EH, Sulej J *et al.* IgA anti-endomysium antibody: A new immunological marker of dermatitis herpetiformis and coeliac disease. *Br J Dermatol* 1984;111:395–402.
211 Beutner EH, Chorzelski TP, Kumar V, Leonard J, Krasny S. Sensitivity and specificity of IgA class antiendomysial antibodies for dermatitis herpetiformis and findings relevant to their pathogenic significance. *J Am Acad Dermatol* 1986;15:464–73.
212 Kapuscinska A, Zalewski T, Chorzelski TP *et al.* Disease specificity and dynamics of changes in IgA class anti-endomysial antibodies in celiac disease. *J Pediatr Gastroenterol Nutr* 1987;6:529–34.
213 Rossi TM, Kumar V, Lerner A, Heitlinger LA, Tucker N, Fisher J. Relationship of endomysial antibodies to jejunal mucosal pathology: Specificity towards both symptomatic and asymptomatic celiacs. *J Pediatr Gastroenterology Nutr* 1988;7:858–63.
214 Kumar V, Lerner A, Valeski JE, Beutner EH, Chorzelski TP, Rossi T. Endomysial antibodies in the diagnosis of celiac disease and the effect of gluten on antibody titers. *Immunol Invest* 1989;18:533–44.
215 Acetta P, Kumar V, Beutner EH, Chorzelski TP, Helm F. Anti-endomysium antibodies: A serological marker of dermatitis herpetiformis. *Arch Dermatol* 1986;122:459–62.
216 Kühn G, Chorzelski TP, Sulej J, Jablonska S. Zur klinischen Bedeutung des Endomysium-Autoantikörpers vom IgA-Typ in der Dermatologie. *Dermatol Monatschr* 1987;173:377–89.
217 Beutner EH, Kumar V, Chorzelski TP, Szaflarska-Czerwionka M. IgG endomysium antibodies in IgA deficient patients with

coeliac disease. *Lancet* 1989;i:1261–2.
218 Chorzelski TP, Rosinska D, Beutner EH, Sulej J, Kumar V. Aggressive gluten challenge of dermatitis herpetiformis cases converts them from seronegative to seropositive for IgA-class endomysial antibodies. *J Am Acad Dermatol* 1989;18:672–8.
219 Doe WF, Booth CC, Brown DL. Evidence for complement-binding immune complexes in adult coeliac disease, Crohn's disease and ulcerative colitis. *Lancet* 1973;i:402–3.
220 Mowbray JF, Hoffbrand AV, Holborow EJ, Seah PP, Fry L. Circulating immune complexes in dermatitis herpetiformis. *Lancet* 1973;i:400–2.
221 Mohammed I, Holborow EJ, Fry L, Thompson BR, Hoffbrand AV, Stewart JS. Multiple immune complexes and hypocomplementaemia in dermatitis herpetiformis and coeliac disease. *Lancet* 1976;ii: 487–90.
222 Husby S, Foged N, Høst A, Svehag SE. Passage of dietary antigens into the blood of children with coeliac disease. Quantification and size distribution of absorbed antigens. *Gut* 1987;28:1062–72.
223 Yancey KB, Cason JC, Russel BS, Hall P, Lawley TJ. Dietary gluten challenge does not influence the levels of circulating immune complexes in patients with dermatitis herpetiformis. *J Invest Dermatol* 1983;80: 468–72.
224 Zone JJ, La Salle BS, Provost TT. Induction of IgA circulating immune complexes after wheat feeding in dermatitis herpetiformis patients. *J Invest Dermatol* 1982;78: 375–80.
225 Hall RP, Lawley T. Characterization of circulating and cutaneous IgA immune complexes in patients with dermatitis herpetiformis. *J Immunol* 1985;135:1760–5.
226 Egelrud T, Bäck O. Dermatitis herpetiformis: Biochemical properties of the granular deposits of IgA in papillary dermis. Characterization of SDS-soluble IgA like material and potentially antigen binding IgA fragments released by pepsin. *J Invest Dermatol* 1985;84:329–45.
227 Lane AT, Huff JC, Weston WL. Detection of gluten in human sera by an enzyme immunoassay: Comparison of dermatitis herpetiformis and coeliac disease patients with normal controls. *J Invest Dermatol* 1982;79:186–9.
228 Maury CPJ, Teppo AM. Demonstration of tissue 90 kD glycoprotein as antigen in circulating IgG immune complexes in dermatitis herpetiformis and coeliac disease. *Lancet* 1984;ii:892–4.
229 Bayless TM, Yardley JH, Hendrix TR. Coeliac disease and possible disease relationships. In: Hekkens WThJM, Pena AS, eds. *Coeliac Disease.* Leiden: Stenfert Kroese, 1974:351–9.
230 Nagy J, Scott H, Brandtzaeg P. Antibodies to dietary antigens in IgA nephropathy. *Clin Nephrol* 1988;29:275–9.
231 Mäki M, Hälström O, Verronen P *et al.* Reticulin antibody, arthritis and coeliac disease in children. *Lancet* 1988;i:479–80.
232 Weiss JB, Austin RK, Scanfield MS, Kagnoff MF. Gluten sensitive enteropathy immunoglobulin G heavy-chain (Gm) allotypes and the immune response to wheat gliadin. *J Clin Invest* 1983;72:96–101.
233 Carbonara AO, DeMarchi M, Van Loghem E, Ansaldi N. Gm markers in celiac disease. *Hum Immunol* 1983;6:91–5.
234 Fredric AJ, Pandey IP, Verkasalo M, Teppo AM, Fudenberg HH. Immunoglobulin allotypes and the immune response to wheat gliadin in a Finnish population with celiac disease. *Exp Clin Immunogenet* 1985;2: 185–90.
235 Kagnoff MF, Weiss JB, Brown RJ, Lee T, Schanfield MS. Immunoglobulin allotype markers in gluten-sensitive enteropathy. *Lancet* 1983;i:952–3.
236 Barbera C, Fusco P, Ansaldi N, De Marchi M, Carbonara A. HLA and antigluten antibodies in children with coeliac disease. *Diagn Clin Immunol* 1987;5:158–61.
237 Mearin ML, Koninckx CR, Biemond I, Polanco I, Pena AS. Influence of genetic factors on the serum levels of antigliadin antibodies in celiac disease. *J Pediatr Gastroenterol Nutr* 1984;3:373–7.
238 Malizia G, Trejdosiewicz LK, Wood GM, Howdle PD, Janossy G, Losowsky MS. The microenvironment of coeliac disease: T cell phenotypes and expression of the T2 'T blast' antigen by small bowel lymphocytes. *Clin Exp Immunol* 1985;60:437–46.
239 Marsh MN. Studies of intestinal lymphoid tissue. XI. The immunopathology of cell mediated reactions in gluten sensitivity and other enteropathies. *Scanning Microsc* 1988;2:1663–84.
240 O'Garra A. Interleukins and the immune system 1. *Lancet* 1989;i:943–6.
241 O'Garra A. Interleukins and the immune system 2. *Lancet* 1989;i:1003–5.

242 MacDonald TT, Spencer J. Evidence that activated mucosal T cells play a role in the pathogenesis of enteropathy in human small intestine. *J Exp Med* 1988;167:1342–9.

243 Madara JL, Stafford J. Interferon γ directly affects barrier function of cultured intestinal epithelial monolayers. *J Clin Invest* 1989; 83:724–7.

244 Scott H, Brandtzaeg P, Solheim BG, Thorsby E. Relation between HLA-DR-like antigens and secretory component (SC) in jejunal epithelium of patients with coeliac disease or dermatitis herpetiformis. *Clin Exp Immunol* 1981;44:233–8.

245 Arnaud-Battandier F, Cerf-Bensussan N, Amsellem R, Schmitz J. Increased HLA-DR expression by enterocytes in children with celiac disease. *Gastroenterology* 1986;91: 1206–12.

246 Scott H, Sollid LM, Fausa O, Brandtzaeg P, Thorsby E. Expression of MHC class II subregion products by jejunal epithelium of patients with coeliac disease. *Scand J Immunol* 1987;26:563–72.

247 Marley NJE, Macartney JC, Ciclitira PJ, HLA-DR, DP and DQ expression in the small intestine of patients with coeliac disease. *Clin Exp Immunol* 1987;70:386–93.

248 Brandtzaeg P, Tolo K. Mucosal penetrability enhanced by serum-derived antibodies. *Nature* 1977;266:262–3.

249 Lim P, Rowley D. The effect of antibody on the intestinal absorption of macromolecules and on intestinal permeability in adult mice. *Int Arch Allergy Appl Immunol* 1982;66:41–6.

250 Ochs HD, Wedgwood RJ. Disorders of the B-cell system. In: Stiehm ER, ed. *Immunologic Disorders in Infants and Children.* Philadelphia: WB Saunders, 1989:226–56.

Chapter 10/T cell-mediated intestinal injury

THOMAS T. MacDONALD

Introduction

The intestinal tract contains large numbers of T cells in the organized lymphoid structures (Peyer's patches, colonic lymphoglandular structures), the lamina propria and between the absorptive epithelial cells [1] (Fig. 10.1). Thus, the cellular apparatus for the induction and expression of a cell-mediated immune response lies in close proximity to the dietary and bacterial antigens of the intestinal lumen, separated only by a single layer of epithelial cells. In general, T cell-mediated immune reactions are frequently accompanied by tissue damage, either due to direct cytotoxicity or the recruitment of non-specific effector cells into the tissues. T cell-mediated hypersensitivity reactions to dietary and bacterial antigens may be responsible for the pathology in

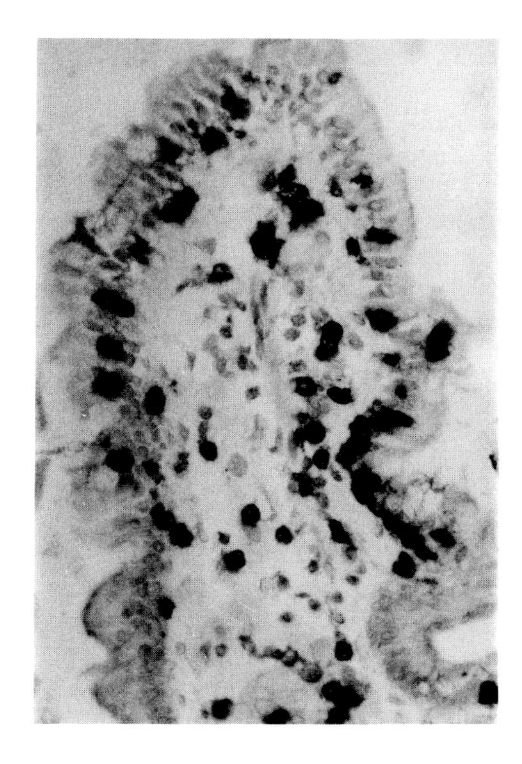

Fig. 10.1 $CD3^+$ T cells in the lamina propria and epithelium of normal human jejunum. (Immunoperoxidase, original magnification ×100.)

a number of important human diseases. In particular it is likely that coeliac disease (CD) is a consequence of a mucosal cell-mediated response to gluten. Although gluten-reactive T cells have not yet been isolated from the mucosa of patients with CD, the striking similarity between the villous atrophy and crypt hypertrophy of untreated coeliac mucosa and the lesions in models of intestinal cell-mediated hypersensitivity is one of the main lines of evidence implicating T cells in the pathogenesis of this disease (see p. 137).

Mechanisms of T cell immunity and tissue injury

T cells mediate immunity and hypersensitivity in two ways. Firstly, antigen stimulated T cells can secrete lymphokines initiating a cascade of cellular and molecular events which result in the recruitment of non-specific effector cells such as macrophages and granulocytes into the tissues. This is usually but not exclusively a property of $CD4^+$, $\alpha\beta$ T cell receptor (TCR) positive T cells. The accessory cells infiltrating the tissues then release mediators (e.g. interleukin 1 and tumour necrosis factor α (TNFα) from macrophages and LTB4 from neutrophils) which damage the surrounding cells and tissues. Secondly, activated T cells (usually $CD8^+$, $\alpha\beta$ TCR^+) can recognize peptides presented on the cell surface in association with major histocompatibility complex (MHC) molecules and lyse the cell (cytotoxicity). Tissue damage in this case is due to direct cell death although cytotoxic cells can also release lymphokines to recruit non-specific effector cells into the tissues. The relative contribution of each of these types of responses is difficult to evaluate in the intestine, but certainly most epithelial $CD8^+$ T cells appear to be cytotoxic cells [2] whereas lamina propria $CD4^+$ T cells can secrete lymphokines [3].

A minority of T cells in the blood and intestine utilize the $\gamma\delta$ form of the TCR [4–7]. The nature of the antigens recognized by these cells is not clearly understood although functionally they usually have non-MHC-linked cytotoxic activity [8,9]. These cells accumulate in chronic infectious lesions such as leishmaniasis and leprosy [10] and in the epithelium in untreated CD but it is not known if they can mediate tissue damage *in vivo*. Mast cells have traditionally been associated with Type 1, IgE-mediated hypersensitivity responses. Recently, however, it has been shown that mast cells can release lymphokines such as interleukin 2 and interleukin 4, and TNFα [11,12]. Thus, mast cells also have the potential to participate in cell-mediated immune responses.

T cell populations in the intestinal mucosa

Phenotypically, there are three main T cell populations in the intestinal

Table 10.1 Cell subpopulations in the normal human intestinal mucosa. (Adapted from [3,6,7,13,61])

	Epithelium (%)	Lamina propria (%)
$CD3^+$, $CD4^+$	10	80
$CD3^+$, $CD8^+$	80	20
$CD3^+$, $CD4^-$, 8^-	6	<1
$CD3^-$, $CD7^+$	12	<1
$CD3^+$, αβ TCR^+	90	>99
$CD3^+$, γδ TCR^+	10	<1

mucosa: $CD4^+$ αβ TCR^+ T cells in the lamina propria; $CD8^+$ αβ TCR^+ T cells in the epithelium; and the γδ TCR^+ T cells in the epithelium which may be $CD8^+$ or $CD8^-$ (reviewed in [1]). The proportion of γδ TCR^+ intraepithelial lymphocytes (IEL) varies considerably between species. In rodents they make up about 30–70% of IEL but in humans they constitute only 0–30% of IEL [13].

The αβ TCR^+ T cells in the mucosa (both $CD4^+$ cells in the lamina propria and $CD8^+$ cells in the epithelium) are derived from T cells in the Peyer's patches. Germ-free adult mice which lack a bacterial flora have virtually no αβ TCR^+ T cells in the intestinal mucosa [14]. After colonization with gut bacteria, there is T cell stimulation in the Peyer's patches and the number of αβ TCR^+ IEL increases dramatically (B. DeGeus, personal communication). Cell transfer and selective depletion experiments have also shown that Peyer's patch and mesenteric lymph node T cell blasts migrate to the gut mucosa [15]. Other experiments have shown that antigen-stimulated T blasts can migrate to the gut epithelium. For instance, after infection of murine Peyer's patch with reovirus, specific cytotoxic αβ TCR^+ T cell precursors can be detected in IEL [16]. The γδ TCR^+ IEL in mice do not come from the thymus but instead migrate from the bone marrow directly to the epithelium [17,18]. Although germ-free mice have only a few IEL, most of them are γδ TCR^+ [14], indicating that the tropism of γδ TCR^+ for the gut epithelium is largely antigen independent. This may also be the case in humans since higher frequencies of γδ TCR^+ IEL are seen in the human foetus than in post-natal intestine [7]. The function of γδ TCR^+ IEL in the gut in health and disease is still unknown. Table 10.1 summarizes the main mucosal T cell populations.

The role of Peyer's patches in intestinal damage

There have been many studies on Peyer's patches in animals, but few studies have been carried out in humans. The reason for this is mainly technical. Peyer's patches, in rodents, are visible as discrete structures from the serosal aspect, whereas in humans they are not readily visualized macroscopically in unfixed tissue [19]. It is not known if Peyer's patch T cells become sensitized to dietary antigens in the food sensitive enteropathies, the cells then migrating to the mucosa and mediating tissue damaging cell-mediated immune reactions when they re-encounter specific antigens. There is, however, some evidence that Peyer's patches and their equivalent in the colon (the lymphoglandular structures) are the site of the early lesion in Crohn's disease [20]. Endoscopically, small aphthous ulcers overlying lymphoid follicles are seen in early Crohn's disease, and in histological sections, the follicle-associated epithelium and dome are the site of the ulceration [21]. Whether the ulceration of Peyer's patches in Crohn's disease is due to an infectious agent or host hypersensitivity response to an enteric antigen is unknown.

Immune deficiency and intestinal injury

One major problem in the interpretation of immunopathological events in the gut is to distinguish between those responses which represent specific primary events and those which are non-specific secondary events. Many antibody responses to luminal food and bacterial antigens may be secondary to the damage effected by a primary cell-mediated immune lesion. Studies of intestinal disease in patients with the common humoral immune deficiencies are useful ways of determining the relative contributions of T cells and humoral events to tissue damage.

The most common immune deficiency is selective IgA deficiency. IgA itself does not appear to play a pathological role in any gut disease. There is a well-established increased incidence of CD in patients with IgA deficiency (see Chapter 9) indicating that IgA, rather than contributing to tissue damage, might protect the gut against gluten sensitization and its consequences, by immune exclusion. Selective IgA deficiency has also been described in association with chronic inflammatory bowel disease [22], but it is probably not a predisposing factor in these disorders.

Of more interest is the occurrence of intestinal disease in patients with common variable immune deficiency. In most of these patients there is a marked deficit in humoral immunity while T cell function is often normal. There is a single well-documented case of a patient with CD and hypogammaglobulinaemia, in whom mucosal plasma cells were absent, and no serum antigliadin antibodies were detectable [23]. Such an observation suggests that humoral immunity is not important in CD, despite the fact that there are strong mucosal and systemic antibody responses to gliadin in most coeliacs (reviewed in [24]). A regional enteritis, with many of the features of Crohn's disease, has been described in a small number of hypogammaglobulinaemic patients

[25]. In a recent case report [26], a patient with agammaglobulinaemia, absent mucosal plasma cells and a regional enteritis-like enteropathy associated with an increase in lamina propria $CD4^+$ T cells was described. The association of antibody deficiency and ulcerative colitis has also been described [27].

A common disorder in hypogammaglobulinaemic patients is a sprue-like disorder which is frequently associated with giardiasis [28]. In severe cases the mucosa becomes as flat as that seen in classical untreated CD. Some patients improve after chemotherapeutic elimination of the *Giardia* but in others broad spectrum antibiotics and passive administration of immunoglobulin is necessary. Unless the passively administered antibody contains specific anti-*Giardia* antibodies it is difficult to understand why this treatment should be effective in eliminating the *Giardia*. Nutritional support may also be needed. Although the pathogenesis of this condition is unknown, it serves to demonstrate that a flat mucosa can occur in the absence of humoral antibody.

Gastrointestinal diseases in patients with T cell defects have not been investigated since T cell deficiency is incompatible with long-term survival. However, some studies of intestinal pathology in T cell-deficient animals have been carried out. Worm infections in mice and rats are associated with villous atrophy and crypt hypertrophy. In T cell-deficient rats infected with *Nippostrongylus brasiliensis* [29] or T cell-deficient mice infected with *Trichinella spiralis* [30], the worms are not expelled from the gut and only minimal intestinal damage ensues. Thus, it is likely that the cell-mediated hypersensitivity response against the worm antigens causes the tissue damage, rather than the direct effects of the worms themselves.

Although it is difficult to tie all of these observations together, the balance of evidence suggests that CD and Crohn's disease can arise in patients with antibody deficiency conditions. It is likely therefore that cell-mediated immunity is of greater importance in the pathogenesis of these diseases than antibody responses which are likely to be secondary, and even inappropriate events.

Intestinal graft-versus-host disease

Mature T cells, injected into a genetically unresponsive recipient (parent→F1) or immunodeficient recipient, react to the host alloantigens and produce a variety of local and systemic disorders (graft-versus-host (GVH) disease). It has long been recognized that intestinal damage is a prominent feature of GVH disease in humans [31] and the mechanisms involved and the types of damage produced in the gut have been the subject of much interest in recent years. It is clear that the number and type of cells transferred to elicit the GVH response, as well as the

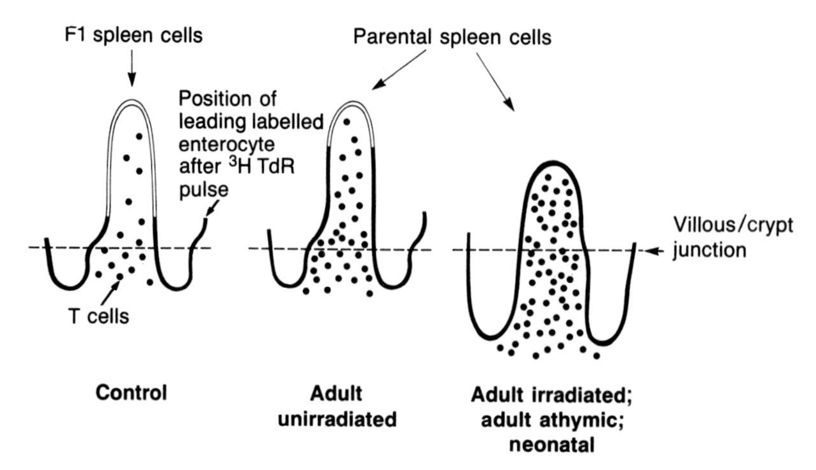

Fig. 10.2 The changes in the mucosa in different types of GVH disease. F1 spleen cells injected into a control F1 recipient produce no changes in mucosal morphology or the rate of epithelial renewal. Parental spleen cells injected into unirradiated adult F1 mice produce little structural change but do increase epithelial cell turnover. In contrast, in adult irradiated recipients, neonatal recipients and athymic recipients, GVH induces villous atrophy, crypt cell hyperplasia and a very large increase in epithelial turnover. ^{3}H-TdR, tritiated thymidine label.

type of recipient (neonate, irradiated adult, immunodeficient adult, normal adult), can influence the type of damage (Fig. 10.2). Injection of parental T cells into irradiated adult F1 recipients, athymic recipients or unirradiated F1 neonates produces an enteropathy consisting of villous atrophy, crypt cell hyperplasia, an increased cell migration along the villi and a mononuclear infiltrate into the lamina propria and epithelium [32–36] (Fig. 10.3). As the enteropathy progresses there is eventual epithelial cell necrosis and apoptosis [37]. There is also increased class 2 MHC expression on intestinal epithelial cells, presumably as the result of the local production of interferon-γ by alloreactive T cells in the mucosa [33].

In unirradiated adult F1 recipients of parental cells the intestinal damage is less pronounced. There is no villous destruction, crypt hypertrophy is not pronounced, but there is still increased crypt cell production and increased epithelial class 2 expression [33]. The epithelial cells which clothe the villus are derived from a number of crypts. During normal neonatal development in mouse intestine the crypt : villus ratio increases. In mice with GVH disease, however, this does not occur and the crypt : villus ratio remains constant, even though each crypt produces 5–10 times more epithelial cells than crypts in control mice [34].

The relative contribution of alloreactive CD4$^+$ and CD8$^+$ T cells to the development of enteropathy in GVH has also been investigated.

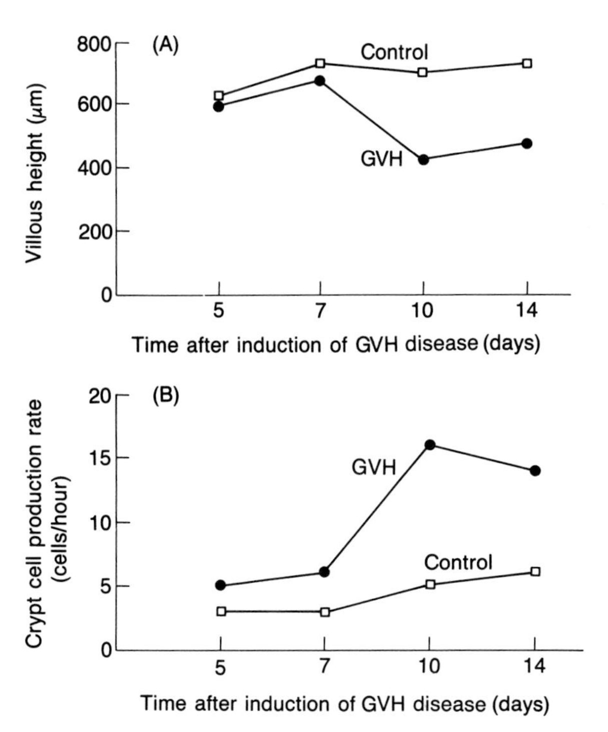

Fig. 10.3 Villous height (A) and crypt cell production rates (B) in baby F1 mice at various times after the induction of GVH disease by injection of parental spleen cells. By 10 days there is profound villous atrophy and crypt cell production rate has trebled. (Data adapted from MacDonald & Ferguson [34].)

Alloreactive $CD4^+$ T cells usually recognize class 2 MHC differences whereas $CD8^+$ T cells usually recognize class 1 MHC alloantigens. When GVH is elicited with unseparated T cells from a donor differing at either the class 1 or class 2 loci, enteropathy is seen only in class 2 incompatible strain combinations. This has been mapped to I-A of the murine MHC [37,38]. Class 1 incompatibility between donor and recipient does not result in intestinal GVH [37]. Since class 2 alloantigenic differences are usually recognized by $CD4^+$ T cells, these results suggest that it is this cell subset which causes gut damage in GVH. This indeed has been formally shown, in that in GVH across a full MHC mismatch, the donor $CD4^+$ T cells are much more effective at inducing gut damage, crypt cell hyperplasia, villous atrophy and an increased intraepithelial cell infiltrate than donor $CD8^+$ T cells [33]. Increasing the numbers of $CD8^+$ T cells injected also results in enteropathy [33] but this may be due to the effects of contaminating $CD4^+$ T cells, since $CD8^+$ T cell anticlass 1 responses need the collaboration of $CD4^+$ lymphokine secreting cells to undergo full clonal expansion.

Table 10.2 Villous atrophy and crypt hypertrophy in parental gut grafts syngeneic to the cells used to elicit the GVH response in an F1 recipient. (Adapted from [41])

	Parental gut graft	
	Villous height (μm)	Crypt depth (μm)
F1 cells → F1 recipient (control)	190±32	77±16
Parental cells → F1 recipient (GVH)	146±28	113±20

The mechanisms of tissue damage in GVH disease

It would seem clear that the gut damage in GVH must be attributable either directly or indirectly to the alloreactive T cells which infiltrate the mucosa. The gut changes could therefore be due to the effects of $CD8^+$ alloreactive cytotoxic cells or $CD4^+$ lymphokine secreting cells. The latter is more likely since this subset is the more effective at inducing intestinal GVH. Epithelial cell damage in GVH may be mediated by cytotoxic T cells, but alternatively it could be the result of cytotoxic lymphokines such as TNFα or β. After eliciting GVH with purified $CD4^+$ or $CD8^+$ T cells, Guy-Grand and Vassalli showed that the donor $CD8^+$ T cells in the gut mucosa were cytotoxic for recipient alloantigens whereas the mucosal $CD4^+$ T cells were not [33]. In addition, the $CD4^+$ T cells secreted lymphokines when stimulated with alloantigens whereas the mucosal $CD8^+$ T cells were relatively poor lymphokine producers [33]. This would suggest that the enteropathy in GVH produced by $CD4^+$ T cells is mediated by soluble factors rather than cytotoxicity. Indeed treatment of mice with anti-TNFα antiserum or anti-interferon-γ prevents GVH [39,40]. These experiments do not show that these mediators are responsible for the intestinal damage since in both cases antibody treatment prevented the intestinal lymphoid infiltrate.

Ingenious experiments to demonstrate that enteropathy could develop in the absence of a cytotoxic T cell response to epithelial cells were devised by Elson *et al.* [41]. Adult C57BL/6 × DBA/2 F1 mice received foetal intestinal grafts under the kidney capsule from C57BL/6 donors. GVH was then elicited with C57BL/6 spleen cells. Surprisingly, mucosal flattening and crypt hypertrophy were produced in the C57BL/6 grafts although the latter were syngeneic to the donor cells (Table 10.2). In this case the recipient target cells against which the donor T cells were reacting, probably comprised recipient blood-borne accessory cells which populate the lamina propria of the transplant [42]. This experiment also suggests that soluble factors, produced during the course of the GVH response, can cause intestinal mucosal damage in the absence of direct epithelial cytotoxicity.

Cell-mediated immune damage in transplanted allografts of intestine

Cell-mediated immune reactions are also responsible for the rejection of intestinal allografts. Transplantation of allografts of the intestine between unrelated dogs has been technically feasible since the 1960s. Twenty-four hours after transplantation, the allografts appear normal. By day 4 however, the lamina propria becomes increasingly infiltrated with mononuclear cells. As rejection progresses, the villi become shorter, the crypts longer with increased mitotic figures, and epithelial cell necrosis is apparent. Without immunosuppression the grafts are rejected with mucosal sloughing by 8 days [43]. Since rejection of first-set allografts is a purely T cell-mediated response with no contribution from humoral immunity, these studies gave credence to the notion that cell-mediated immunity might also be responsible for the villous atrophy and crypt hyperplasia seen in the jejunum in tropical and non-tropical sprue. More recent studies on intestinal allografts in children with short-bowel syndrome have shown similar findings to those in dogs (N. Cerf-Bensussan and N. Brousse, personal communication). During rejection phases, the mucosa becomes infiltrated with T cells and villous atrophy and crypt hypertrophy are seen. Successful immunotherapy to inhibit the rejection process reduces the mucosal infiltrate and mucosal morphology returns to near-normal.

Allograft rejection of foetal mouse small intestine heterotopically implanted under the kidney capsule provides a system wherein mucosal changes in transplanted intestine can be followed in detail. Since the transplanted intestine is foetal, it is antigen and bacteria-free [44], so that any changes seen may be entirely attributed to the rejection process and not to secondary infection. Mouse foetal intestine lacks T and B cells [45] so that any graft infiltrating cells must therefore be of recipient origin. In addition, strain combinations of MHC-compatible mice can be used in which rejection through minor transplantation antigens proceeds over an extended period, allowing detailed analysis of the evolution of epithelial changes.

Acute rejection between MHC disparate strains takes 8 days and shows many of the features seen in allograft rejection of transplanted canine intestine described above [46]. By day 4 of rejection, crypt hypertrophy is apparent in the allograft mucosa which increases until final rejection on day 8 (Fig. 10.4). There is also a progressive villous atrophy. Between MHC identical mouse strains, rejection takes 20 days [46]. This process is also characterized by crypt hypertrophy and a progressive villous atrophy in the allograft. Notable histological features

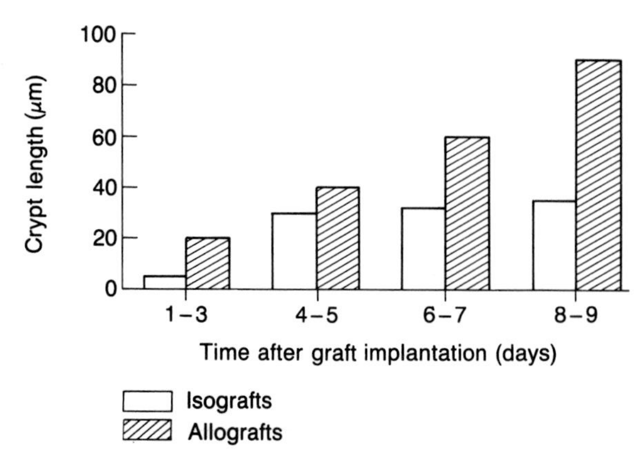

Fig. 10.4 Crypt hypertrophy during allograft rejection of foetal mouse small intestine. Balb/c mice received either isografts (Balb/c) or allografts (CBA) of foetal mouse small intestine implanted under the kidney capsule. At the times indicated tissues were sampled and crypt depth measured on histological sections. (Adapted from MacDonald & Ferguson [46].)

of rejection include a massive lamina propria mononuclear cell infiltrate and increase in IEL, some epithelial cell damage, absence of mucosal plasma cells, and absence of a neutrophil infiltrate. Intestinal allograft rejection is accompanied by a 10-fold increase in the rate of crypt epithelial cell proliferation [34].

These studies unequivocally show that a local cell-mediated response to histocompatibility antigens can result in the tissue changes of crypt hypertrophy and villous atrophy which characterize a number of bowel diseases, including CD, tropical sprue and giardiasis. The altered mucosal morphology and increased crypt cell proliferation are clearly adaptive responses to local cell-mediated tissue injury mediated by T cells infiltrating the transplanted tissue and responding to alloantigens on lamina propria cells.

Cell-mediated immune injury in foetal human small intestine

In order to extend the studies in experimental animals into human tissues a new *in vitro* system has recently been developed [47]. T cells migrate into foetal human intestine at about 12–14 weeks gestation [48] (Fig. 10.5). Until 19 weeks gestation the T cells are present as aggregates within the lamina propria and as single cells in the lamina propria and epithelium. Peyer's patches with organized T cell and B cell follicles do not develop until 19–20 weeks gestation [49]. As in post-natal intestine $CD8^+$ cells are found mostly in the epithelium and $CD4^+$ cells predominate in the lamina propria [48].

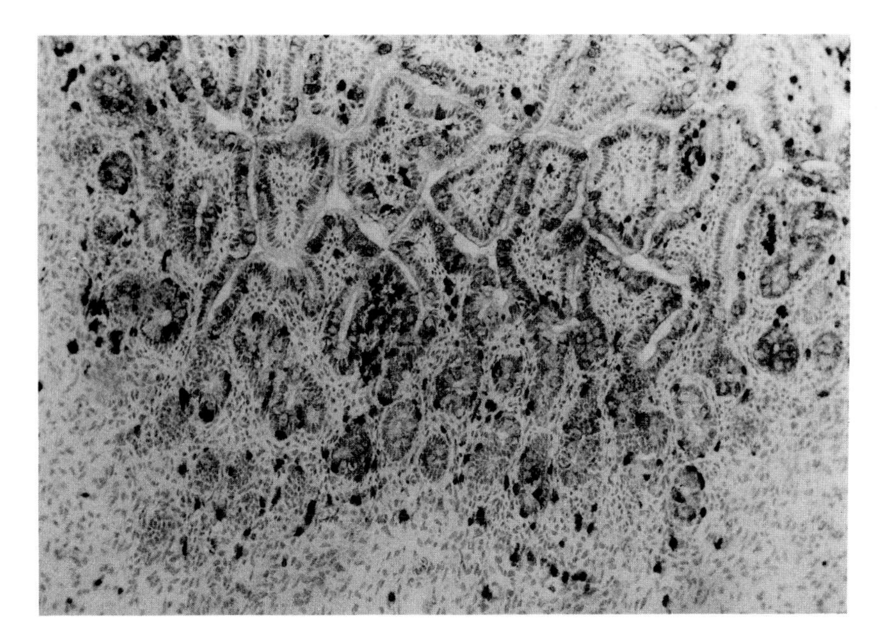

Fig. 10.5 $CD3^+$ T cells in the gut epithelium and lamina propria of a 20-week-old human foetal intestine. (Immunoperoxidase, original magnification ×100.)

Explants of human foetal small bowel can also be maintained in culture for extended periods [50]. Explants of foetal human intestine, containing T cells (usually from 17–20-week-old foetuses), were therefore cultured with the lectin pokeweed mitogen (PWM) or monoclonal anti-CD3 antibody (which activates T cells by crosslinking the CD3 complex associated with the TCR), in an attempt to polyclonally activate the T cells *in situ*. T cell activation was measured by immunohistochemical staining of frozen sections for T cell activation antigens and by the measurement of lymphokines in the culture supernatants.

Frozen sections of explants cultured for 1 or 3 days with PWM or anti-CD3 were stained with anti-CD25 by the peroxidase method. Numerous $CD25^+$ cells were apparent in the lamina propria of stimulated cultures (Fig. 10.6), but not control cultures [47]. The $CD25^+$ cells were morphologically diverse; some were small and round (probably T cells), whereas many were large and macrophage-like [51]. Activated epithelial $CD8^+$ T cells were rarely seen. The activated T cells in the lamina propria are $CD4^+$ and use the $\alpha\beta$ TCR (T.T. MacDonald, unpublished observations).

Supernatants of control and PWM-treated explants were also tested for the presence of the T cell products, IL-2 and interferon-γ. No activity was detected in control supernatants or supernatants from PWM-stimulated 14-week-old explants (which contain few T cells). In

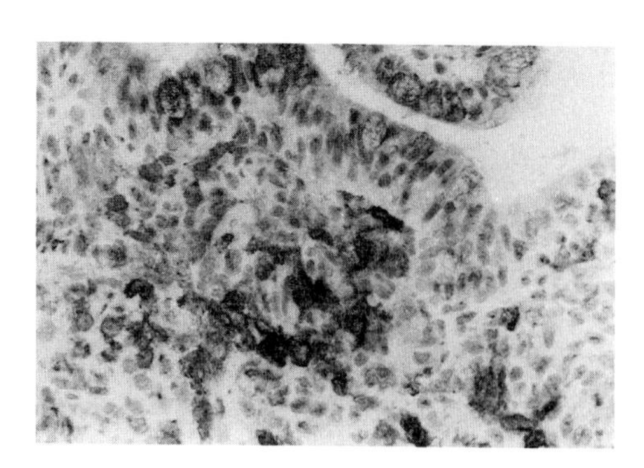

Fig. 10.6 $CD25^+$ cells in the lamina propria of a foetal gut explant 24 hours after the addition of anti-CD3 monoclonal antibody. (Immunoperoxidase, original magnification ×400.)

contrast, supernatants from older tissues stimulated with PWM contained low levels of both IL-2 and interferon-γ [3]. Thus, both immunohistologically and functionally, lamina propria T cells are activated after the addition of anti-CD3 or PWM to the explant cultures.

The consequences of T cell activation in foetal small intestine

The most dramatic effects of T cell activation are on explant morphology. After 3 days in culture with PWM or anti-CD3 there is a variable degree of villous flattening and profound crypt hypertrophy [47]. With the monoclonal antibody Ki67 which identifies a nuclear antigen on all dividing human cells, it can be demonstrated that these morphological changes are associated with a profound crypt cell hyperplasia (Fig. 10.7). These effects are mediated by lamina propria T cells and not through non-specific effects on epithelium by the T cell mitogens since they do not occur when foetal gut (14 weeks old and with few T cells) is stimulated with PWM. The effects in older foetal gut are inhibited by cyclosporin A (Table 10.3) while the degree of crypt cell hyperplasia is related to the amount of anti-CD3 added to the cultures.

Other features of the *in vitro* enteropathy

The addition of T cell mitogens to cultures of foetal intestine causes an increase in the numbers of lamina propria and epithelial T cells. Increased HLA-DR expression on epithelial cells and lamina propria accessory cells is observed, probably secondary to the effects of T cell derived lymphokines [52]. Finally, after 7 days in culture, aggregates of strongly $HLA\text{-}DR^+$ cells are present in the lamina propria [53]. These are probably aggregates of macrophages. The resemblance between *in vitro* enteropathy in foetal intestine and food sensitive enteropathy is shown in Table 10.4.

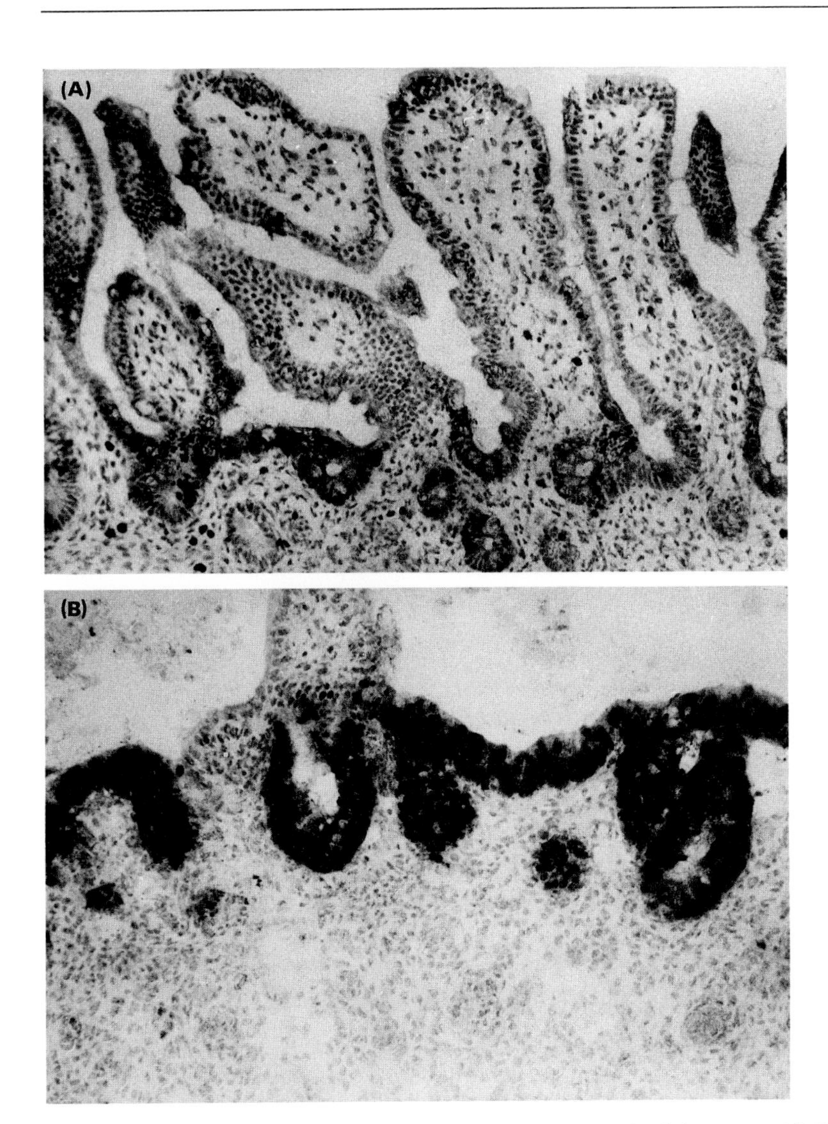

Fig. 10.7 The change in gut structure and cell proliferation (proliferating epithelial cells identified immunohistochemically by Ki67 staining) by the addition of PWM to explants of foetal human intestine. In (A) foetal gut at the onset of culture is shown with long villi and short crypts. In (B) after 3 days in culture with PWM the villi have disappeared and there is intense crypt cell proliferation. (Immunoperoxidase, original magnification ×100.)

The relationship between CD and *in vitro* enteropathy

The most striking feature of the *in vitro* enteropathy produced by polyclonal activation of lamina propria T cells in foetal gut is the resemblance to the mucosa in untreated CD and other food sensitive enteropathies (Table 10.4). One major difference, however, is that

Table 10.3 Cyclosporine A inhibits cytokine production by activated T cells in foetal gut and also prevents crypt cell hyperplasia. (Adapted from [47] and author's unpublished observations)

	20-week-old foetal gut after 3 days in culture	
	IL-2 in culture supernatant (units/ml)	Ki67 cells/crypt
Control	<1	5.6
PWM*	22.2	30.2
Cyclosporine A†	<1	4.1
PWM + cyclosporine A	1.6	6.2

* Added to the explant cultures at a concentration of 7 μg/ml.
† Added to the explant cultures at 10 μg/ml.

Table 10.4 Comparison of the changes to the gut mucosa in CD compared to *in vitro* enteropathy. (Data from [47,51–54])

	In vitro enteropathy	CD
Villous atrophy	Yes	Yes
Crypt hypertrophy	Yes	Yes
Crypt cell hyperplasia	Yes	Yes
Increased IEL	Yes	Yes
Enterocyte damage	No	Yes
Epithelial HLA-DR	Yes	Yes

whereas damaged surface epithelial cells are characteristic of untreated CD, the epithelial cells in the foetal gut model appear morphologically normal [54] despite the profound structural changes to the explant mucosa (Fig. 10.8).

A long-held view to explain the pathogenesis of the flat mucosa in CD is that crypt cell proliferation is negatively regulated by villus columnar cells, or the rate of cell loss from the villus. Thus in untreated CD, which is characterized by damage to surface enterocytes and a reduction in the number of villus enterocytes, it is thought that epithelial cell damage and cell loss are primary events and that crypt cell hyperplasia is secondary and compensatory in an effort to maintain villus height, and/or the normal numbers of epithelial cells [55]. Efforts to isolate the local factors which are produced by mature villus cells and which inhibit crypt cell proliferation have, however, been disappointing [56,57].

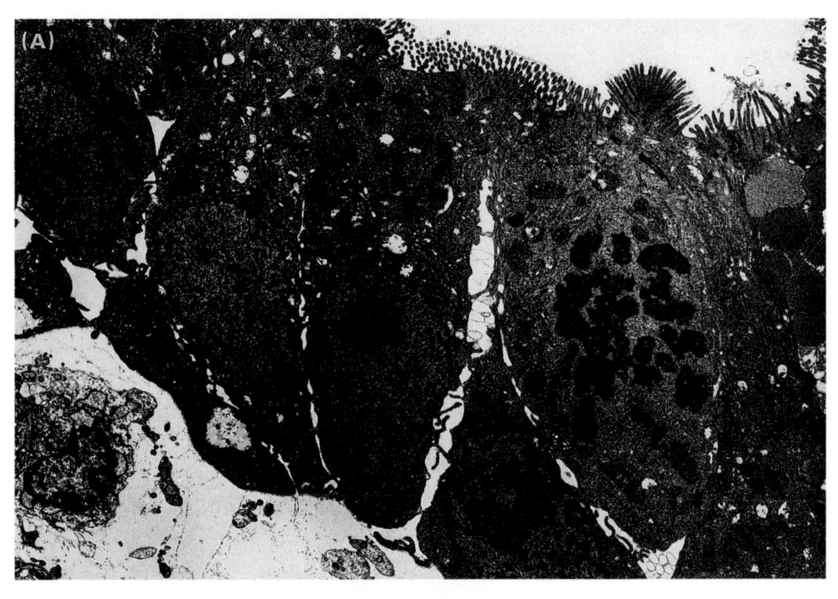

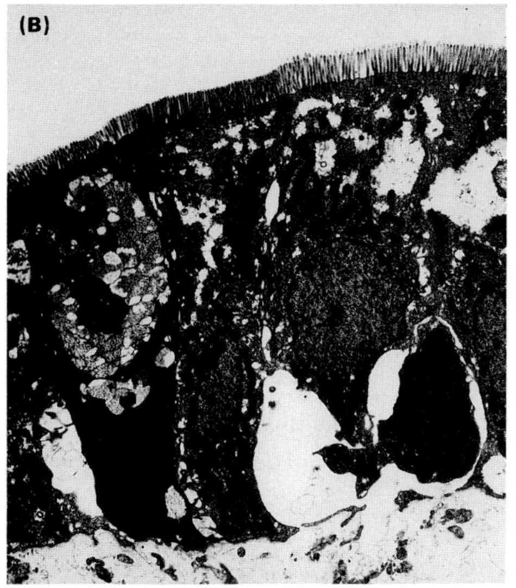

Fig. 10.8 Electron microscopy of the gut epithelium in foetal gut explants stimulated for 3 days with PWM. In (A) a region of the crypt is shown with a dividing enterocyte. In (B) surface epithelium is shown. The cells have tall microvilli and appear normal. Note the motile granulated lymphocyte within epithelium.

The observations derived from the foetal gut model would, in contrast, suggest that gut epithelial damage is not important in the pathogenesis of the coeliac lesion and that crypt cell hyperplasia is a more important, earlier event. Indeed in the foetal gut model, an increase in crypt cell proliferation occurs 18 hours after T cell activation, and before the onset of villus atrophy [54]. A usual consequence of crypt cell hyperplasia is crypt hypertrophy, and if the total mucosal thickness remains the same, crypt hypertrophy must produce an 'apparent' loss of villi. Lengthening of the crypts to almost full mucosal thickness will produce a flat, non-villus-bearing mucosa. Changes in crypt size will change the position of the villus/crypt junction, which in turn will influence the 'apparent' length of the villus.

The mechanism of T cell-mediated changes in the *in vitro* enteropathy

The molecular mechanisms whereby the activated $CD4^+$ T cells in the foetal gut mediated changes in epithelial proliferation are still unknown. The activated T cells secrete interleukin 2 and interferon-γ, but neither of these cytokines is enteropathogenic when added to foetal intestinal explants. Enteropathy cannot be mimicked by most of the known mediators, nor can it be neutralized by antibodies to cytokines. It is likely that the enteropathy involves the participation of subepithelial mesenchymal cells which are known to be responsible for maintaining normal epithelial cell proliferation and differentiation [58].

The role of $\gamma\delta$ TCR^+ IEL in cell-mediated intestinal injury

One of the most interesting new developments in CD has been the demonstration that the density of $\gamma\delta$ TCR^+ T cells is increased in the jejunal epithelium in untreated CD [6,7,59]. These cells are relatively uncommon (10% of $CD3^+$ IEL) in normal individuals. Since the best characterized function of $\gamma\delta$ TCR^+ T cells is that of non-specific cytotoxicity [8,9], it seemed that $\gamma\delta$ TCR^+ IEL might be responsible for the profound surface epithelial cell damage seen in untreated CD. It seems unlikely however that these cells are responsible for the gut damage, since in other diseases associated with a flat mucosa including tropical sprue, giardiasis and autoimmune enteropathy, there is no increase in $\gamma\delta$ TCR^+ IEL [7]. The $\gamma\delta$ TCR^+ IEL are also increased in the crypts of Lieberkuhn in untreated CD [59] where there is no epithelial damage [60]. Furthermore, there is no evidence that these cells are gluten reactive.

Cell-mediated immune injury in inflammatory bowel disease

The mucosa in Crohn's disease and ulcerative colitis becomes extensively infiltrated with T cells [61] and although the lesions in Crohn's disease are much more destructive than those in CD, in areas adjacent to ulcers there is villus atrophy and crypt hypertrophy [62]. Recent work from the author's laboratory supports the notion that cell-mediated immunity is important in Crohn's disease and may be re-

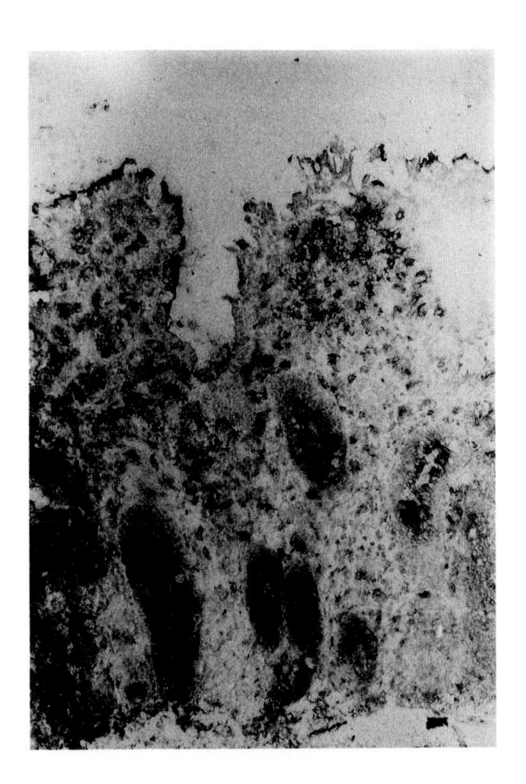

Fig. 10.9 $CD25^+$ cells in the ileal lamina propria of a child with active Crohn's disease. The cells are clustered below the surface epithelium and scattered throughout the lamina propria. (Immunoperoxidase, original magnification ×100.)

sponsible for the flat mucosa adjacent to Crohn's ulcers. Using alkaline phosphatase immunohistochemistry, we demonstrated that the mucosa in both Crohn's disease and ulcerative colitis contains large numbers of $CD25^+$ cells [63]. In Crohn's disease the $CD25^+$ cells are mostly $CD3^+$ T cells (Fig. 10.9) whereas in ulcerative colitis they are mostly macrophages. The antigenic stimulus which activates mucosal T cells to express CD25 in Crohn's disease is unknown. Further circumstantial evidence that cell-mediated immune injury is important in inflammatory bowel disease is shown by the therapeutic effect of cyclosporin A in Crohn's disease [64].

Antigen-specific cell-mediated immune damage in the intestine

Despite the clear evidence that activated T cells in the gut mucosa can cause tissue damage in model systems, the evidence that T cells which recognize intestinal antigens mediate tissue injury *in vivo* in patients is still circumstantial. For example, even though CD is an antigen-specific, HLA-linked disorder, and the degree of intestinal damage and mucosal lymphocytic infiltrate is related to the dose of gluten ingested [65,66], there is still no clear evidence for gluten-reactive T cells, either within the mucosa or in the blood of these patients. Fifteen years ago it was demonstrated that challenge of coeliac biopsies in organ culture with α-gliadin resulted in lymphokine secretion into the organ culture supernatant [67]. This still remains the only evidence for the existence of gluten-specific T cells in the mucosa of coeliacs. Recently, serum interleukin 2 receptor levels have been shown to be raised in untreated CD [68]. These decrease to normal levels on a gluten-free diet and increase on gluten challenge. The origin of circulating interleukin 2R is almost certainly the intestine but the cell source is unclear since interleukin 2R are present on T cells, accessory cells and B cells.

The evidence that cytokines can directly alter epithelial cell differentiation and proliferation is scant. Interferon-γ inhibits the proliferation of rodent intestinal epithelial cell lines and also increases HLA-DR expression on these cells [69]. Interferon-γ stimulates increased HLA-DR expression and secretory component synthesis by human epithelial cell lines [70]. An important recent observation is that interferon-γ, but not interleukin 1, interleukin 2 or TNFα, decreases epithelial tight junction permeability [71], and thus may play a role in protein-losing enteropathy.

Contact sensitizing haptens such as dinitrochlorobenzene (DNCB) are effective in eliciting cell-mediated immune responses. These agents have been used extensively as a means of generating cell-mediated inflammation in the bowel. Pigs sensitized topically to DNCB were subject to repeated challenge in the colon with DNCB in an inert carrier. This treatment elicited mucosal inflammation consisting of a lymphoid infiltrate, haemorrhage and mucosal giant cells [72]. It was considered that DNCB intestinal hypersensitivity might be a useful model of ulcerative colitis. These studies have been repeated many times in a variety of species. Feeding of DNCB to sensitized pigs also produces an inflammatory response in the small intestine. It is, however, a destructive type of inflammation and bears no resemblance to that of the human small bowel enteropathies [72,73]. More recently it has been demonstrated that a single colonic infusion of the hapten trinitrobenzene sulphonic acid (TNB) in ethanol into rats results in chronic intestinal inflammation with some of the features of Crohn's disease [74]. Within the inflamed colonic mucosa there is increased production of myeloperoxidase, interleukin 1 and leukotriene B4 activity [75]. It is assumed that in this model, the ethanol damages the colonic epithelium allowing hapten to penetrate mucosal tissues, bind to self antigens and chronically stimulate a local delayed-type hypersensitivity response.

The functional role of cell-mediated tissue injury in the intestine

Helminth and protozoan infection in rodent and human small bowel can be associated with villus flattening and crypt cell hyperplasia [76,77]. In rodents, these changes are thymus dependent which would indicate that it is the host response to the parasite, rather than direct mechanical damage which is responsible for the gut damage [29]. T cells are essential for rejection of helminth parasites in rodents [78] and rejection is associated with changes in mucosal morphology [30]. Teleologically, it would make sense to have, as a component of a host intestinal antiparasite immune response, a mechanism to produce a reduction in villus surface area and an increase in crypt cell proliferation, thus making the microenvironment more hostile to parasites which live in and on the epithelium [79].

The morphological changes in the intestinal mucosa seen in CD, if these are indeed a result of local cell-mediated immune responses, may thus be a consequence of inappropriate expression of the host intestinal antiparasite response to a cereal product which has formed a major part of the human diet only in the last 4 millenia.

References

1 MacDonald TT, Parrott DMV. Mucosal lymphoid tissue. In: Lachmann PJ, Peters DK, Rosen FS, Walport MJ, eds. *Clinical Aspects of Immunology*. 5th edn. Oxford: Blackwell Scientific Publications, 1993: in press.

2 Viney JL, Kilshaw PK, MacDonald TT. Cytotoxic α/β+ and γ/δ+ T cells in murine intestinal epithelium. *Eur J Immunol* 1990;20: 1623–6.

3 MacDonald TT. The role of activated T lymphocytes in gastrointestinal disease. *Clin Exp Allergy* 1990;20:247–52.

4 Borst J, Van Dongen JJM, Bolhuis RLH *et al.* Distinct molecular forms of the human T cell receptor γδ detected on viable T cells by a monoclonal antibody. *J Exp Med* 1988;167: 1625–44.

5 Groh V, Porcelli S, Fabbi M *et al.* Human lymphocytes bearing the T cell receptor γδ are phenotypically diverse and evenly distributed throughout the lymphoid system. *J Exp Med* 1989;169:1277–94.

6 Halstensen TS, Scott H, Brandtzaeg P. Intraepithelial T cells of the TCRγ/δ+ CD8− and Vδ1/Jδ1+ phenotypes are increased in coeliac disease. *Scand J Gastroenterol* 1989; 30:665–72.

7 Spencer J, Isaacson PG, Diss TC, MacDonald TT. Expression of disulphide linked and non-disulphide linked forms of the T cell receptor gamma/delta heterodimer in human intestinal intraepithelial lymphocytes. *Eur J Immunol* 1989;19:1335–8.

8 Nowill A, Moingeon P, Ythier A *et al.* Natural killer clones derived from fetal (25wk) blood. Probing the human T cell receptor with WT31 monoclonal antibody. *J Exp Med* 1986;163:1601–6.

9 Ferrini S, Zarcone D, Viale M *et al.* Morphologic and functional characterization of human peripheral blood T cells expressing the T cell receptor γ/δ. *Eur J Immunol* 1989; 19:1183–8.

10 Modlin RL, Pirmez C, Hofman FM *et al.* Lymphocytes bearing antigen-specific γδ T-cell receptors accumulate in human infectious disease lesions. *Nature* 1989;339: 544–8.

11 Plaut M, Pierce JH, Watson CJ, Hanley-Hyde J, Nordan RP, Paul WE. Mast cell lines produce lymphokines in response to cross-linkage of Fc ε or to calcium ionophores. *Nature* 1989;339:64–7.

12 Gordon JR, Galli SJ. Mast cells as a source of both preformed and immunologically inducible TNF-α/cachectin. *Nature* 1990;346: 274–6.

13 Viney JL, Spencer J, MacDonald TT. Gamma/delta T cells in the gut epithelium. *Gut* 1990;31:841–4.

14 Bandeira A, Mota-Santos T, Itohara S *et al.* Localisation of γ/δ T cells to the intestinal epithelium is independent of normal

microbial colonisation. *J Exp Med* 1990;172: 239–44.
15 Guy-Grand D, Griscelli C, Vassalli P. The mouse gut T lymphocyte, a novel type of T cell. Nature, origin, and traffic in mice in normal and graft-versus-host conditions. *J Exp Med* 1978;148:1661–77.
16 London SD, Cebra JJ, Rubin DH. Intraepithelial lymphocytes contain virus-specific MHC-restricted cytotoxic cell precursors after gut mucosal immunization with reovirus serotype 1/Lang. *Reg Immunol* 1989; 2:99–105.
17 Viney J, MacDonald TT, Kilshaw PJ. T cell receptor expression in intestinal intraepithelial lymphocyte subpopulations of normal and athymic mice. *Immunology* 1989;66: 583–7.
18 Bonneville M, Itohara S, Krecko EG *et al.* Transgenic mice demonstrate that epithelial homing of γ/δ T cells is determined by cell lineages independent of T cell receptor specificity. *J Exp Med* 1990;171:1015–26.
19 MacDonald TT, Spencer J, Viney JL, Williams CB, Walker-Smith JA. Selective biopsy of Peyer's patches during ileal endoscopy. *Gastroenterology* 1987;93:1356–62.
20 Rickert RR, Carter HW. The 'early' ulcerative lesion of Crohn's disease: correlative light- and scanning electron- microscopic studies. *J Clin Gastroenterol* 1980;2:11–9.
21 Walker-Smith JA. *Diseases of the Small Intestine in Childhood.* 3rd edn. London: Butterworths, 1988.
22 Hodgson HJF, Jewell DP. Selective IgA deficiency and Crohn's disease: report of 2 cases. *Gut* 1977;18:644–6.
23 Webster ADB, Slavin G, Shiner M, Platts-Mills TAE, Asherson G. Coeliac disease with severe hypogammaglobulinaemia. *Gut* 1981; 22:153–7.
24 Brandtzaeg P. The B cell system. In: Brostoff J, Challacombe SB, eds. *Food Allergy and Intolerance.* London: Bailliere Tindall, 1987: 118–55.
25 Soltoft J, Petersen L, Kruse P. Immunoglobulin deficiency and regional enteritis. *Scand J Gastroenterol* 1972;7:233–6.
26 Abramowsky CR, Sorensen RU. Regional enteritis-like enteropathy in a patient with agammaglobulinaemia: Histologic and immunocytologic studies. *Hum Pathol* 1988;19:483–6.
27 Kirk BW, Freedman SO. Hypogammaglobulinemia, thymoma and ulcerative colitis. *Can Med Assoc J* 1967;96:1272–7.
28 Ross IN. Primary immunodeficiency and the small intestine. In Marsh MN, ed. *Immunopathology of the Small Intestine.* Chichester: John Wiley, 1987:283–332.
29 Ferguson A, Jarrett EEE. Hypersensitivity reactions in the small intestine. I. Thymus dependence of experimental 'partial villous atrophy'. *Gut* 1975;16:114–7.
30 Manson-Smith DF, Bruce RG, Parrott DMV. Villous atrophy and expulsion of intestinal *Trichinella spiralis* are mediated by T cells. *Cell Immunol* 1978;47:285–92.
31 Glucksberg H, Storb R, Fefer A *et al.* Clinical manifestations of graft-versus-host disease in human recipients of marrow from HLA-matched sibling donors. *Transplantation* 1974;18:295–303.
32 Felstein MV, Mowat AM. Experimental studies of immunologically mediated enteropathy. IV. Correlation between immune effector mechanisms and type of enteropathy during a GVHR in neonatal mice of different ages. *Clin Exp Immunol* 1988;72:108–12.
33 Guy-Grand D, Vassalli P. Gut injury in mouse graft-versus-host disease. *J Clin Invest* 1986;77:1584–95.
34 MacDonald TT, Ferguson A. Hypersensitivity reactions in the small intestine. III. The effect of allograft rejection and graft-versus-host disease on epithelial cell kinetics. *Cell Tissue Kinet* 1977;10:301–12.
35 Mowat AM, Felstein MV, Baca ME. Experimental studies of immunologically mediated enteropathy. III. Severe and progressive enteropathy during a graft-versus-host reaction in athymic mice. *Immunology* 1987; 61:185–8.
36 Mowat AM, Felstein MV, Borland A, Parrott DMV. Experimental studies of immunologically mediated enteropathy: Development of cell mediated immunity and intestinal pathology during a graft-versus-host reaction in irradiated mice. *Gut* 1988; 29:949–56.
37 Piguet P-F. GVHR elicited by products of Class I or Class II loci of the MHC: Analysis of the response of mouse T lymphocytes to products of Class I and Class II loci of the MHC in correlation with GVHR-induced mortality, medullary aplasia, and enteropathy. *J Immunol* 1985;135:1637–43.
38 Mowat AM, Borland A, Parrott DMV. Hypersensitivity reactions in the small intestine. VII. Induction of the intestinal phase of murine graft-versus-host reaction by Lyt2- T cells activated by I-A alloantigens. *Trans-*

plantation 1986;41:192–8.
39 Piguet PF, Grau GE, Allett B, Vassalli P. Tumor necrosis factor 1 Cachectin is an effector of skin and gut lesions of the acute phase of graft-versus-host disease. *J Exp Med* 1987;166:1280–9.
40 Mowat AM. Antibodies to IFN-γ prevent immunologically mediated intestinal damage in murine graft-versus-host reaction. *Immunology* 1989;68:18–23.
41 Elson CO, Reilly RW, Rosenberg IH. Small intestinal injury in the graft versus host reaction: an innocent bystander phenomenon. *Gastroenterology* 1977;72:886–9.
42 Mayrhofer G, Pugh CW, Barclay AN. The distribution, ontogeny and origin in the rat of Ia-positive cells with dendritic morphology and of Ia antigen in epithelial, with special reference to the intestine. *Eur J Immunol* 1983;13:112–22.
43 Holmes JT, Klein MS, Winawer SJ, Fortner JG. Morphological studies of rejection in canine jejunal allographs. *Gastroenterology* 1971;61:693–706.
44 Ferguson A, Parrott DMV. Growth and development of antigen-free grafts of foetal mouse intestine. *J Pathol* 1972;106:95–101.
45 Parrott DMV, MacDonald TT. Ontogeny of the mucosal immune system in rodents. In: MacDonald TT, ed. *Ontogeny of the Intestinal Immune System*. Boca Raton: CRC Press, 1990:51–68.
46 MacDonald TT, Ferguson A. Hypersensitivity reactions in the small intestine. II. The effect of allograft rejection on mucosal architecture and lymphoid cell infiltrate. *Gut* 1976;17:81–91.
47 MacDonald TT, Spencer J. Evidence that activated mucosal T cells play a role in the pathogenesis of enteropathy in human small intestine. *J Exp Med* 1988;167:1341–9.
48 Spencer J, Dillon SB, Isaacson PG, MacDonald TT. T cell sub-classes in fetal human ileum. *Clin Exp Immunol* 1986;65:553–9.
49 Spencer J, MacDonald TT, Finn T, Isaacson PG. Development of Peyer's patches in human fetal terminal ileum. *Clin Exp Immunol* 1986;64:536–43.
50 Menard D, Arsenault P. Explant culture of human fetal small intestine. *Gastroenterology* 1985;88:691–7.
51 Monk TJ, Spencer J, Cerf-Bensussan N, MacDonald TT. Activation of mucosal T-cells *in situ* with anti-CD3 antibody: phenotype of the activated T cells and their distribution within the mucosal micro-environment. *Clin Exp Immunol* 1988;74: 216–22.
52 MacDonald TT, Weinel A, Spencer J. HLA-DR expression in human fetal intestinal epithelium. *Gut* 1988;29:1342–8.
53 MacDonald TT, Spencer JM. The consequences of T cell activation in human small intestine. In: McDermott RM, ed. *Inflammatory Bowel Disease: Current Status and Future Approaches*. New York: Elsevier Science Publishers, 1988:107–12.
54 Ferreira R daC, Forsyth LA, Richman P, Wells C, Spencer J, MacDonald TT. Changes in mucosal morphology and the rate of epithelial cell renewal induced by a T cell mediated immune response in human small intestine *in vitro*. *Gastroenterology* 1990;98:1255–63.
55 Booth CC. Enteropoesis: structural and functional relationships of the enterocyte. *Postgrad Med J* 1968;44:12–16.
56 May RJ, Quaroni A, Kirsch K, Isselbacher K. A villus cell-derived inhibitor of intestinal cell proliferation. *Am J Physiol* 1981;241: G520–7.
57 Rampal P, Nano JL, Zunino C. Inhibition of intestinal cell proliferation by villus cell extract. *Gut* 1987;28:109–15.
58 Haffen K, Kedinger M, Simon-Assman P. Mesenchyme-dependent differentiation of epithelial progenitor cells in the gut. *J Paediatr Gastroenterol Nutr* 1987;6:14–23.
59 Savilahti E, Arato A, Verkasalo M. Increased numbers of T cell receptor gamma/delta bearing lymphocytes in the epithelium of coeliac patients. In: MacDonald TT, Challacombe SJ, Bland PW, Stokes CR, Heatley RV, Mowat AM, eds. *Advances in Mucosal Immunology*. Dordrecht: Kluwer Academic Publishers, 1990:61–6.
60 Padykula HA, Strauss EW, Ladman AJ, Gardner FH. A morphologic and histochemical analysis of the human jejunal epithelium in nontropical sprue. *Gastroenterology* 1961;40:735–65.
61 Selby WS, Janossy G, Bofill M, Jewell DP. Intestinal lymphocyte subpopulations in inflammatory bowel disease: an analysis by immunohistological and cell isolation techniques. *Gut* 1984;25:32–40.
62 Entrican JH, Busuttil A, Ferguson A. Focal microscopical jejunal lesions in Crohn's disease suggestive of a T cell mediated immune response. *Scand J Gastroenterol* 1987;22:1071–5.
63 Choy M-Y, Richman PI, Walker-Smith JA, MacDonald TT. Differential expression of

CD25 on mucosal T cells and macrophages distinguishes the lesions in ulcerative colitis and Crohn's disease. *Gut* 1990;31:1365–70.
64 Brynskov J, Freund L, Rasmussen SN *et al.* A placebo-controlled, double blind, randomized trial of cyclosporine therapy in active Crohn's disease. *New Engl J Med* 1989;321:845–50.
65 Marsh MN. Coeliac disease. In: Marsh MN, ed. *Immunopathology of the Small Intestine.* Chichester: John Wiley, 1987:371–99.
66 Leigh RJ, Marsh MN, Crowe P, Kelly C, Garner V, Gordon D. Studies of intestinal lymphoid tissue. IX. Dose-dependent, gluten-induced lymphoid infiltration of coeliac jejunal epithelium. *Scand J Gastroenterol* 1985;20:715–9.
67 Ferguson A, MacDonald TT, McClure JP, Holden RJ. Cell-mediated immunity to gliadin within the small intestinal mucosa in coeliac disease. *Lancet* 1975;i:895–901.
68 Crabtree JE, Heatley RV, Juby LD, Howdle PD, Losowsky MS. Serum interleukin-2-receptor in coeliac disease: response to treatment and gluten challenge. *Clin Exp Immunol* 1989;77:345–8.
69 Cerf-Bensussan N, Quaroni A, Kurnick JT, Bhan AK. Intraepithelial lymphocytes modulate Ia expression by intestinal epithelial cells. *J Immunol* 1984;132:2244–52.
70 Sollid LM, Kvale D, Brandtzaeg P, Markussen G, Thorsby E. Interferon-γ enhances expression of secretory component, the epithelial receptor for polymeric immunoglobulins. *J Immunol* 1987;138:4303–6.
71 Madara JL, Stafford J. Interferon-τ directly affects barrier function of cultured intestinal epithelial monolayers. *J Clin Invest* 1989;83:724–7.
72 Bicks RO, Azar MM, Rosenberg EW, Dunham WG, Luther J. Delayed hypersensitivity reactions in the intestinal tract. I. Studies of 2,4 dinitrochlorobenzene-caused guinea pig and swine colon lesions. *Gastroenterology* 1967;53:422–36.
73 Bicks RO, Azar MM, Rosenberg EW. Delayed hypersensitivity reactions in the intestinal tract. II. Small intestinal lesions associated with xylose malabsorption. *Gastroenterology* 1967;53:437–43.
74 Morris GP, Beck PL, Herridge MS *et al.* Hapten-induced model of chronic inflammation and ulceration in the rat colon. *Gastroenterology* 1989;96:795–803.
75 Rachmilewitz D, Simon PL, Schwartz LW *et al.* Inflammatory mediators of experimental colitis in the rat. *Gastroenterology* 1989;97:326–37.
76 Kotcher E, Mario Miranda G, Rodrico Esquivel R *et al.* Intestinal malabsorption and helminthic and protozoan infections of the small intestine. *Gastroenterology* 1988;50:366–71.
77 Symons LEA. Kinetics of the epithelial cells and morphology of villi and crypts in the jejunum of the rat infected by the nematode *Nippostrongylus brasiliensis. Gastroenterology* 1965;49:158–68.
78 Ogilvie BM, Love RJ. Co-operation between antibodies and cells in immunity to a nematode parasite. *Transplant Rev* 1974;19:147–68.
79 Miller HRP. Immunopathology of nematode infestation and expulsion. In: Marsh MN, ed. *Immunopathology of the Small Intestine.* Chichester: John Wiley, 1987:177–208.

Chapter 11/Cereal proteins and coeliac disease

PETER R. SHEWRY, ARTHUR S. TATHAM AND DONALD D. KASARDA

Introduction

The consumption of wheat and related cereals (barley, rye) is such an important and accepted part of the lifestyle of developed countries that it is difficult for most people to imagine the problems encountered by those who suffer from coeliac disease (CD), or gluten sensitivity.

The pervasiveness of our cereal-based diet is due to two factors. First, as a result of their immense success in agricultural terms, cereal crops provide high yields over a wide range of climatic and geographical conditions. In 1987, for example, about 510 × 10^6 tonnes of wheat were harvested worldwide, while barley and rye production yielded about 170 × 10^6 and 30 × 10^6 tonnes, respectively [1]. Second, the inherent physical properties of cereal proteins are uniquely suited to their use in food production; in particular, the cohesive viscoelasticity of wheat gluten permits the baking of leavened bread while its binding properties allow flour and isolated gluten to fulfil many other roles in the preparation of foodstuffs. Thus, cereals are present where expected (in breads, biscuits, cakes and pastas) but also in beverages (beer, malted drinks) and in a range of other products, such as processed meats, thickenings and those coated with bread crumb or batter.

In this chapter, current knowledge of gluten and other related cereal proteins is reviewed, including data on their conformations and role in food systems. Their relationship to the pathogenesis of CD is discussed, with particular emphasis on studies of the A-gliadin group of α-gliadins.

The classification and evolutionary relationships of cereals

Cereals are a species of grasses (Gramineae) that are cultivated for their seeds. Although many species are grown in different parts of the world, three account for about 80% of the total production. These are wheat (510 × 10^6 tonnes in 1987), maize (405 × 10^6 tonnes) and rice (483 × 10^6 tonnes) [1]. Others are Triticale (a 'man made' cereal produced by crossing wheat and rye), rye, barley, oats, sorghum, Job's

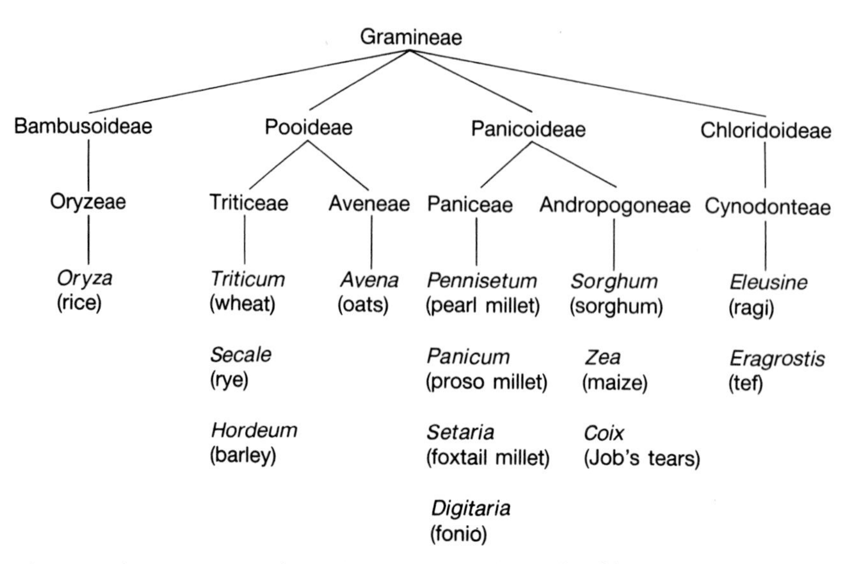

Fig. 11.1 The taxonomic relationships of cereals. (From [174].)

tears, tef and a number of small-seeded species collectively termed millets.

The cereals are classified into four groups (Fig. 11.1). The subfamily Pooideae comprises two tribes, the Triticeae which embraces the major temperate cereals barley, wheat and rye and the Aveneae, or oats. The subfamily Panicoideae has within it the major tropical cereals: maize and sorghum, and most millets. Rice is not closely related to the other cereals. It is sometimes classified in the subfamily Pooideae but in a tribe (the Oryzeae) distant from the Aveneae or Triticeae, but more usually in a separate subfamily, the Bambusoideae. Finally, the subfamily Chloridoideae comprises two minor cereals, ragi (finger millet) and tef.

These taxonomic relationships, to a large extent reflect the chemical structure of their seed storage proteins, should be borne in mind when their relative effects in activating CD are compared.

Characteristics of prolamins; chemical and biological

Wheat gluten can be defined as the cohesive mass that remains when dough is washed to remove starch granules. It was first described by Beccari in 1745 [2] and was subsequently divided into two fractions that were either soluble or insoluble in aqueous alcohol [3,4]. Similar alcohol-soluble fractions were also demonstrated in rye and barley [5,6]. Osborne coined the name prolamin for the alcohol-soluble proteins of these and other cereals [7], while the alcohol-insoluble fractions were termed glutelins. Such fractions are usually given trivial names in different species, for example gliadins (alcohol-soluble) and glutenins (alcohol-insoluble) in wheat (Fig. 11.2).

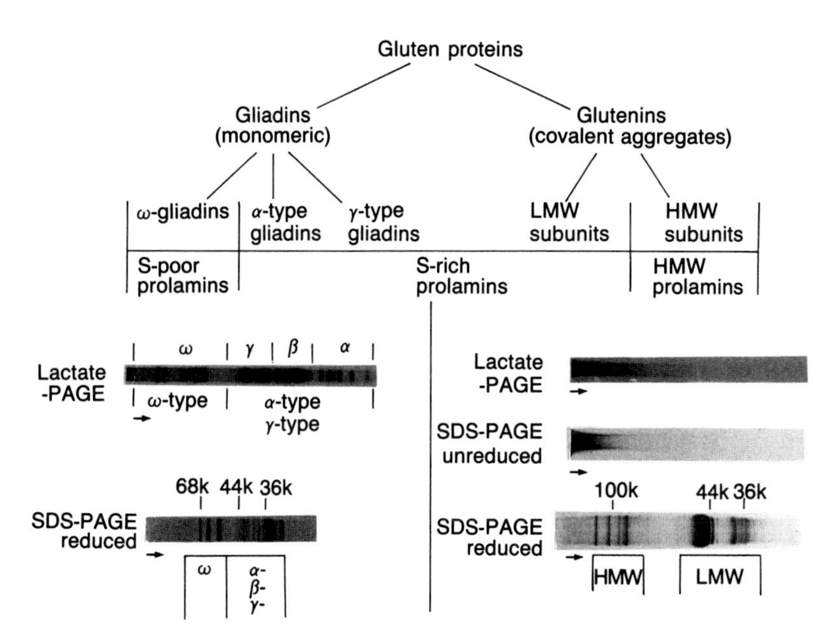

Fig. 11.2 The classification and nomenclature of wheat gluten proteins. Separations of total gliadins and glutenins by electrophoresis with aluminium lactate buffer at pH 3.2 (Lactate-PAGE) (unreduced only) and SDS-PAGE (reduced and unreduced) are also shown.

Alcohol-solubility remains the most widely used diagnostic characteristic of prolamins, but we now know that not all prolamins are alcohol-soluble (similarly, not all alcohol-soluble proteins are prolamins, even in cereal grains). Many proteins present in the glutelin fraction of wheat (i.e. the glutenins) and other cereals are closely related to the alcohol-soluble prolamins, but are not soluble in aqueous alcohols because they form aggregates of high relative molecular mass (M_r) stabilized by intermolecular disulphide bonds linking the protein subunit chains. It is now usual to consider that these are also prolamins.

The second diagnostic property of the prolamins is amino acid composition. Obsborne [7] coined the name 'prolamin' to reflect their high content of proline and amide nitrogen (now known to be derived from glutamine). Although this is true for all groups of prolamins, the combined proportions of these amino acids vary from about 30 to 70 mol%. There is also variation in the proportions of other residues, for example, phenylalanine (0–9 mol%), glycine (2–20 mol%) and histidine (0–8 mol%) [8] (Table 11.1). There is a similarly high degree of variation in their molecular weights, from about 14 000 for one group of maize prolamins to almost 90 000 for some high molecular weight subunits of wheat glutenin.

All prolamin fractions are complex mixtures of proteins, which may vary in their M_r, isoelectric point (pI) and amino acid composition.

Table 11.1 Amino acid compositions (expressed as mol%) of HMW, S-poor and S-rich prolamins of wheat, rye and barley. (Data from [15, 23, 152, 176, 179, 181–183])

	HMW			S-poor			S-rich						
	Wheat sub-unit 1By9	Rye HMW secalin	Barley D-hordein	Wheat ω-gliadin	Rye ω-secalin	Barley C-hordein	Wheat α-gliadin	Wheat γ-gliadin	Wheat LMW sub-unit	Barley γ-hordein	Barley B-hordein	Rye 40K γ-secalin	Rye 75K γ-secalin
Asx	0.9	1.3	1.3	0.6	0.5	1.0	3.0	2.9	1.3	2.9	1.4	3.0	1.5
Thr	3.2	2.7	8.1	1.7	1.0	1.0	1.6	1.7	2.7	3.1	2.1	3.2	1.6
Ser	7.0	5.0	9.7	5.7	4.1	4.6	5.2	5.3	7.7	5.5	4.7	5.2	5.7
Glx	36.2	34.0	29.6	42.9	42.9	41.2	37.2	41.7	38.4	32.4	35.4	34.8	40.3
Pro	9.9	13.7	11.6	29.2	30.6	30.6	15.5	15.1	15.0	16.5	20.6	18.4	23.5
Gly	18.9	16.5	15.7	1.1	1.4	0.3	2.5	2.4	3.3	5.9	1.5	2.4	1.7
Ala	2.9	6.4	2.5	0.6	0.6	0.7	2.9	3.4	2.3	2.6	2.2	2.8	2.2
Cys	1.0	1.4	1.5	0	0	0	1.9	1.8	2.7	2.7	2.5	2.5	1.8
Val	2.5	2.8	4.5	0.4	1.0	1.0	4.0	3.8	4.7	3.7	5.6	4.7	4.5
Met	0.4	0.3	0.2	0	0.1	0.2	1.2	0.9	0.6	1.2	0.6	1.0	0.6
Ile	1.3	1.6	0.7	1.6	2.4	2.6	4.1	3.9	3.7	2.9	4.1	4.8	2.8
Leu	4.4	4.4	3.3	4.1	3.9	3.6	8.1	6.9	7.0	8.6	7.0	7.4	4.9
Tyr	5.6	4.1	3.9	1.5	1.4	2.3	3.1	3.1	1.5	1.7	2.5	0.7	0.9
Phe	0.3	0.9	1.4	8.9	7.4	8.8	3.9	3.7	4.7	4.7	4.8	5.3	5.4
His	1.6	2.2	3.4	0.7	0.5	1.1	2.5	1.5	1.6	2.0	2.1	1.7	1.4
Lys	0.9	0.2	1.1	0.3	0.3	0.2	0.5	0.1	0.5	1.6	0.5	0.7	0.4
Arg	2.3	2.3	1.5	0.6	1.8	0.8	2.4	1.6	2.4	2.0	2.4	1.3	0.8
Trp	0.6	nd	nd	nd	nd	nd	0.3	0.2	nd	nd	nd	nd	nd

This polymorphism exists both within individual plants and between genotypes of the same species. These proteins are usually, although probably not exclusively, the products of individual genes, and the degree of post-translational modification (with the exception of signal peptide cleavage) is very low. There is no conclusive evidence that glycosylation either occurs or contributes to the observed polymorphism. Despite the high degree of polymorphism, the prolamins present within a species can be classified into a small number of groups or families, encoded by clustered or dispersed families of genes.

Prolamins have only one known function which is to act as stores of nitrogen, sulphur and carbon that are mobilized during germination to support sprouting and seedling growth. Because of this vital role the biosynthesis of prolamins is strictly regulated, and occurs only in the starchy endosperm (not in any other tissues) and at a specific stage of development. Prolamin genes have, therefore, proved to be an attractive and valuable system for studies of the control of gene expression [9].

The synthesized protein accumulates within the starchy endosperm in discrete membrane-bound deposits called protein bodies. There has been some dispute and uncertainty about the precise origin of these deposits and of their surrounding membrane, which may reflect at least two different mechanisms of formation. Cereal prolamins are synthesized by polysomes bound to endoplasmic reticulum (ER), and have a signal peptide which directs the protein into the lumen of the ER. In young developing endosperms of wheat and barley, the protein is transported via the Golgi apparatus to the vacuole to form protein bodies with a surrounding membrane of vacuolar origin [10]. In maize, and probably also in older endosperms of wheat and barley, the protein bodies form directly within the lumen of the ER, and are surrounded by a membrane of ER origin [11,12]. The requirements for deposition and packaging within protein bodies may have placed constraints on the evolution of prolamins, and at least some of their unusual properties (e.g. solubility, conformation) may reflect this. Similarly, the prolamins must also be readily mobilized (digested and transported) during germination.

Methods of prolamin analysis; chemical and molecular

Cereal proteins have been extensively investigated by a wide range of methods concerned with separation, purification and characterization [13], including sophisticated physicochemical methods which permit study of their molecular size, shape, conformation and dynamics [14]. However, no detailed three-dimensional information, comparable to that available since the 1950s from X-ray diffraction patterns of crystals of various globular proteins of animal origin, has been obtained.

Similarly, until recently, little was known of their amino acid sequences. Only one prolamin has been studied in detail by direct protein sequencing, A-gliadin of wheat [15], and it was not possible to determine the complete sequence by this approach, although 260 of the 266 residues were obtained. A dramatic increase in our knowledge of amino acid sequences came in the 1980s from the application of molecular cloning techniques, and we now know complete sequences of members of almost all the major groups of prolamins. The amino acid sequences are deduced from the nucleotide sequences of cloned cDNAs or genes, and the application of this technology allowed Kasarda *et al.* [15] to complete their sequence of A-gliadin, and subsequently provided the sequences of several other α-type gliadins of wheat. The availability of extensive sequence data enables us to determine the structural and evolutionary relationships of prolamins to each other and to other proteins [16], and also facilitates studies of the physicochemical properties of purified proteins [14].

The prolamins of wheat, barley and rye

Classification and families

It is traditional to classify the prolamins of wheat into two groups, on the basis of their solubility (gliadins) or insolubility (glutenins) in alcohol : water mixtures. The gliadins consist predominantly of mono-

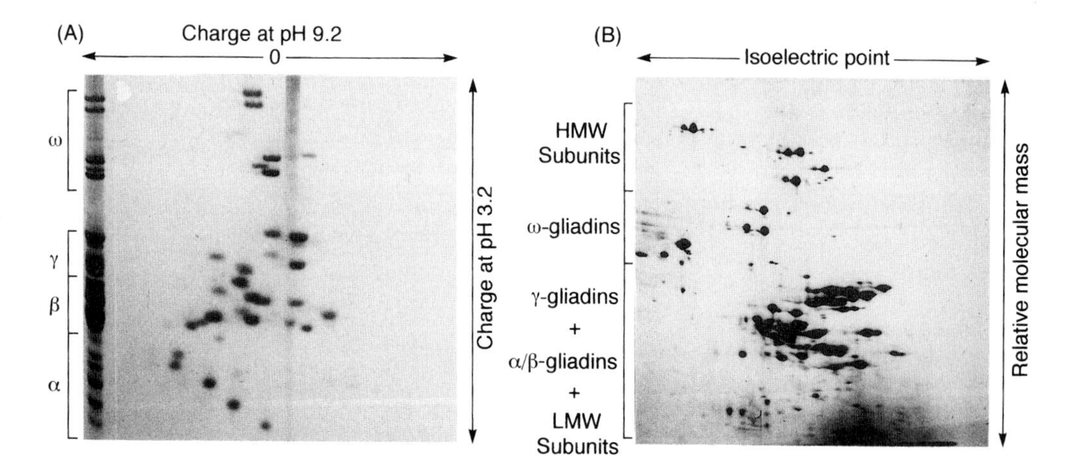

Fig. 11.3 Two-dimensional electrophoresis of gluten proteins from wheat cv. Chinese Spring. (A) gliadins separated on the basis of charge by electrophoresis at pH 3.2 followed by electrophoresis at pH 9.2. A one-dimensional separation at pH 3.2 is also shown. (B) total reduced gluten protein (gliadins and glutenins) separated firstly on the basis of isoelectric point (by isoelectric focusing) and secondly on the basis of relative molecular mass (by SDS-PAGE).

meric proteins, which can be separated by electrophoresis at low pH into four groups designated α-, β-, γ- and ω-gliadins (in order of decreasing mobility) (Figs 11.2, 11.3). Whereas the α-, β- and γ-gliadins contain intrachain disulphide bonds, the ω-gliadins contain no cysteine and therefore no disulphide bonds. The gliadin fraction also contains a small proportion of polymeric proteins, related to those which comprise the glutenins. The glutenins consist of alcohol-soluble subunits which form alcohol-insoluble polymers stabilized by interchain disulphide bonds. The subunits are classified into two groups, the high molecular weight (HMW) and low molecular weight (LMW) subunits, based on their mobility by sodium dodecylsulphate-polyacrylamide gel electrophoresis (SDS-PAGE).

The availability of extensive amino acid sequence data permits an alternative classification, based on molecular relationships. Three groups of prolamins can be recognized, which are called sulphur-rich (S-rich), sulphur-poor (S-poor), and HMW (intermediate-S) prolamins (Figs 11.2, 11.3) (Table 11.1). The HMW and S-poor groups of prolamins comprise the HMW glutenin subunits and ω-gliadins, respectively. The remaining group, the S-rich prolamins, consists of at least three discrete families: the γ-type (γ-gliadins), α-type (α- and β-gliadins) and aggregated type (with intermolecular disulphide bonds). The aggregated type corresponds to the major group of LMW glutenin subunits, although this complex also contains some α-type, γ-type [17,18] and possibly also S-poor (ω-type) [19] subunits.

S-rich, S-poor and HMW prolamins are also present in barley and rye (see Table 11.2, Fig. 11.4), but neither species appears to contain α-type S-rich prolamins. Rye contains two types of γ-type S-rich prolamin, differing in their M_r and aggregation behaviour; the M_r 40 000

Table 11.2 Homologous groups of S-rich, S-poor and HMW prolamins present in wheat, rye and barley

	Wheat	Rye	Barley
S-rich prolamins			
γ-type	γ-gliadins	M_r 40 000 M_r 75 000 γ-secalins	γ-hordein
α-type	α- and β-gliadins	—	—
Aggregated type	LMW subunits of glutenin	—	B hordein
S-poor prolamins	ω-gliadins	ω-secalins	C hordein
HMW prolamins	HMW subunits of glutenin	HMW secalin	D hordein

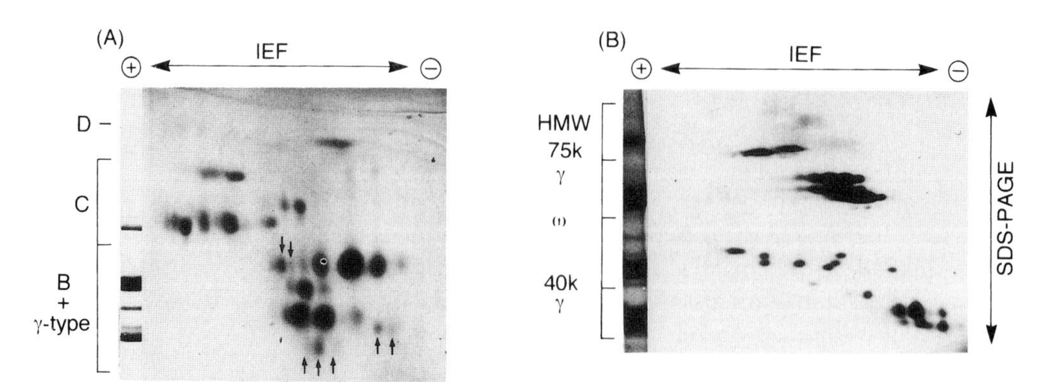

Fig. 11.4 Two-dimensional analyses of total prolamins from barley and rye. (A) barley, cv. Carlsberg II. The arrows indicate γ-hordeins. (B) rye, inbred line MPI 109. (From Shewry & Tatham [8].)

γ-secalins are monomers, whereas the M_r 75 000 γ-secalins form polymers stabilized by interchain disulphide bonds. The major S-rich prolamins of barley, called B hordeins, are of the aggregated type, but small amounts of γ-type hordeins are also present. The groups of prolamins present in wheat, barley and rye, with their trivial names, are summarized in Table 11.2.

The S-rich, S-poor and HMW prolamins also have characteristically different M_rs. The HMW prolamins have true M_rs of about 65 000–90 000 [20], although these may be overestimated by SDS-PAGE [21,22]. The S-poor prolamins have M_rs, determined by SDS-PAGE or hydrodynamic measurements, of between 40 000 and 70 000, with many components around 50–60 000 [23,24]. The S-rich prolamins generally have M_rs of between about 30 000 and 45 000, the M_r 75 000 γ-secalins being an exception.

Amino acid sequences

The amino acid sequences of representative prolamins from wheat, rye and barley are summarized in Fig. 11.5 and their detailed sequences presented in Figs 11.6, 11.7 and 11.8. Their amino acid compositions are given in Table 11.1. Despite great variation in sequence and composition, they have two features in common. First, they all consist of two or more distinct regions, sometimes called domains. Second, in all cases one of these domains is composed of repeated blocks of amino acids (Fig. 11.9).

The S-rich prolamins are diverse in sequence, but each consists of an N-terminal repetitive domain (which in some cases is preceded by a short unique sequence) and a C-terminal non-repetitive domain (Figs 11.5, 11.6). The latter contains most, or all, of the cysteines, methionines and charged residues. The repetitive domains consist of single or inter-

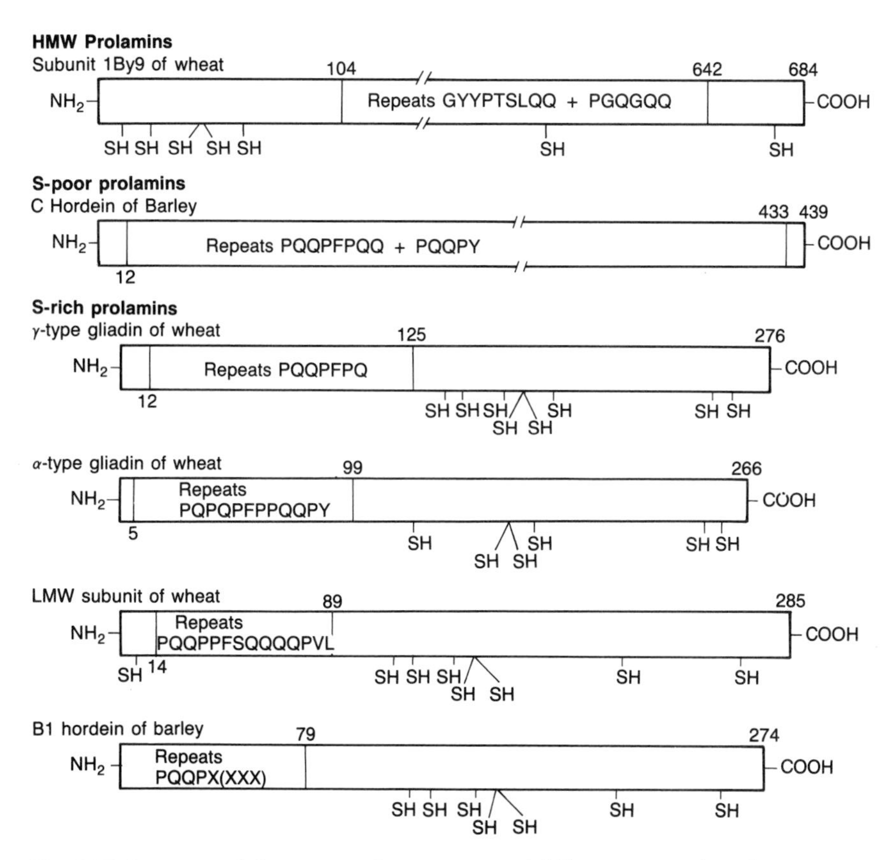

Fig. 11.5 Summary of the structural organization of different types of S-rich, S-poor and HMW prolamins. Single letter code for amino acids: A, alanine; C, cysteine; D, aspartate; E, glutamate; F, phenylalanine; G, glycine; H, histidine; I, isoleucine; K, lysine; L, leucine; M, methionine; N, asparagine; P, proline; Q, glutamine; R, arginine; S, serine; T, threonine; V, valine; W, tryptophan; X, unidentified; Y, tyrosine. (Sequences and data reported in [15,24,173–178].)

spersed repeats which vary in length and consensus sequence, but all are rich in proline and glutamine (Figs 11.5, 11.6, 11.9). In addition all groups have repeat motifs which contain the tetrapeptide PQQP which is related to the pentapeptide (PQQPY) and octapeptide (PQQPFPQQ) motifs of C hordein. However, there is no homology between the repeat motifs of the S-rich and S-poor prolamins compared with those of the HMW prolamins (Fig. 11.9).

Comparisons of the C-terminal domains of α-, γ- and aggregated types of S-rich prolamin reveal regions of related sequence, although these are separated by divergent regions [16,25,26]. The latter include two glutamine-rich regions (called poly-gln) in the α-type gliadins (Fig. 11.6), which are discussed in more detail below.

The complete amino acid sequences of S-poor prolamins are unknown, although the general structure of a typical C hordein has been

B1 hordein

```
  1  QQQPFPQQPIPQQPQPYPQQPQPYPQQPFPPQQPFPQQPV.PQQPQPYPQQPFPPQQPFPQ   60
 61  QPPFWQQKPFPQQPPFGLQQPILSQQQPCTPQQTPLPQGQLYQTLLQLQIQYVHPSILQQ  120
121  LNPCKVFLQQQCSPVPVPQRIARSQMLQQSSCHVLQQQCCQQLPQIPEQFRHEAIRAIVY  180
181  SIFLQEQPQQLVEGVSQPQQQLWPQQVGQCSFQQPQPQQVGQQQQVPQSAFLQPHQIAQL  240
241  EATTSIALRTLPMMCSVNVPLYRILRGVGPSVGV  274
```

***α*-gliadin**

```
  1  VRFPVPQLQPQNPSQQQPQEQVPLVQQQFLGQQQPFPPQQPYPQPQPFPSQLPYLQLQP   60
 61  FPQPQLPYSQPQPFRPQQPYPQPQPQYSQPQQPISQQQQQQQQQQQQQQQQQILQQILQ  120
121  QQLIPCMDVVLQQHNIAHGRSQVLQQSTYQLLQELCCQHLWQIPEQSQCQAILKVVHAII  180
181  LHQQQKQQQQPSSQVSFQQPLQQYPLGQGSFRPSQQNPQAQGSVQPQQLPQFEEIRNLAL  240
241  QTLPAMCNVYIPPYCTIAPFGIFGTN  266
```

***γ*-gliadin**

```
  1  NMQVDPSSQVQWPQQQPVPQPHQPFSQQPQQTFPQPQQTFPHQPQQQFPQPQQPQQQFLQ   60
 61  PQQPFPQQPQQPYPQQPQQPFPQTQQPQQLFPQSQQPQQQFSQPQQQFPQPQQPQQSFPQ  120
121  QQPPFIQPSLQQQVNPCKNFLLQQCKPVSLVSSLWSMIWPQSDCQVMRQQCCQQLAQIPQ  180
181  QLQCAAIHTVIHSIIMQQEQQQGMHILLPLYQQQQVGQGTLVQGQGIIQPQQPAQLEAIR  240
241  SLVLQTLPTMCNVYVPPECSIIKAPFSSVVAGIGGQ  276
```

LMW subunit

```
  1  MKTFLVFALIAVVATSAIAQMETSCISGLERPWQQQPLPPQQSFSQQPPFSQQQQQPLPQ   60
 61  QPSFSQQQPPFSQQQPILSQQPPFSQQQQPVLPQQSPFSQQQQLVLPPQQQQQQLVQQQI  120
121  PIVQPSVLQQLNPCKVFLQQQCSPVAMPQRLARSQMWQQSSCHVMQQQCCQQLQQIPEQS  180
181  RYEAIRAIIYSIILQEQQQGFVQPQQQQPQQSGQGVSQSQQQSQQQLGQCSFQQPQQQLG  240
241  QQPQQQQQQVLQGTFLQPHQIAHLEAVTSIALRTLPTMCSVNVPLYSATTSVPFGVGTG  300
301  VGAY  304
```

Fig. 11.6 The amino acid sequences of typical S-rich prolamins. All are shown as mature proteins except the LMW glutenin. This is shown with a signal peptide, with the predicted (but unconfirmed) cleavage site indicated by a small arrow. The large arrows indicate the junctions between N-terminal (repetitive) and C-terminal (non-repetitive) domains. The sequence repeats in all the proteins are underlined and the poly–gln regions in the α-type gliadins are underlined twice. See Fig. 11.5 for standard single letter abbreviations for amino acids. (Sequences taken from [152,175,177,180].)

Protein N-terminus

NH_2-RQLNPSSQELQSPQQSY
LQQPY
PQNPY
L

Chymotryptic peptides

XFXQQ	PNQQ
PQQPFPLQ	PQQIIPQQ
PQQPFPQQ	PQQPFPQQ
PQQI	PQQPFPQQ

Partial cDNA (pcP387)

PQQSYPVQ
PQQPFPQ
PQPVPQQ
PQQASPLQ
PQQPFQG
SEQII
PQQPFPLQ
PQQPFPQQ
PQQPLPQ
PQQPFRQQ
AELIIPQQ
PQQPLPLQ
PHQPYTQQ
TIWSMV-COOH

Fig. 11.7 Summary of available amino acid sequences of C hordein (S-poor) of barley. See Fig. 11.5 for standard single letter abbreviations for amino acids. (Sequences from [40,176].)

deduced from data obtained from various sources [24] (Fig. 11.7). It consists almost entirely of repeats, with only short unique regions at the N and C termini (totalling 18 residues). The repetitive domain consists predominantly of octapeptides, with several pentapeptides close to the N terminus. The high proportions of proline, glutamine and phenylalanine in these motifs (Fig. 11.7) account for the presence of about 80 mol% of these residues in the whole protein. Comparisons between the amino acid compositions (Table 11.1), and N-terminal amino acid sequences (Fig. 11.8), of ω-gliadins and ω-secalins indicate that most have similar sequences to C hordein [23].

The HMW subunits of wheat glutenin consist of a central repetitive domain flanked by shorter non-repetitive domains which contain most or all of the cysteine residues (Fig. 11.5). The repetitive domain consists of tandem and interspersed repeats of two or, in some subunits, three motifs (see Figs 11.9, 11.10), which are rich in glycine and account for the unusually high proportion of this amino acid in the whole protein. Less is known about the HMW prolamins of barley and rye, but they probably have similar sequences to the HMW subunits of wheat (Fig. 11.11) [27].

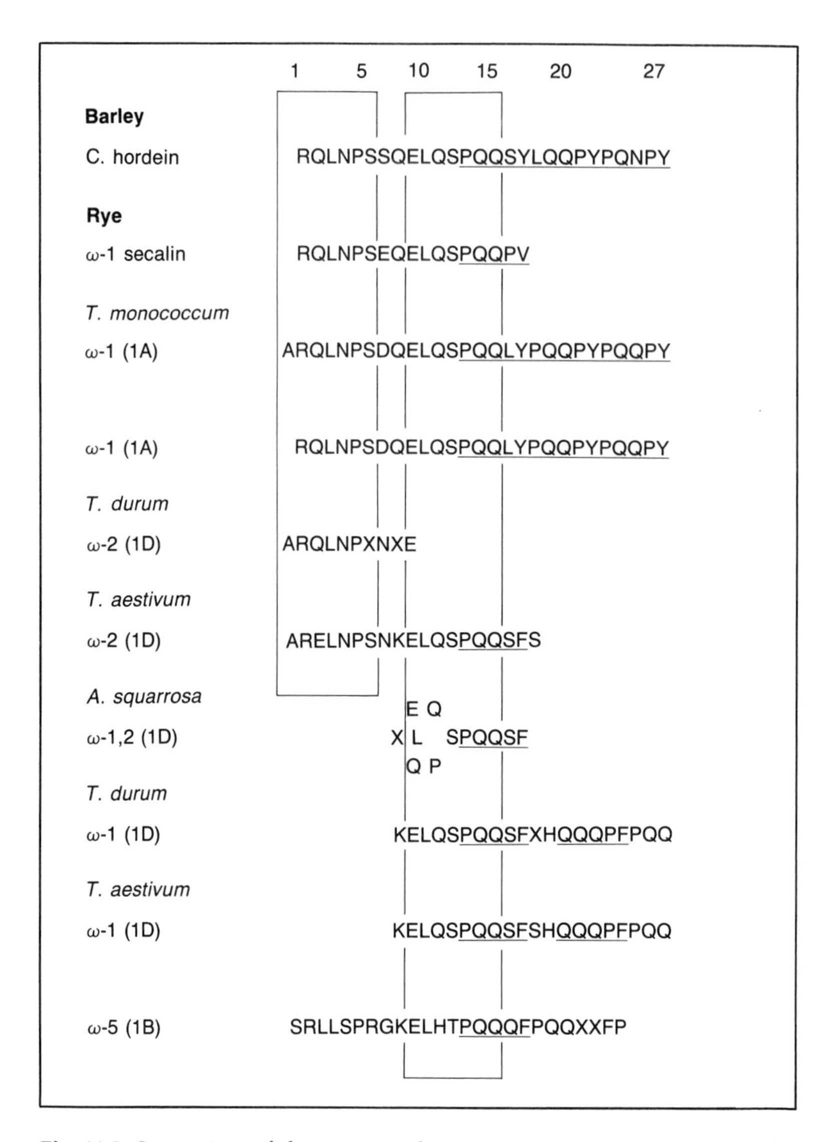

Fig. 11.8 Comparison of the N-terminal amino acid sequences of S-poor prolamins from barley (C hordein), rye (ω-secalins) and diploid, tetraploid and hexaploid species of wheat (ω-gliadins). Repeated blocks of five residues are underlined. See Fig. 11.5 for standard single letter abbreviations for amino acids. (Sequences taken from [23].)

The folding and subunit interactions of wheat, rye and barley prolamins

Levels of protein structure

Four levels of protein structure are recognized, the first being the amino acid sequence or primary structure. Secondary structure refers

S-rich prolamins	
γ-gliadin γ-secalins	PQQPFPQ(Q)
γ-hordeins	PQQPFPQQ
α-gliadins	PQPQPFPPQQPY*
LMW subunits	PQQPPPFSQQQQPVL*
B1 hordein	PQQPX(X)(X)
S-poor prolamins	
C hordein	PQQPFPQQ + PQQPY
HMW prolamins	
HMW subunits	PGQGQQ (+GQQ) + GYYPTS$^{P}_{L}$QQ

Fig. 11.9 The consensus repeat motifs of S-rich, S-poor and HMW prolamins. (These motifs can also be interpreted as interspersed repeats of two shorter motifs, see [25].) See Fig. 11.5 for standard single letter abbreviations for amino acids.

Sequence of subunit 1By9

```
                                    N
1 EGEASRQLQCERELQESSLEACRQVVDQQLAGRLPWSTGLQMRCCQQLRDVS
  AKCRPVAVSQVVRQYEQTVVPPKGGSFYPGETTPLQQLQQVIFWGTSSQTVQ
  GYYPSVSSPQQ GPYYPGQASPQQ PGQGQQ PGKWQE LGQGQQ GYYPTSLHQ
  SGQGQQ GYYPSSLQQ PGQGQQ IGQGQQ GYYPTSLQQ PGQGQQ IGQGQQ
  GYYPTSPQH PGQRQQ PGQGQQ IGQGQQ LGQGRQ IGQGQQ SGQGQQ GYYPTSPQQ
  LGQGQQ PGQWQQ SGQGQQ GYYPTSQQQ PGQGQQ GQYPASQQQ PGQGQQ
  GQYPASQQQ PGQGQQ GQYPASQQQ PGQGQQ GHYLASQQQ PGQGQQR RHYPASLQQ
  PGQGQQ GHYTASLQQ PGQGQQ GHYPASLQQ VGQGQQ IGQ LGQRQQ PGQGQQ
  TRQGQQ LEQGQQ PGQGQQ TRQGQQ LEQGQQ PGQGQQ GYYPTSPQQ SGQGQQ
  PGQSQQ PGQGQQ GYYSSSLQQ PGQGLQ GHYPASLQQ PGQGH PGQRQQ PGQGQQ
  PEQGQQ PGQGQQ GYYPTSPQQ PGQGKQ LGQGQQ GYYPTSPQQ PGQGQQ PGQGQQ
  GHCPTSPQQ TGQAQQ PGQGQQ IGQVQQ PGQGQQ GYYPISLQQ SGQGQQ SGQGQQ
                                               C
  SGQGHQ LGQGQQ SGQEQQ GYD NPYHVNTEQQTASPKVAKVQQPATQLPIMCRMEGGDALSASQ
                                                                  684
```

Fig. 11.10 The amino acid sequence of a typical γ-type HMW subunit of wheat glutenin, arranged to show the repeated blocks of six and nine residues. N and C indicate the non-repetitive N-terminal and C-terminal domains, respectively. See Fig. 11.5 for standard single letter abbreviations for amino acids. (Sequence from [177].)

to the regular local arrangement of the peptide backbone, and is stabilized by hydrogen bonds between peptide amide and carbonyl groups. Three major types are recognized: α-helix, β-sheet and β-turns (Fig. 11.12).

Tertiary structure refers to the three-dimensional structure of the protein, which is stabilized by disulphide bonds, hydrophobic inter-

```
              -3  1          10    15   16   20           30        40
D hordein     NIFLDSRSRQLQCERELQ---XSXLEACRRVVDQQLVGQLPSS*
HMW secalin          EGEASGQLQCERELQ---QSSLEACRQVVDQQLAGRLPWSTGL*
1Ay(silent)          EGEASKQLQCERELQ---ESSLEACRLVVDQQLASRLPWSTGL
1By9                 EGEASRQLQCERELQ---ESSLEACRQVVDQQLAGRLPWSTGL
1Dy10                EGEASKQLQCERELQ   ESSLEACRQVVDQQLAQRLPWSTGL
1Dy12                EGEASKQLQCERELQ---ESSLEACRQVVDQQLAGRLPWSTGL
                                                                **
1Ax2*                EGEASGQLQCERELQ---EHSLKACQQVVDQQL----------
T.monococcum         EGEASGQLQCEXELQ---EXXLKACQQV*
                                                                **
1Bx7                 EGEASGQLQCEHELE---------ACQQVVDQQL----------
                                                                **
1Dx2                 EGEASEQLQCERELQELQERELKACQQVMDQQL----------
                                                                **
1Dx5                 EGEASEQLQCERELQELQERELKACQQVMDQQL----------
T.tauschii           EGEASEQLQCERELQELQEXELKAC*
```

Fig. 11.11 Comparison of the N-terminal amino acid sequence of HMW prolamins from barley (D hordein), rye (HMW secalin), diploid wheats (*T. monococcum* and *T. tauschii*) and hexaploid bread wheat (subunits 1Ax2*, 1Dx2, 1Dx5, 1Bx7, 1By9, 1Dy10 and 1Dy12). Variant residues are boxed. *Indicates last residue determined by automated Edman degradation, **indicates deleted region present in protein encoded by genomic clone. (From Shewry *et al.* [20].)

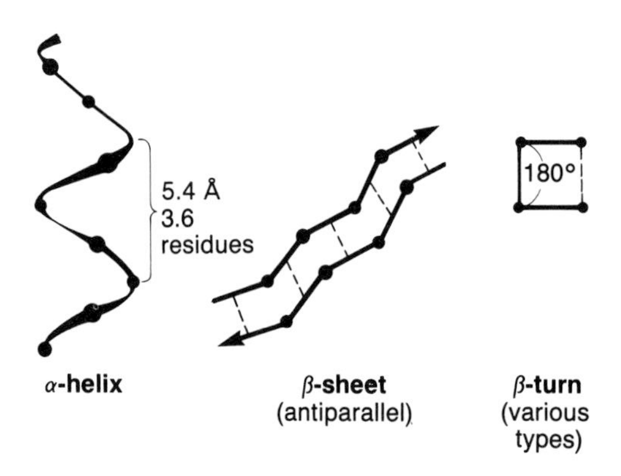

Fig. 11.12 Schematic diagram of the three major elements of protein secondary structure: α-helix, β-sheet and β-turn. Dashed lines indicate hydrogen bonds, which are often (but not always) present between residues one and four of a β-turn.

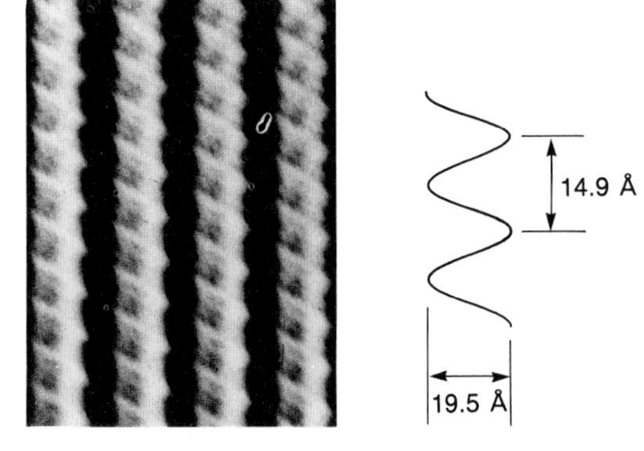

Fig. 11.13 Scanning tunnelling microscopy (STM) of a wheat glutenin subunit shows a novel helical super-secondary structure. (The STM image is taken from Miles *et al.* [44].)

actions, hydrogen bonding and electrical forces. The ω-gliadins of wheat and related S-poor prolamins lack cysteine residues, and their tertiary structures are stabilized solely by non-covalent forces. The α-type and γ-type gliadins of wheat are examples of monomeric proteins in which intramolecular disulphide bonds contribute to stabilization of the tertiary structure.

Quaternary structure refers to the assembly of individual proteins to form a polymer or aggregate. These structures may again be stabilized by covalent disulphide bonds and/or by non-covalent forces. For example, A-(α-)gliadins form fibrils stabilized by non-covalent forces [28,29], while the glutenins of wheat are stabilized additionally by disulphide bonds.

Secondary and tertiary structures

The secondary structures of cereal prolamins have been determined directly by circular dichroism and optical rotary dispersion (ORD) spectroscopy, but also predicted from their amino acid sequences with computer algorithms. In addition, the shapes and dimensions of some individual prolamins have been determined by a range of methods, most recently by viscometric analyses [30,31,32].

The repetitive domains of the S-rich prolamins are predicted to form β-turns, and this has been confirmed for γ-gliadins and α-gliadins by direct spectroscopic analyses of peptides [33,34,35]. A β-turn results in a 180° change in the direction of the polypeptide backbone, and involves four amino acid residues (Fig. 11.12). The regularity of the predicted turns varies with the degree of degeneracy of the repeat motifs, but they may be sufficiently regular to form a helical structure in the γ-gliadins [34] and γ-secalins (A.S. Tatham and P.R. Shewry, unpublished results), as described below for the S-poor and HMW proteins.

The non-repetitive domains of the S-rich and HMW prolamins appear to be globular with compact tightly folded conformations and elements of α-helix and β-sheet [30,33,36–38].

Recent studies suggest that the repetitive domains of the HMW subunits of wheat, and of C hordein of barley, adopt an unusual super-secondary structure based on β-turns (Fig. 11.13). Regular β-turns are predicted to form within the repetitive domains of both proteins, and this is supported by direct spectroscopic (circular dichroism, infrared and nuclear magnetic resonance) analyses of whole proteins and of synthetic peptides based on the repeat motifs [39–43]. The C hordein and HMW subunit molecules are rod-shaped [31,32] and it was proposed that this resulted from the formation of a loose spiral structure based on regularly repeated β-turns. In fact, scanning tunnelling microscopy (STM) of an HMW subunit has recently provided direct visual evidence for such a structure [44]. Preliminary spectroscopic analyses of other HMW and S-rich prolamins indicate that they have essentially similar structures to those of the HMW subunits, and C hordein, respectively [33,37,42].

Subunit interactions

The classification of wheat gluten proteins into gliadins and glutenins is based on whether the individual subunits are present as monomers or form polymers stabilized by interchain disulphide bonds; similar distinctions can be made in barley and rye. It is not, however, so easy to define these groups at the molecular level; whereas the HMW prolamins occur only in polymers in all three species, the other polymeric prolamins do not fall into distinct groups. In wheat they consist predominantly of aggregated-type S-rich prolamins, but also include some α-type and γ-type and probably also ω-type subunits [17,18,19]. In barley they consist predominantly of B hordeins [45], but it is not known whether some γ-type hordeins are also present (similarly some B hordeins may be monomeric). In rye most, if not all, of the M_r 75 000 γ-secalins form polymers, but not the M_r 40 000 γ-secalins [45,46], which are monomeric and consist of single polypeptide chains.

In addition to covalent disulphide bonds, prolamins also interact by strong non-covalent forces. The most intensively studied interactions of this type occur in the A-gliadin group of α-type S-rich gliadins. The individual α-gliadin monomers are globular molecules [30] and these aggregate under certain conditions of pH and ionic strength to form

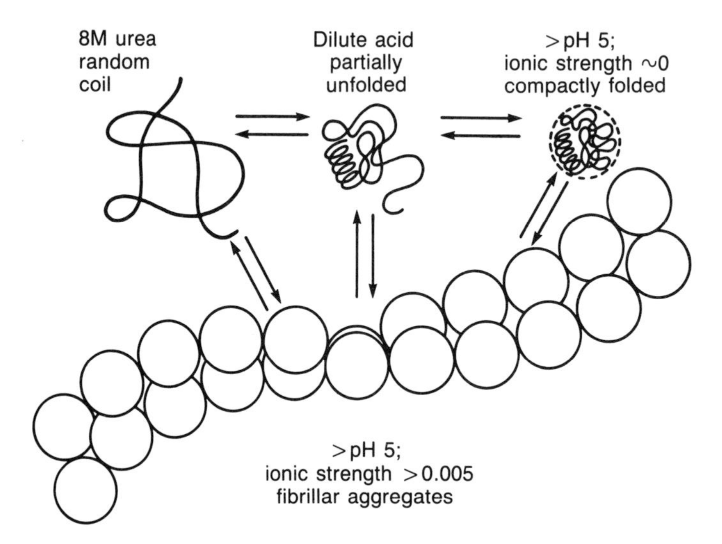

Fig. 11.14 Schematic diagram of the conformational structure and aggregation state of A-gliadin under various conditions. (From Kasarda *et al.* [180].)

fibrils with diameters up to 8 nm and lengths up to 300–400 nm [29,47] (Fig. 11.14). These fibrils are probably stabilized mainly by hydrogen bonding but contributions from ionic interactions and hydrophobic forces are likely to be present.

Role of wheat, rye and barley prolamins in food systems and effects of processing

The major use of wheat in Europe and the USA is for baking leavened bread. Its suitability for this purpose is determined by the amounts and properties of the glutenin polymers, and their interactions with each other and with the gliadin monomers. In order to understand how these interactions are established it is necessary to return to our account of protein deposition.

The prolamin-containing protein bodies deposited in the developing wheat endosperm become disorganized during the later stages of grain maturation and grain drying, forming part of a matrix surrounding the starch granules [48]. The adding of water to flour, and the kneading to form dough, may serve to rearrange these proteins to form the gluten network, allowing the establishment of strong non-covalent interactions.

Disulphide-stabilized prolamin polymers with similar polypeptide compositions to those prepared from gluten are present in protein bodies isolated from developing endosperms [49], demonstrating that interchain disulphide bonds are formed during grain development. Their formation may be catalysed by the enzyme protein disulphide isomerase, which is associated with the ER in developing endosperms of wheat [50] and in other tissues [51]. This enzyme also catalyses *in vitro* disulphide bond formation in a number of proteins, including wheat gliadins and glutenins [52,53,54]. The extent to which rearrangement of the disulphide bonds in gluten occurs both during dough formation and the later stages of the breadmaking process is unknown, but some commonly used dough 'improvers', for example cysteine, are able to catalyse such reactions.

The properties of wheat gluten are also important in determining its suitability for other purposes, such as the baking of flat breads, biscuits and cakes, the making of pasta and noodles (whether using bread or durum wheat) as well as other usages in the food industry. In all these applications processing may affect the structures and properties of the gluten proteins. Chemical agents are used to adjust (via effects on disulphide bonds) the strength of wheat doughs for biscuits.

In the breadmaking process, carbon dioxide, produced by yeast fermentation, is trapped in the dough gluten–starch matrix, to form a light porous crumb structure. It is generally accepted that this structure is 'fixed' by starch gelatinization and protein modification/denaturation

[55]. In the oven the temperature at the surface of the loaf, the crust, often exceeds 200°C, which leads to decomposition of the protein to produce non-volatile compounds, with a consequent loss of extractable protein [56,57]. The dough to crumb transformation takes place around 70°C [58] and further heating to 95–100°C fixes the crumb structure [59]. Gliadins can be extracted from the bread crumb without the use of reducing agents, though less are extracted than from flour; in addition, they appear to be largely unmodified [56,57,60,61]. Similar results are reported for cooked noodles, spaghetti and macaroni [62].

Studies on the thermal properties of whole gluten have shown that protein denaturation is not an important factor in the baking process and that the proteins do not show marked enthalpy transitions [63]. Isolated gliadins in solution show reversible temperature effects up to about 80–90°C, as judged by their structure contents [37]. Thus, during processing it appears that the gliadins, the principal coeliac-active components of wheat, undergo little change apart from aggregation via disulphide bonds. This view is supported by binding studies of wide-specificity monoclonal and polyclonal antibodies raised against proteins associated with starch granules and against HMW subunits of glutenin. All types of antibody recognized proteins in flour, dough and bread; indicating that the antigenic sites are not destroyed by heat [64]. However, antibodies to the gluten proteins did not recognize the proteins after extrusion cooking at high temperature, shear rate and pressure [64]. This combination of processes destroyed the antigenic sites, possibly due to racemization and decomposition of the amino acid side chains and cleavage of the protein backbone.

Structural studies of synthetic peptides show that some sequences that appear to be associated with coeliac activity are found in the proline-rich repetitive domains, and are conformationally flexible [35,43]. Their structures change with temperature (heating or cooking) but are not irreversibly affected by these processes and regain their initial conformations at ambient temperature. Thus, coeliac-active sequences should be unaffected by these milder forms of processing and heating and hence remain active in wheat-based foodstuffs.

Although some barley is used in the food industry or is ingested as whole grain (for example in soups and stews), most of the barley consumed by humans is in the form of beer and whisky. In both cases the basic raw material is malt, consisting of grains which have been allowed to germinate under carefully controlled conditions of temperature and hydration and then dried. The malt provides enzymes for the degradation of starch, which comes partly from the malt itself, but also from other added sources, for example, unmalted barley or other cereals. The use of such adjuncts depends on their relative cost and on regulations governing beer and spirit production. The fate of the cereal prolamins during these processes is unknown.

Malting of barley is accompanied by partial proteolysis of the prolamins [65], and further digestion of these and the prolamins present in added grain undoubtedly occurs during the fermentation stage. It is known that beer contains a complex mixture of peptides which vary in their M_r, amino acid composition, and hydrophobicities [66–68]. These may be detrimental in forming hazes on chilling, but also contribute positively to head formation and lacing (the cling of the beer to the glass) [69,70]. Some of these peptides could derive from prolamins, especially from the N-terminal repetitive domains of the S-rich and S-poor prolamins whose high contents of proline might be expected to inhibit proteolysis. It is much less likely that appreciable amounts of prolamin-derived peptides would be present in distilled liquors such as whisky.

Rye is used directly for human nutrition as bread (sometimes mixed with wheat to give a lighter crumb structure) and crispbread, and is also used for whisky production. Processing can be expected to have effects on the grain prolamins similar to those described above for wheat and barley.

The prolamins of other cereals

The prolamins of oats (avenins) and rice

Oats and rice differ from other cereals in that prolamins account for only about 5–15% of the total seed proteins. In both cases the major seed storage proteins are related to the 11S legumin-type globulins of legumes and other dicotyledonous plants.

Avenin consists of about 12 components with M_rs by SDS-PAGE of about 22–37 000 [71], and contains about 36 mol% glutamate + glutamine, and 10 mol% each of proline and leucine [72]. Bietz [73] submitted a total avenin fraction to automated Edman degradation and demonstrated a single major sequence starting with the unusual sequence thr–thr–thr. Related or identical N-terminal amino acid sequences have since been reported for a number of purified components with M_rs ranging from 23 to 34 000 [71,74], while Egorev [75] determined the complete sequence of a single component (Fig. 11.15). This consisted of 182 residues, with a true M_r of 21 000. A unique N-terminal sequence of 20 residues had limited homology with those of γ-type prolamins of the Triticeae [76], and was followed by three repeated sequences consisting of pro–phe–val with three, four and five glutamines. The unique C-terminal domain contained three conserved regions corresponding to regions A, B and C of the S-rich and HMW prolamins of wheat, barley and rye. It differed from other prolamins of the Triticeae, however, in having three imperfect glutamine-rich repeats between regions B and C. More recently Chesnut *et al.* [77] have reported the

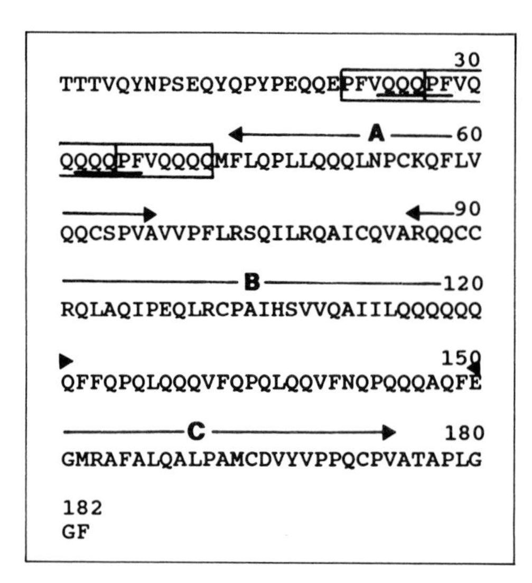

Fig. 11.15 The amino acid sequence of a major 'fast' avenin taken from Egorev [75]. A, B and C indicate conserved regions which are homologous with regions present in the prolamins of barley, wheat and rye. Three sequence repeats are boxed, while two copies of the pentapeptide motif QQQPF are underlined. See Fig. 11.5 for standard single letter abbreviations for amino acids.

sequences of three cloned cDNAs encoding avenins of M_rs 18 441 (162 residues), 23 276 (201 residues) and 23 538 (203 residues). They are essentially similar in structure to the avenin studied by Egorev [75], differing mainly in the numbers of repeats in the N-terminal repetitive domain and between regions B and C (five and five, respectively, in two of the proteins; two and three, respectively, in the third protein).

Fabijanski *et al.* [78] recently reported the N-terminal amino acid sequence and complete cDNA sequence of an avenin of M_r about 18 000. This consisted of 186 residues, and contained no sequence repeats. The spacing of cysteine residues in the N-terminal part of the protein, and in particular the presence of a double cysteine, indicates that it may be distantly related to the C-terminal domain of the more typical avenin studied by Egorev [75]. However, the C-terminal third of the protein showed unexpected homology with the oat 12S globulin [79], including an identical sequence of 21 residues. Pernollet *et al.* [74] have also purified a protein of M_r 16 000 with an N-terminal amino acid sequence related to that of the protein encoded by this cDNA clone.

SDS-PAGE analyses of rice prolamins show a major band with an M_r reported as between 11 000 and 14 000 and minor bands of lower M_r [73,80–83]. Kim and Okita [84,85] reported the nucleotide and deduced amino acid sequences of three cDNAs and one gene related to the major prolamin group. They encoded mature proteins of about 145 residues, with M_r of about 15 200. The clones could be classified into two subclasses, the encoded proteins differing most notably in their contents of cysteine (0.7 compared to 5.9 mol% in typical examples). A sequence of the low cysteine type is shown in Fig. 11.16. They did not contain repeated sequences, and had no significant homology with

```
        10     ↓   20          30
MKIIFVFALLAIAACRPLPSLMFLGQSYRQ
        40         50          60
YQLQSPVLLQQQVLSPYNEFVRQQYGIAAS
        70         80          90
PFLQSAAFQLRNNQVWQHQAGGQQSRYQDI
       100        110         120
NIVQAIAYELQLQQFGDLYFDRNQAQAQAL
       130        140        149
LAFNVPSRYGIYPRYYGAPSTITTLGGVL
```

Fig. 11.16 The amino acid sequence of a rice prolamin taken from [84]. The sequence is deduced from the nucleotide sequence of a cloned cDNA, and includes a signal peptide. The predicted site of signal peptide cleavage is indicated by an arrow. See Fig. 11.5 for standard single letter abbreviations for amino acids.

prolamins from other species. Because non-prolamin proteins, for example wheat albumins, may also be alcohol-soluble, there may be no true equivalents of the prolamins of wheat, rye, barley and oats present in rice.

More recently Matsumura *et al.* [86] reported the characterization of a cDNA encoding a minor S-rich rice prolamin of M_r 10 000. Part of the sequence around two adjacent cysteine residues was homologous with the conserved region B present in the S-rich prolamins of the Triticeae, but proline-rich repeats were not present.

The prolamins of maize and related species

The zeins of maize consist of four groups of proteins with M_rs by SDS-PAGE ranging from 10 000 to 28 000. All are rich in glutamine and proline and lack lysine and tryptophan, but they differ considerably in their contents of other amino acids (notably histidine, cysteine and methionine).

Two of these groups, the α- and δ-zeins, do not appear to be related to any other proteins. The α-zeins account for about 75–80% of the total fraction [87] and consist of multiple components with M_rs by SDS-PAGE of about 19 000 and 22 000 (true M_rs 23 000–24 000 and 26 000–27 000, respectively). The individual components have a similar structure with between 60 and 97% sequence identity [87]. They consist of unique domains of 36–37 and 10 residues at the N and C termini, respectively, separated by a repetitive domain consisting of blocks of about 20 residues. The repeats are degenerate in sequence, and it is not possible to recognize an unambiguous consensus motif. They are rich in leucine and alanine residues, and have no apparent relationship to the repeat motif present in the prolamins of wheat,

N-Terminal

36
FIIPQCSLAPSASIPQFLPPVTSMGFEHPAVQAYRL

Repeats

50
1 QLALAASALQQPIA

67
2 QLQQQSLAHLTLQTIAT

90
3 QQQQQQFLPSLSHLAMVNPVTYL

108
4 QQQLLASNPLALANVAAY

133
5 QQQQQLQQFMPVLSQLAMVNPAVYL

150
6 QLLSSSPLAVGNAPTYL

174
7 QQQLLQQIVPALTQLAVANPAAYL

192
8 QQLLPFNQLAVSNSAAYL

213
9 QQRQQLLNPLAVANPLVATFL

232
10 QQQQQLLPYNQFSLMNPAL

C-Terminal

242
QQPIVGGAIF

Fig. 11.17 The amino acid sequence of an M_r 22 000 α-zein (cZZZA1) of maize arranged to show the repeat structure. The underlining indicates glutamine-rich regions discussed in the text. See Fig. 11.5 for standard single letter abbreviations for amino acids. (From Rubenstein & Geraghty [156].)

barley and rye. The size difference between the M_r 19 000 and M_r 22 000 components appears to result from the insertion of an additional repeat motif in the latter, resulting in 10 repeats compared to nine in the M_r 19 000 group. The sequence of a typical M_r 22 000 α-zein is shown in Fig. 11.17.

The δ-zein is a minor component with an M_r by SDS-PAGE of 10 000 (true M_r 14 400). It is methionine-rich (about 22 mol%), but not related to the other group of methionine-rich zeins, the β-zeins [88]. The latter consist of components with M_rs by SDS-PAGE of 14 000 and 16 000, and account for about 10–15% of the total fraction [87]. Their true M_rs are about 17 500, and they are rich in methionine (~11 mol%) and cysteine (~4 mol%). They do not contain repeated sequences, but do have three conserved regions which are related to those present in the S-rich and HMW prolamins of the Triticeae.

Regions related to A, B and C are also present in the γ-zeins, which have M_rs by SDS-PAGE of about 28 000 and true M_rs of about 22 000. They also contain repeated sequences, eight conserved hexapeptides with the sequence pro–pro–pro–val–his–leu (PPPVHL). These are not related to the repeated sequences present in the Triticeae, and there is evidence that they adopt a poly-L-proline II structure rather than a β-turn rich structure when dissolved in non-polar solvents [89].

The prolamins of sorghum, millets and Job's tears (*Coix lachryma-jobi*) have been less well-studied, but available information indicates that those species have similar groups of prolamins to those present in maize [73,90–92].

Cereal proteins and CD

As described by Anderson (p. 8) it was shown in a series of investigations beginning in 1950 [93–96] that wheat, rye and oats are harmful to coeliac patients, whereas rice flour, maize (corn) flour, buckwheat flour, potatoes and wheat starch are not; barley was soon added to that list [97] on the basis of its ability to interfere with fat absorption. Weijers *et al.* [96] emphasized that 'wheat does not cause the disease, but may trigger the appearance of what are probably constitutionally determined abnormalities'.

It now seems reasonably certain that only the prolamins of these grains are responsible for triggering mucosal damage in coeliac patients, and that they comprise a complex mixture of components. In order to better understand the results of more recent experiments that attempt to define which of these components is active, or most active, or whether all have some effect, and which specific amino acid sequences cause mucosal damage, it may be useful to consider the conclusions of earlier workers in the light of present criteria and knowledge.

Because the technique of intestinal biopsy was not introduced until c. 1960, workers up to that time relied on the production of symptoms or of fat malabsorption; other tests, such as the degree of xylose malabsorption, were also employed, although none are considered satisfactory by all physicians. The early data on wheat and rye are beyond doubt; however, some studies carried out in controlled scientific studies, but with relatively few patients included work on the effects of rice flour and maize flour. Simoons [98] considered that maize flour used in early studies was possibly maize starch and thus essentially free of protein; there have been no controlled scientific studies on maize proteins. Rice and maize have come to be regarded as safe for coeliac patients, presumably because no contradictory evidence was encountered by physicians over the years; conclusions regarding the effect of wheat have been backed up in recent years by considerable testing in which the state of the intestinal epithelium was monitored by mucosal biopsies.

For other grains the body of clinical evidence for a pathogenic role is much less, and controlled scientific studies are relatively few. Furthermore, the results of certain studies are conflicting. Although oats were considered harmful by Weijers *et al.* [96] based on their ability to induce fat malabsorption, at least four subsequent studies

[99] did not incriminate oats including that of Dissanayake *et al.* [100]. This last study seems well done and in accordance with most modern criteria. Four patients were studied, all diagnosed to have CD with intestinal biopsy to demonstrate a flat mucosa, and rapid improvement on a strict gluten-free diet. (There was no indication in the paper, however, that these patients had undergone subsequent gluten challenge to determine how readily they were affected by wheat.) A baseline intestinal biopsy was taken and the patients were fed 40–60 g/day of oats. The patients remained symptom-free for 4 weeks and all tests, including biopsy, indicated that no harm had been done. On this basis Dissanayake *et al.* [100] concluded that oats are not harmful.

Two years later, Baker and Read [99] reported that oats were damaging. However, they did not use intestinal biopsy, but relied on the xylose absorption test and the appearance of symptoms for their conclusions. Nevertheless, they included more patients in their study and carried out the test over a longer period than Dissanayake *et al.* [100], which is an important difference.

Controversy in regard to the coeliac toxicity of oats is likely to result in part from the relatively lesser amounts of avenins (4–14% of total protein) in this grain [101] as compared with gliadin in wheat (approximately 40% of total protein). Thus, even if the prolamins of oats were equivalent in their activity to the gliadin of wheat (which has not been established), it would most likely take a considerably greater intake of oats to bring about equivalent effects. Because there are so many apparent conflicts in the literature on CD in regard to grain toxicity, it is often impossible to draw rigorous scientific conclusions. To some extent, it is only the studies of wheat and wheat proteins that are based on a truly solid foundation.

Speculations on the pathogenicity of untested grains

Wheat, rye, barley, oats, maize, rice and buckwheat have all been subjected to some degree of testing in CD. Concerning the role of other grains or seeds in this regard, about the best that can be done is to make some educated guesses on the basis of taxonomy, which classifies plants into degrees of relationship based on morphology and other factors.

In Fig. 11.1, it may be seen that wheat, rye and barley fall within the same tribe, whereas oats belongs to a neighbouring tribe; these are the only known toxic cereal grains. On the other hand, rice and maize are not harmful. It seems reasonable to assume that grains related closer to maize than wheat, such as sorghum, millet, and Job's tears are unlikely to be harmful. Furthermore, grains or seeds of plants that do not belong to the grass family are even less worthy of concern; these include buckwheat, amaranth and quinoa. Conversely, all grains that belong to the tribe Triticeae (sometimes Hordeae) should be approached with some caution by coeliac patients, especially close relatives of wheat within the same genus (*Triticum*). Examples are the diploid wheat *Triticum monococcum*, the tetraploid durum wheats (used for pasta making), and hexaploid relatives of *Triticum aestivum* (common bread wheat), such as *Triticum spelta* and *Triticum macha*. *Triticum monococcum* and durum wheats have been shown by amino acid sequencing to contain proteins belonging to all the major prolamin types of bread wheats [23,102] and the electrophoretic pattern of the proteins *Triticum spelta* along with chromosomal assignments of these proteins indicate that they are virtually identical to those of bread wheats [103,104]. Auricchio *et al.* [105] found that durum wheat gliadins are toxic by *in vivo* testing, although they did not find toxicity by *in vitro* testing.

Amino acid sequences suggest that certain wild grasses of the genera *Phleum, Dactylis, Lolium, Festuca, Elytrigia (Agropyron)* and *Haynaldia* contain proteins fairly closely related to the prolamines of wheat and oats [106,107,108] although seeds of these grasses would not ordinarily be eaten by humans.

Fractionation of wheat

Once it had been established that wheat flour is largely responsible for the symptoms of CD [93], attempts to pinpoint the active fraction began immediately. Gluten, prepared by washing the starch from a dough was demonstrated to be harmful, whereas wheat starch was not [94,95,109]. When gluten was extracted with 50% aqueous ethanol to yield gliadin (the soluble fraction) and glutelin (the residue fraction also called glutenin), the gliadin fraction was shown to cause malabsorption in coeliac patients; the glutenin fraction, tested on one patient, gave only a slight reaction [95].

This glutenin test deserves further comment. The patient studied was known to give a violent reaction to even a small piece of bread, causing vomiting and abdominal pain within a few hours and this reaction was used by van de Kamer *et al.* [95] as a screening test. It is surprising to find that the residue from a 50% ethanol extraction of gluten, which would normally contain at least small amounts of gliadin, had little effect. This same patient was also used to screen the solutions used to wash gluten from doughs, as well as the ash, crude fibre and fat fractions of flour. When gluten was washed from flour with water, the washwater caused slight reaction; however, when the gluten was washed out of the latter with 10% sodium chloride, no effect was noted. These last results were taken as an indication that wheat albumins and globulins that would be extracted in both cases are not harmful, the slight reaction in the case of the water wash resulting presumably from slight solubility of gliadin in the lower ionic strength solution. The patient showed no reaction to other fractions. It is not at all clear that patients who have violent, almost 'immediate' reactions to wheat are representative of coeliac patients, since this response is very atypical. This patient could have had an IgE-mediated allergy to wheat. Thus, little confidence can be placed in results based on one patient. Furthermore, Sheldon [110] reported no differences between his gliadin and glutenin fractions; both were active.

The conclusion that wheat starch is not harmful to patients also deserves some comment. The fat absorption experiments were not likely to pick up the effects of tiny amounts of harmful proteins as too little of the intestinal epithelium may have been damaged to cause malabsorption or obvious symptoms. Wheat starch has been shown to contain small amounts of gliadins [111] and although it has not been demonstrated to damage the intestinal epithelium in studies involving biopsies and relatively short-term feeding of wheat starch products [112], the long-term effects of even small amounts of gliadin might be undesirable in view of the increased prevalence of cancer in coeliac patients, which appears to be diminished by a strict gluten-free diet [113].

Van de Kamer and Weijers [114] recognizing the predominance of the amino acid glutamine in the composition of the gliadin fraction of wheat, tested patients with 2–4 g of glutamine/day, which corresponds to 125–150 g of wheat flour. They found no effects and thus concluded that glutamine as a free amino acid is without effect. In order to test the effect of glutamine bound into the polypeptide chains of gliadins, the same authors [114] hydrolysed gliadin for 2 hours with 1 N HCl at 37°C. They estimated that only 3% of the glutamine was left unhydrolysed to glutamic acid and that peptide chains were largely intact with about 15% of the peptide bonds hydrolysed. The resulting gliadin appeared free of activity as judged by an immediate improvement in fat absorption when fed to a patient. Because the principal effect of the hydrolysis was to hydrolyse glutamine to glutamic acid, these authors suggested that glutamine incorporated into the peptide chains of gliadins is responsible for their tissue damaging effects. The small amount of polypeptide chain cleavage reported could, however, have cleaved the chains in the middle of a key sequence, thus rendering the peptides inert. The possibility remains that glutamine incorporated into the polypeptide chain, particularly as part of a specific sequence involving other amino acids, such as proline, might produce pathological effects and it is unfortunate that further work along these lines has not been carried out. An obvious extension would have been to test the effects of polyglutamine, polyproline, and copolymers of these two amino acids (which are both predominant in gliadins) on coeliac patients by examining biopsied intestinal tissues after challenge.

The non-toxic nature of albumins first indicated by Van de Kamer [95] was supported by an 18-day feeding study carried out by Auricchio *et al.* [115] in which xylose excretion, faecal fat excretion, and intestinal biopsies were used as indicators of intestinal damage. The wheat albumins are a complex group of proteins that are substantially different in structure from the wheat gluten proteins (although they have small regions of similar amino acid sequence; see Kreis *et al.* [26]), and on this basis are highly unlikely to be relevant to CD.

Enzymatic digestion of gliadin

In an attempt to study the effect of the normal digestion process on gluten toxicity, Frazer *et al.* [116] digested gluten with pepsin and trypsin and showed that the ultrafiltrate comprising highly soluble peptides with M_rs <15 000 retained activity, even after autoclaving. These results established that intact proteins are not essential for disease. They also reported that activity could be abolished by treatment with a fresh extract of pig intestinal mucous membrane [116], but no details of how the extract was prepared, or the peptides treated, were given; this experiment has never been repeated.

Bronstein *et al.* [117] fractionated, by ion exchange chromatography, ultrafiltrates of peptic–tryptic digests and similar preparations digested with crude pancreatic enzyme. They concluded that an acidic fraction rich in glutamine and proline, in which N-terminal glutamine had been cyclized to N pyrrolidone, is the active moiety based on faecal fat measurements. This hypothesis was not supported by subsequent work [118,119], but Woodley [120] found that the enzyme capable of hydrolysing such pyrrolidone residues is present in coeliac mucosae. It thus seems likely that the active 'acidic peptides' of Bronstein *et al.* [117] correspond to amino acid sequences containing glutamine and proline, and that the presence of N-pyrrolidone terminal amino acids in their preparation was a coincidental phenomenon.

Cornell *et al.* [121–126] also digested a crude gliadin fraction with pepsin, trypsin and pancreatin, followed by ultrafiltration and ion-exchange chromatography and identified a fraction (no. 9) that appeared to be active when monitored by xylose absorption, organ culture of challenged intestinal tissue and ability to disrupt rat liver lysosomes.

Further fractionation of fraction 9, followed by 'digestion' with treated coeliac mucosae led to the conclusion that the latter was less capable of digesting gliadin peptides of fraction 9 (or certain subfractions of fraction 9) than normal mucosae. Two resistant peptides (M_r = 700) were subjected to amino acid analysis [126] yielding the compositions Glx_3 Pro_2 Ser_1 and Glx_3 Pro_2 Tyr_1, and corresponding apparently to amino acid sequences found in the primary structure of A-gliadin [15], i.e. amino acid residues 13–18 (PSQQQP) and 40–45 (QQPYPQ); the latter sequence is repeated at residues 77–82. The former sequence is highly similar to residues 213–218, (PSQQNP). Cornell *et al.* [125] considered an enzyme defect, or at least an enzyme deficiency, to be the most likely explanation for their results, but admitted that no evidence for this view has ever been obtained.

Furthermore, in a careful study by Bruce *et al.* [127] in which brush border preparations were made from biopsied tissues rather than from homogenates, no evidence of deficient (in terms or rate of completeness) digestion of gliadin peptides from a peptic–tryptic digest of α-gliadin was obtained. The brush border cleaves oligopeptides to amino acids or dipeptides, whereas cytosolic peptidases act only on dipeptides, which presumably arise from the digestive action of brush border peptidases [128]. It would appear that brush border peptidases are the key for gliadin digestion, but are not the fundamental defect predisposing to CD. The apparent conflict between the results of Cornell *et al.* [125] and Bruce *et al.* [127] remains unresolved.

In the studies of enzymatic digests of gliadin just described, peptides linked by intramolecular disulphide bonds would have remained intact. Van Roon *et al.* [129] oxidized peptides of a peptic–tryptic digest with performic acid and then bromine, confirmed the absence of cysteine in hydrolysates, and fed the resulting peptides to three subjects, two with CD in remission, and one control. Only the two coeliac patients responded with an increase in non-absorbed fat. It was thus concluded [129] that gliadin 'toxicity' is independent of intramolecular cysteine residues, or of peptides combined through such crosslinks.

Fractionation of gliadin

In the 1960s, the development of gel electrophoresis showed that the gliadin fraction of wheat could be resolved into at least 20 components in a high resolution one-dimensional gel [130], but we know that there are about 40 gliadin components resolvable by two-dimensional gel electrophoresis [55,104,131]. The differences in amino acid sequences among the major electrophoretic mobility groups (α-, β-, γ- and ω-gliadins) and even among the components in a given group are sufficiently large [8] that digestion of a crude gliadin fraction with mixtures of enzymes, such as pepsin and trypsin, gives rise to enormously complicated mixtures of peptides. As the complexity of the gliadin fraction itself became apparent, the question arose whether all these different gliadin components were active in CD or whether this was limited to a particular component(s).

Hekkens and coworkers [132] were first to answer this question. They prepared an α-gliadin fraction characterized as 80% pure, with impurities corresponding mainly to β-gliadin, but also some γ-gliadins and albumins. The β-gliadins have since been shown to be structurally close to α-gliadin and have been grouped with them as α-type gliadins [24]. The α-gliadin fraction of Hekkens *et al.* [132] probably comprised ~90% α-type gliadins. Instillation of this fraction into the small intestine of a gluten-sensitive patient (but with mucosa not completely returned to normal) on a wheat-free diet produced changes in the mucosa. In subsequent work, Hekkens and coworkers [132–134] have made a reasonably good case for the pathogenicity of α-gliadin, especially the A-gliadin fraction (a type of α-gliadin [135]).

Following this Kendall *et al.* [136] carried out an ion-exchange fractionation of crude gliadin and fed a fraction described as 'α-gliadin' to patients. They concluded that the α-fraction was clearly active in a study involving five patients, whereas changes in xylose absorption for other fractions were not significant, thus proposing that other gliadins are irrelevant. Unfortunately, no gel electrophoresis patterns were shown in this paper so it is difficult to assess the nature and purity of their pre-α, γ-, and post-α-gliadin fractions. Kumar *et al.* [137] also reported *in vivo* toxicity in an α-gliadin fraction, but not with other gliadin types.

Strober's group [138–140] pioneered the *in vitro* organ culture of intestinal mucosal tissues obtained by biopsy as a model for CD. Damaged tissues from patients with active CD (wheat included in the diet) showed improvement in enzyme levels and morphology when cultured in the absence of gliadin, but not when gliadin was present [141]. The gliadin used in these studies was highly purified by the method of Bernardin *et al.* [47] and their results support the view that α-gliadin damages coeliac mucosa. Levels of gliadin that prevented recovery of damaged tissues had no effect on mucosae that were essentially normal following a gluten-free diet [138], which does not seem to be in accord with any direct effect towards epithelial cells.

Jos *et al.* [142] fractionated gliadins into the classical electrophoretic groups (α-, β-, γ- and ω-) and tested peptic–tryptic digests of the fractions on *in vitro* organ cultured mucosal fragments from patients with active disease. In later work, Jos *et al.* [143] fractionated peptic–tryptic digests of these groups and tested a particular fraction (fraction V) obtained by gel filtration, by the same method. They concluded that fraction V, derived from all classes of gliadins even ω-gliadins, damaged coeliac mucosa, a finding later substantiated by Howdle *et al.* [144] who also used the organ culture approach with intact gliadins, rather than fraction V.

The damaging effect of all gliadin protein components on post-challenge mucosae was supported by Ciclitira *et al.* [145] who instilled 1 g portions of α-, β-, γ- and ω-gliadins, prepared by ion exchange chromatography, into the duodenum of three patients. In all studies, the α-, β-, γ- and ω-gliadin fractions represented groups of components that had the appropriate range of electrophoretic mobilities. Such traditional mobility groupings, however, do not necessarily correspond to structural types [23]. Most notably, components that are apparently structurally identical to α-gliadins are found in the γ-gliadin mobility fraction [146]. Although it is difficult to say how much (if any) α-type gliadin was present in the γ-mobility fractions of Ciclitira *et al.* [145], it is possible that disease activity of the γ-gliadin fractions resulted from such α-type gliadins. In the case of their ω-gliadins, however, the ω-mobility grouping has only ω-type (by structure) gliadins [23]. Because ω-type gliadins are farthest removed structurally from α-type gliadins mucosal activity in this fraction provides support for the contention that all gliadins are damaging to coeliac patients.

In experiments where peptides (obtained by enzymic digestion of purified gliadin fractions) containing multiple protein components are further fractionated by ion-exchange chromatography, gel-permeation chromatography, or reverse phase high-performance liquid chromatography (HPLC), as in the experiments of Cornell [118,126] and Jos *et al.* [143], the use of a common peak from each separation makes it more likely that structures in common are being used for testing. Thus, if a chromatogram peak resulting from subfractionation of a γ-gliadin peptide mixture is eluted under the same solvent conditions that produces a peak in the separation of peptides from an α-gliadin preparation, it is quite possible that the peptides from the γ-mixture will be close in structure to components derived from α-type structures. Furthermore, if an active peptide sequence should appear many times in the proteins of one type, but only once in the proteins of another type, testing of equivalent amounts of the equivalent peptide fractions would tend to indicate equal damaging potential for both types of proteins. It appears therefore that no results to date provide meaningful information about γ-gliadins with γ-type structure relative to the activity of γ-gliadins (and β-gliadins and α-gliadins) with α-type structure.

Testing of gliadin peptides of known amino acid sequence

Jos *et al.* [146] carried out further purification of fraction V from a β-gliadin by reverse phase (RP) HPLC. They found clear evidence in the organ culture test of activity at very low concentration (0.01 mg/ml) for one of their purified peptides (peptide b). Although they did not report amino acid sequences other than N-terminal amino acids, the derivation of their peptide b from a peptic–tryptic digest of a β-gliadin (which is almost certain to have α-type structure) combined with its having an N-terminal valine residue and an appropriate amino acid composition, makes it fairly likely that their peptide corresponded to residues 3–24 of α-type gliadins (see Figs 11.6, 11.18).

Jos *et al.* [146] reported MWs of 5500 for two peptides a and b. This

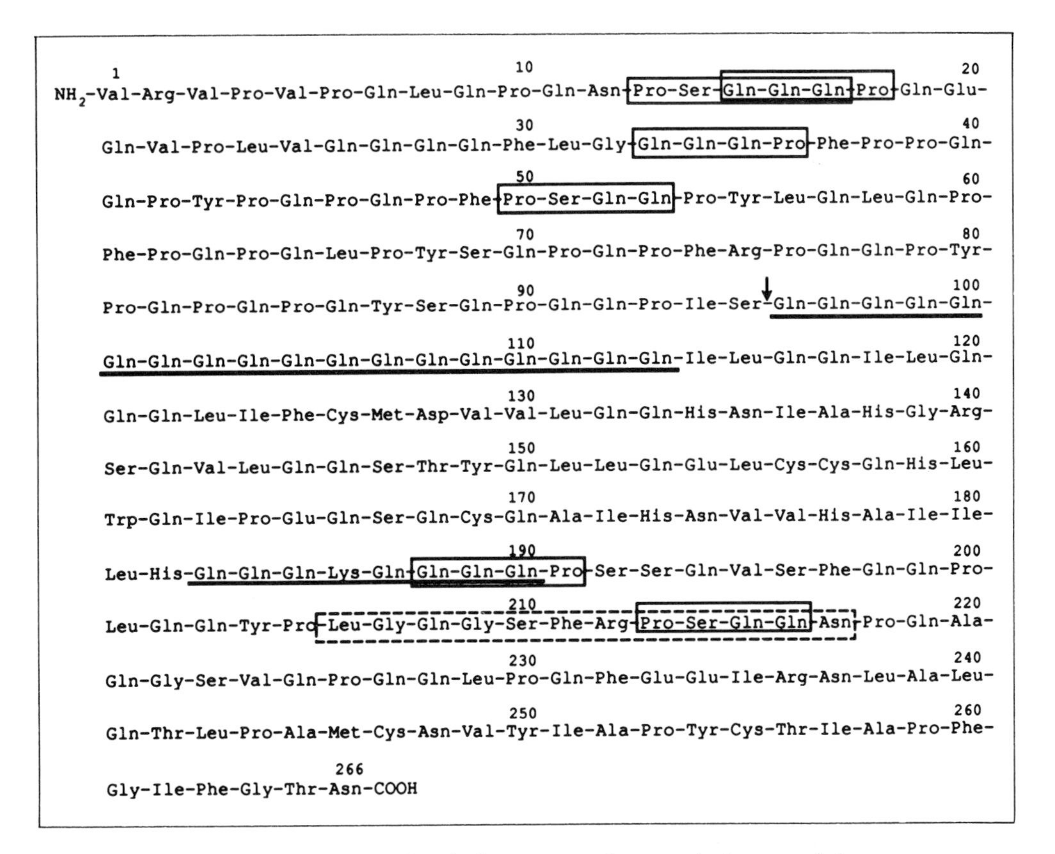

Fig. 11.18 The amino acid sequence of A-gliadin, a group of α-type gliadins encoded by genes on chromosome 6A in some wheat cultivars such as Scout 66. Most of the sequence was determined by direct protein sequencing, and therefore represents a consensus sequence for the whole group of proteins. Standard three letter abbreviations for amino acids are used. The boxes indicate putative toxic tetrapeptide motifs (gln–gln–gln–pro and pro–ser–gln–gln). The polyGln regions are underlined and the junction between domain 1 and 2 indicated by an arrow. (From Kasarda *et al.* [15].)

MW is too large for a peptide corresponding to residues 3–24, but de Ritis *et al.* [147] found that small gliadin peptides seem to give anomalous results in SDS-PAGE. For example, a peptide corresponding to residues 31–55 of an α-type gliadin, which has a calculated MW of 2900 actually migrated more slowly in SDS-PAGE than a ribonuclease standard with a MW of 13 700.

Jos *et al.* [146] noted that β-gliadins were somewhat more damaging than α-gliadins in their experiments. β-gliadins are usually of the same structural type as α-gliadins, but some are greater in MW [148] probably either from insertion of additional repeating sequences into the N-terminal region of the polypeptide chain or because of an amplification of the polyglutamine stretch in the N-terminal half of α-gliadins (O.D.

Anderson, personal communication). The former mechanism might result in an increase in the copy number of an active sequence associated with the gln–pro repeats, with a consequent increased potential over α-gliadins for mucosal damage.

Wieser *et al.* [149–151] purified a peptide from a peptic–tryptic digest of crude gliadin and subsequently degraded it into two fragments with chymotrypsin. Each peptide was shown to be active by the organ culture test and the leucocyte migration inhibition factor (LIF) test. Their amino acid sequences corresponded to regions of gliadins with α-type structure; the equivalent residues in the A-gliadin structure (Fig. 11.18) being 3–55 (B 3142), 3–24 (CT-1) and 25–55 (CT-2) with one difference of a substitution of proline at position 31 for the leucine of A-gliadin [15], which is a known variant of the A-gliadin sequence [152]. Wieser *et al.* [151] noted that the largest sequence in common to their peptides was a four-residue sequence pro–ser–gln–gln (PSQQ), which occurred three times in the sequence of A-gliadin but which was not present in proteins, such as zeins, that do not exacerbate CD.

de Ritis *et al.* [147] degraded the A-gliadin molecule which consists of 266 amino acid residues [15] into a series of peptides that covered the entire sequence (Fig. 11.19) and whose activity was investigated by the organ culture technique. The three intramolecular disulphide bonds of the protein were first cleaved by reduction and the resulting cysteine residues were S-methylated to stabilize them. The protein was next subjected to cleavage by cyanogen bromide, which broke the molecule into two large peptides and one small peptide.

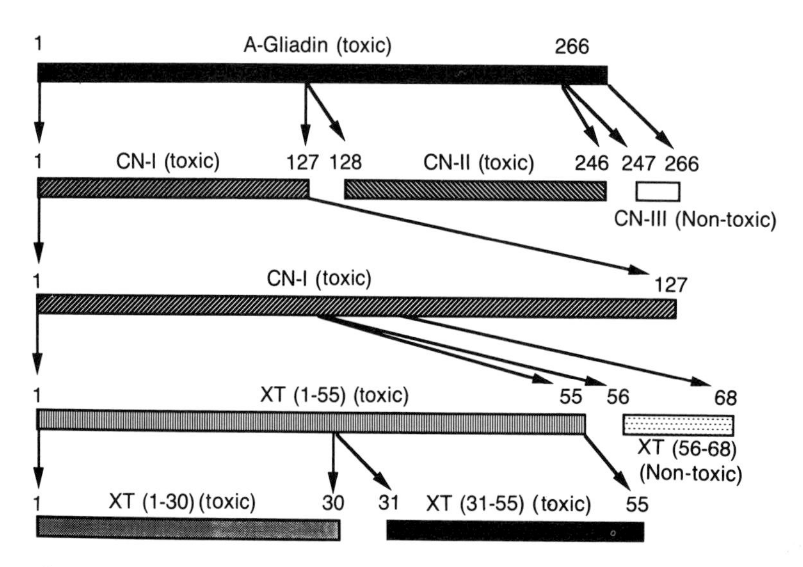

Fig. 11.19 Summary of the toxicity of A-gliadin peptides tested by [147] using the organ culture technique.

The two larger peptides prevented restitution of enterocyte cell height, while the smaller one did not. The latter peptide contained no glutamine and only two proline residues in its 20-residue primary structure. The large N-terminal peptide was then further degraded by limited chymotryptic digestion and two peptides, corresponding to residues 1–55 and 56–68 of A-gliadin were purified and tested. Only the larger peptide prevented cell recovery despite the smaller peptide having glutamine and proline in interesting combinations such as pro–phe–pro–gln–pro–gln (PFPQPQ). Complete digestion of peptide 1–55 by further chymotryptic digestion yielded two smaller peptides corresponding to residues 1–30 and 31–55. Both peptides prevented mucosal recovery in organ culture and are almost identical to active peptides CT-1 and CT-2 of Wieser *et al.* [151].

In addition to the sequence PSQQ recognized as the largest sequence common to peptides CT-1 and CT-2 by Wieser *et al.* [149], de Ritis *et al.* [147] noted that the sequence QQQP was also common to all of their active peptides, along with PSQQ. This commonality does not necessarily signify that these four-residue sequences constitute the immunogenic sequence in CD, but obviously they should receive high priority in further testing. Devery *et al.* [153] as reviewed in Skerritt *et al.* [154] found no activity for the tetrapeptide PSQQ when tested in a macrophage procoagulant assay (MPC assay). Devery *et al.* also found no activity for the peptide ser–phe–arg–pro–ser–gln–gln–asn–pro–gln–ala–gln–gly (SFRPSQQNPQAQG) that corresponds to gliadin residues 210–222 (Fig. 11.18) and which includes the PSQQ sequence, whereas they found high activity for the peptide pro–gln–pro–phe–pro–ser–gln–gln–pro–tyr–leu–gln (PQPFPSQQPYLQ), which corresponds to gliadin residues 46–57. It remains to be established, however, that the MPC assay is a valid measure of coeliac-active peptides. The results apparently conflict, for example, with organ culture test results [147]. *In vivo* testing ultimately will be necessary to evaluate conclusions based on *in vitro* testing.

Kagnoff *et al.* [155] found a 12 residue sequence of gliadin that was similar to a sequence found in the E1b protein produced as a consequence of infection by adenovirus 12, a human gastrointestinal tract virus. The E1b protein is not an integral viral protein, but is expressed early in infection, presumably playing a role in controlling gene transcription through another protein, E1a. The gliadin sequence (residues 206–217) leu–gly–gln–gly–ser–phe–arg–*pro–ser–gln–gln*–asn, which shows homology with the E1b protein sequence, also includes the PSQQ motif. Kagnoff *et al.* [155] suggested that sequence homology between a viral protein and gliadins might result in viral infection being an environmental factor involved in the pathogenesis of CD. The well-documented cases of discordance for the disease in identical twins [140] has been taken as an indication that an environmental factor may be necessary to trigger the development of CD in genetically susceptible individuals. Once the immune system has been primed by viral infection and exposure to the E1b protein, subsequent encounters with the related protein sequence found in α-type gliadins might trigger an adverse immune response capable of damaging the absorptive mucosal cells of the small intestinal epithelium.

The sequence QQQP appears to be common to many wheat gluten proteins (α-type gliadins, γ-gliadins, LMW-glutenin subunits, some ω-gliadins and some HMW-glutenin subunits) and their equivalents in rye and barley, and also in the avenins or prolamins of oats [75,77] (Fig. 11.15). Although not a proof of toxicity in oats, the presence of this sequence in avenins, but not in zeins [156] or in rice prolamins (Fig. 11.16) and glutenins [84,85,157], provides indirect evidence to support disease activity for oats.

Pavone *et al.* [158] synthesized the pentapeptide tyr–gln–gln–gln–pro (YQQQP) and characterized its NMR spectrum. In later, unpublished work (S. Auricchio, personal communication) Pavone and coworkers repeated this fundamental motif four times within a peptide comprising 20 residues and tested it by the organ culture approach. Unfortunately, the results were ambiguous in that one lot of the peptide was highly active, but two other independently prepared lots were not.

Although zeins are presumably inactive in coeliac patients, maize prolamins nevertheless contain sequences that are gliadin-like, gln–gln–pro (QQP), gln–gln–leu–leu–pro–phe (QQLLPF) and gln–gln–gln–gln–gln–gln–phe (QQQQQQF) [156] (Fig. 11.17). The occurrence of six adjacent glutamine residues in zein makes it seem likely that stretches of gln alone, such as that in the N-terminal half of A-gliadin, where 18 adjacent glutamine residues can be found (Fig. 11.18), are irrelevant to the pathogenesis of CD. There appear to have been no controlled tests of zein peptide fractions, for example by the organ culture technique. It might be interesting to reinvestigate them under more rigorous conditions than those employed in the early 1950s, particularly in the light of Simoons' [98] query about the nature of the maize flour used and his suggestion that maize starch may have been employed rather than complete maize endosperm.

Can the active pathogenic factor in wheat be removed?

Kasarda and coworkers noted in 1976 [159] that only α-gliadins, especially the α-gliadin group known as A-gliadin [28,135] had been clearly implicated in the pathogenesis of CD [132,133,136]. It had also been shown by Kasarda's laboratory that the A-gliadin genes are located on chromosome 6A [159] in certain cultivars e.g. Scout 66 but not in

Chinese Spring. Because satisfactory lines of the suitable cultivars were not available, it was decided to grow sufficient amounts of a Chinese Spring line from which the chromosome 6A had been deleted (nullisomic 6A-tetrasomic 6B was chosen) for feeding tests, even though fewer α-gliadin genes were coded for by chromosome 6A of this variety [159].

Although it was recognized that other α-gliadins, coded on chromosomes other than 6A (chromosome 6D, especially) remained, it was felt that testing was warranted on the chance that only the 6A-coded proteins might be damaging. Initial studies, based on xylose and fat absorption, showed no effect, and the two patients who received about 65 g of bread made from nullisomic 6A flour daily for 16 days remained asymptomatic [160]. Further studies in which three additional patients (and one of the original two in a retest) were fed about 130 g of bread per day and in which intestinal biopsies were taken before and after feeding demonstrated, however, that definite tissue damage occurred by the end of the test periods, even though the patients remained asymptomatic (D.M. Goodenberger, D.D. Kasarda, C.O. Qualset, D.K. Mecham and W. Strober, unpublished results). Thus, it became clear that simply deleting the genes coding for α-gliadins on chromosome 6A from the cultivar Chinese Spring did not remove its tissue damaging effects. The point was also established by Ciclitira *et al.* [161].

Because we are now fairly certain that all gliadins, and possibly glutenins, can cause mucosal damage in susceptible patients, is it feasible to construct a new cultivar from which the responsible genes have been deleted? If all the genes encoding for gliadins and glutenins could be deleted or silenced, the flour would almost certainly lose its ability to form a dough with desirable elasticity and extensibility. It could not therefore be processed into leavened breads or other forms in which it is normally consumed without addition of a synthetic gluten substitute such as methyl cellulose. Breads made from such a cultivar would probably be no more desirable to coeliac patients than rice breads or potato breads.

Despite the paucity of available information, it is a distinct possibility that different cultivars do differ in their potential to evoke symptoms or mucosal damage. Furthermore, despite the conflicting evidence, the α-type gliadins may be more potent in this respect compared with γ- or ω-species; certainly many studies appear to point in that direction. Autran *et al.* [102] measured the relative proportion of α-type gliadins to γ-type gliadins in two different wheat cultivars and in some of the diploid species related to the A, B and D genomes of hexaploid bread wheats by an amino acid sequencing method. They found that the ratio of α-type to γ-type gliadins was 1.6 for the cultivar 'Scout 66', a cultivar that has the A-gliadin cluster of α-gliadin genes and which appeared to produce symptoms more readily in patients studied by D.M. Goodenberger *et al.* (unpublished results). The ratio was 0.9 for the cultivar 'Justin', which does not carry the A-gliadin cluster and which appears similar in protein electrophoretic pattern to Chinese Spring [135], the cultivar used to produce the nullisomic 6A line used by D.M. Goodenberger *et al.*

It is at least possible, therefore, that different wheat varieties might have intrinsically different pathogenic activities and that the tetraploid durum wheats used in the making of pasta might be less active than bread wheats (*Aegilops squarrosa*, the contributor of the third (D) genome that distinguishes bread wheats from pasta wheats, had large amounts of α-type gliadins [102]). These differences in activity, should they exist, would not justify eating bread from cultivars of lower toxicity by coeliac patients, because it is clear that even the nullisomic 6A line of Chinese Spring produced damage to the intestinal mucosa of coeliac patients (D.M. Goodenberger *et al.*, unpublished results) [160] and that such intestinal damage, in the longer term, could conceivably lead to the development of certain malignancies associated with gluten sensitivity [113].

Comments on the nature of the active factor in wheat in relation to possible mechanisms of mucosal damage

The active factor seems to be a simple polypeptide without covalently bound carbohydrate [28], derived from the degradation of gluten proteins. Furthermore, cyclization of N-terminal glutamine residues to form a pyrrolidone ring does not seem to be responsible for toxicity [120]. At present, the most likely possibility is that the factor consists of a relatively small peptide that includes a specific sequence made up of glutamine and proline residues, and, possibly, tyrosine, phenylalanine or serine residues. The size is uncertain although it seems likely that fewer than 25 amino acid residues are required, on the basis of organ culture studies, and perhaps only four to six key residues may be important [117,147].

There seems to be little doubt that immunological factors are central to the production of intestinal damage in coeliac patients [140,162,163]. Other workers cling to older hypotheses and suggest that one or other of these mechanisms is a necessary prelude for a secondary immunological process to be initiated.

That the primary defect may be a brush border membrane hydrolase (peptidase) defect [119,126] has been considered above and felt to be inadequate an explanation; furthermore, such a view contravenes current ideas about protein digestion in the mammalian intestine [164,165]. Secondly, the proposal that an inherited defect in mucosal permeability

[166] could be the necessary predisposing factor is unlikely because no abnormality could be demonstrated in first degree coeliac relatives, despite villous lymphoid infiltrates [163,165,166]. Thirdly, it has been advanced that gliadin has lectin-like properties and binds to enterocyte membranes [167]. However, there is little evidence for binding of intact gliadin proteins to enterocytes, while an additional difficulty stems from the small size of active gliadin oligopeptides compared with the fairly large MWs of known lectins; the active gliadin peptides with MWs as small as about 2500 do not seem large enough to contain the specific carbohydrate binding sites characteristic of lectin proteins.

Finally, we note the similarity between gliadin amino acid sequences and those of the proline-rich and glutamine-rich domains of various transcription controlling proteins [168–171]. If gliadin peptides could gain entry into cells (by some unspecified mechanism) and then enter the nucleus (small proteins seems to pass freely into the nucleus [173]), they might mimic the effects of such control proteins and thus interfere with important processes such as transcription of genes necessary for cell proliferation and differentiation, expression of cell surface receptors, or replication of latent adenovirus (e.g. adenovirus 12). There is at present, however, no experimental evidence for this hypothesis.

To date, certain *in vitro* tests have produced clues about possible peptide sequences that might be specific in their ability to trigger mucosal damage in CD. Synthesis of peptides corresponding to those sequences and their use in controlled feeding tests are likely to produce unambiguous identification of one or more active sequences concerned with CD pathogenesis. The identification of clearly defined active peptides should then facilitate the discovery of the mechanisms by which mucosal damage occurs.

References

1 *Production Yearbook*. Food and Agricultural Organisation, Rome, 1988:41.
2 Beccari JB. *De Frumento. De Bononiensi Scientarium et Artium*. Instituto atque Academia Commentarii 2 (Part 1). Bologna: L. Vulpe, 1745: 122–7.
3 Parmentier AA. Examin chimique des pommes de terre, dans lequel on traite des parties contistuantes du ble. *Didot de Jeune*. Paris, 1773.
4 Taddei G. Richerche sul glutine del frumento. Giornale di fisia, chemica e storia naturale. *Brugnatelli* 1819;2:360–1.
5 Einhof H. Chemical analysis of rye (*Secale cereale*). *Neues Allgem J Chem* 1805;5: 131–53.
6 Einhof H. Chemical analysis of small barley (*Hordeum vulgare*). *Neues Allgem J Chem* 1806;6:62–98.
7 Osborne TB. *The Vegetable Proteins*. 2nd edn. London: Longmans, Green and Co., 1924.
8 Shewry PR, Tatham AS. The prolamin storage proteins of cereal seeds: structure and evolution. *Biochem J* 1990;267:1–12.
9 Halford NG, Forde J, Shewry PR, Kreis M. Functional analysis of the upstream regions of a silent and expressed member of a family of wheat seed protein genes in transgenic tobacco. *Plant Sci* 1989;62:207–16.
10 Kim WT, Franceschi VR, Krishnan H, Okita TW. Formation of wheat protein bodies:

involvement of the Golgi apparatus in gliadin transport. *Planta* 1988;176:173–82.
11 Larkins BA, Hurkman WJ. Synthesis and deposition of zein in protein bodies of maize endosperm. *Plant Physiol* 1978;62:256–63.
12 Miflin BJ, Burgess SR, Shewry PR. The development of protein bodies in the storage tissues of seeds. *J Exp Bot* 1981;32:199–219.
13 Shewry PR. Methods of the analysis of cereal prolamins. In: Pattakou V, ed. *Protein Evaluation in Cereals and Legumes*. EEC Report EUR 10404 EN. Luxembourg: EEC, 1987:5–19.
14 Tatham AS, Shewry PR, Belton PS. Structural studies of cereal prolamins, including wheat gluten. In: Pomeranz Y, ed. *Advances in Cereal Science and Technology*. X. St Paul, Minnesota: American Association of Cereal Chemists, 1990:1–78.
15 Kasarda DD, Okita TW, Bernardin JE *et al.* Nucleic acid (cDNA) and amino acid sequences of α-type gliadins from wheat (*Triticum aestivum*). *Proc Natl Acad Sci USA* 1984;81:4712–16.
16 Kreis M, Shewry PR. Unusual features of seed protein structure and evolution. *Bioessays* 1989;10:201–7.
17 Shewry PR, Miflin BJ, Lew EJL, Kasarda DD. The preparation and characterization of an aggregated fraction from wheat. *J Exp Bot* 1983;34:1403–10.
18 Tao HP, Kasarda DD. Two dimensional gel mapping and N-terminal sequencing of LMW glutenin subunits. *J Exp Bot* 1989; 40:1015–20.
19 Payne PI, Holt LM, Lister PG. *Gli*-A3 and *Gli*-B3, two newly designated loci coding for omega-type gliadins and D subunits of glutenin. In: Miller TE, Koebner RMD, eds. *Proceedings of the International Wheat Genetics Symposium*. Cambridge: Institute of Plant Science Research, 1988:999–1002
20 Shewry PR, Halford NG, Tatham AS. The high molecular weight subunits of wheat, barley and rye: genetics, molecular biology, chemistry and role in wheat gluten structure and functionality. In: Miflin BJ, ed. *Oxford Surveys of Plant Cell and Molecular Biology*. Oxford: Oxford University Press, 1989:163–219.
21 Bunce NAC, White RP, Shewry PR. Variation in estimation of molecular weights of cereal prolamins by SDS-PAGE. *J Cereal Sci* 1985;3:131–42.
22 Ng PKW, Bushuk W. Concerning the nomenclature of high molecular weight glutenin subunits. *J Cereal Sci* 1989;9:53–60.
23 Kasarda DD, Autran JC, Lew EJL, Nimmo CC, Shewry PR. N-Terminal amino acid sequences of ω-gliadins and ω-secalins: implications for the evolution of prolamin genes. *Biochem Biophys Acta* 1983;747: 138–50.
24 Shewry PR, Tatham AS. Recent advances in our understanding of cereal seed protein structure and functionality. *Comments Agric Food Chem* 1987;1:71–93.
25 Kreis M, Forde BG, Rahman S, Miflin BJ, Shewry PR. Molecular evolution of the seed storage proteins of barley, rye and wheat. *J Mol Biol* 1985;183:499–502.
26 Kreis M, Shewry PR, Forde BG, Forde J, Miflin BJ. Structure and evolution of seed storage proteins and their genes, with particular reference to those of wheat, barley and rye. In: Miflin BJ, ed. *Oxford Surveys of Plant Cell and Molecular Biology*. Oxford: Oxford University Press, 1985:253–317.
27 Shewry PR, Kreis M. The development and composition of barley grain: relationship to end use, and the potential for manipulation. In: Sparrow DHB, Lance RCM, Henry RJ eds. *Alternative End Uses of Barley*. Parkville, Victoria, Australia: Cereal Chemistry Division, Royal Australian Chemical Institute, 1989:61–6.
28 Bernardin JE, Saunders RM, Kasarda DD. Absence of carbohydrate in celiac-toxic A-gliadin. *Cereal Chem* 1976;53:612–14.
29 Kasarda DD, Bernardin JE, Thomas RS. Reversible aggregation of A-gliadin to fibrils. *Science* 1967;155:203–5.
30 Cole EW, Kasarda DD, Lafiandra D. The conformational structure of A-gliadin. Intrinsic viscosities under conditions approaching the native state and under denaturing conditions. *Biochem Biophys Acta* 1984;787:244–51.
31 Field JM, Tatham AS, Baker A, Shewry PR. The structure of C hordein. *FEBS Lett* 1986;200:76–80.
32 Field JM, Tatham AS, Shewry PR. The structure of a high molecular weight subunit of wheat gluten. *Biochem J* 1987;247: 215–21.
33 Purcell JM, Kasarda DD, Wu CSC. Secondary structures of wheat α- and ω-gliadin proteins: fourier transform infrared spectroscopy. *J Cereal Sci* 1988;7:21–32.
34 Tatham AS, Masson P, Popineau Y. Conformational studies of peptides derived from the enzymic hydrolysis of a gamma-type gliadin. *J Cereal Sci* 1990;11:1–13.
35 Tatham AS, Marsh MN, Wieser H, Shewry

PR. Conformational analysis of peptides corresponding to the coeliac active regions of A-gliadin. *Biochem J* 1990;270:313–18.
36 Kasarda DD, Bernardin JE, Gaffield W. Circular dichroism and optical rotatory dispersion of α-gliadin. *Biochemistry* 1968;7: 3950–57.
37 Tatham AS, Shewry PR. The conformation of wheat gluten proteins. The secondary structures and thermal stabilities of α-, β-, γ- and ω-gliadins. *J Cereal Sci* 1985;3: 103–13.
38 Tatham AS, Field JM, Smith SJ, Shewry PR. The conformation of wheat gluten proteins. 2. Aggregated gliadins and low molecular weight subunits of glutenin. *J Cereal Sci* 1987;5·203–14.
39 Tatham AS, Shewry PR, Miflin BJ. Wheat gluten elasticity: a similar molecular basis to elastin? *FEBS Lett* 1984;177:205–8.
40 Tatham AS, Drake AF, Shewry PR. A conformational study of C hordein, a glutamine and proline-rich cereal seed protein. *Biochem J* 1985;226:557–62.
41 Tatham AS, Drake AF, Shewry PR. Conformational studies of a synthetic peptide corresponding to the repeat motif of C hordein. *Biochem J* 1989;259:471–6.
42 Tatham AS, Drake AF, Shewry PR. Conformational studies of synthetic peptides corresponding to the repetitive regions of the high molecular weight (HMW) glutenin subunits of wheat. *J Cereal Sci* 1990;11:189–200.
43 Tatham AS, Miflin BJ, Shewry PR. The β-turn conformation in wheat gluten proteins: relationship to gluten elasticity. *Cereal Chem* 1985;62:405–12.
44 Miles MJ, Carr HJ, McMaster TJ *et al.* Scanning tunneling microscopy of a wheat seed storage protein reveals details of an unusual supersecondary structure. *Proc Natl Acad Sci USA* 1991;88:68–71.
45 Field JM, Shewry PR, Miflin BJ. Aggregation states of alcohol-soluble storage proteins of barley, rye, wheat and maize. *J Sci Food Agric* 1983;34:362–9.
46 Shewry PR, Parmar S, Miflin BJ. The extraction, separation and polymorphism of the prolamin storage proteins (secalins) of rye. *Cereal Chem* 1983;60:1–6.
47 Bernardin JE, Kasarda DD, Mecham DK. Preparation and characterization of α-gliadin. *J Biol Chem* 1967;242:445–50.
48 Parker ML. Protein body inclusions in developing wheat endosperms. *Ann Bot* 1980; 46:29–36.
49 Field JM, Shewry PR, Burgess SR, Forde J, Parmar S, Miflin BJ. The presence of high molecular weight aggregates in the protein bodies of developing endosperms of wheat and other cereals. *J Cereal Sci* 1983;1:33–41.
50 Roden LT, Miflin BJ, Freedman RB. Protein disulphide isomerase is located in the endoplasmic reticulum of developing wheat endosperm. *FEBS Lett* 1982;138:121–4.
51 Munro S, Pelham HRB. A C-terminal signal prevents secretion of luminal ER proteins. *Cell* 1987;48:899–907.
52 Bulleid NJ, Freedman RB. The transcription and translation *in vitro* of individual cereal storage protein genes from wheat (*Triticum aestivum*, cv. Chinese Spring). *Biochem J* 1988;254:805–10.
53 Bulleid NJ, Freedman RB. Defective co-translational formation of disulphide bonds in protein disulphide-isomerase-deficient microsomes. *Nature* 1988;335:649–51.
54 Freedman RB. Protein disulphide isomerase: multiple roles in the modification of nascent secretary proteins. *Cell* 1989;57:1069–72.
55 Shewry PR, Tatham AS. New light on an old technology: the structure of wheat gluten and its role in breadmaking. *Outlooks on Agriculture* 1989;18:65–71.
56 Ziderman II, Friedman M. Thermal and compositional changes of dry wheat gluten-carbohydrate mixtures during simulated crust baking. *J Agric Food Chem* 1985;33: 1096–102.
57 Menkovska M, Lookhart GL, Pomeranz Y. Changes in gliadin fraction(s) during bread-making: isolation and characterization by high performance liquid chromatography and polyacrylamide gel electrophoresis. *Cereal Chem* 1987;64:311–14.
58 Bloksma AH, Nieman WJ. The effects of temperature on some rheological properties of wheat flour doughs. *J Texture Stud* 1975; 6:343–8.
59 Krist-Spit CE, Sluimer P. Heat transfer in ovens during the baking of bread. In: Morton ID, ed. *Cereals in A European Context.* Chichester: Ellis Horwood, 1987:344–63.
60 Menkovska M, Pomeranz Y, Lookhart GL, Shogren MD. Gliadin in crumb of bread from high-protein wheat flours of varying bread-making potential. *Cereal Chem* 1988;65: 198–201.
61 Meier P, Windeman H, Baumgartner E. Auftrennung von Gesamtgliadin aus unterschiedlich hitzebelasteten weizenmehlen mittels phasenumkehar-hochdruchflussig-chromatographie. *Z Lebensm Unters Forsch* 1985;180:467–73.

62 Fujii T, Danno G. Extractability of wheat flour proteins in cereal products. *Kaseigaku Zasshi* 1986;37:419–24.
63 Eliasson AC, Heg PO. Thermal stability of wheat gluten. *Cereal Chem* 1986;57:436–7.
64 Ariss AJ. *Immunocytochemical studies of wheat proteins.* PhD Thesis, CNAA: 1986.
65 Shewry PR, Faulks AJ, Parmar S, Miflin BJ. Hordein polypeptide pattern in relation to malting quality and the varietal identification of malted grain. *J Inst Brew* 1980;86: 138–41.
66 Sorenson SB, Ottesen M. Fractionation and characterization of beer proteins. *Carlsberg Res Commun* 1978;43:133–44.
67 Dale CJ, Young TW, Brewer S. Amino acid analysis of beer polypeptides. *J Inst Brew* 1989;95:89–97.
68 Dale CJ, Young TW. Fractionation of small peptides from beer. *J Inst Brew* 1989;95: 35–41.
69 Asano K, Hashimoto N. Isolation and characterization of foaming proteins of beer. *ASBC J* 1980;38:129–37.
70 Slack PT, Bamforth CW. The fractionation of polypeptides from barley and beer by hydrophobic interaction chromatography; the influence of their hydrophobicity on foam stability. *J Inst Brew* 1983;89:397–401.
71 Pernollet JC, Huet JC, Galle AM, Salentin M. N-Terminal sequences of oat avenins compared to other cereal prolamins. *Biochimie* 1988;69:683–9.
72 Kim SI, Charbonnier L, Mosse J. Heterogeneity of avenin, the oat prolamin. Fractionation, molecular weight and amino acid composition. *Biochem Biophys Acta* 1978; 537:22–30.
73 Bietz JA. Cereal prolamin evolution and homology revealed by sequence analysis. *Biochem Genet* 1983;20:1039–53.
74 Pernollet JC, Potier B, Galle AM, Huet JC, Beauvais F, Salentin M. 2D-HPLC separation, electrophoretic characterization and N-terminal sequences of oat seed prolamins. *Phytochem* 1989;28:2565–70.
75 Egorev TsA. The amino acid sequence of the 'fast' avenin component (*Avena sativa* L.). *J Cereal Sci* 1988;8:289–92.
76 Burgess SR, Festenstein GN, Hay FC, Shewry PR. The immunochemical relationships of prolamins of temperate meadow grasses and cereals. *J Exp Bot* 1986;38:247–53.
77 Chesnut RS, Shotwell MA, Boyer SK, Larkins BA. Analysis of avenin proteins and the expression of their mRNAs in developing oat seeds. *The Plant Cell* 1989;1: 913–24.
78 Fabijanski S, Chang SC, Dukiandjev S, Bahramian MB, Ferrera P, Altosaar I. The nucleotide sequence of a cDNA for a major-prolamin (avenin) in oat (*Avena sativa* L. cv. Hinoat) which reveals homology with oat globulin. *Biochem Physiol Pflanzen* 1988;183:143–52.
79 Walburg G, Larkins BA. Isolation and characterization of cDNAs encoding oat 12S globulin mRNAs. *Plant Mol Biol* 1986;6: 161–9.
80 Padhye VW, Salunkhe DK. Extraction and characterization of rice proteins. *Cereal Chem* 1979;56:389–93.
81 Tanaka K, Sugimoto T, Ogawa M, Kasai Z. Isolation and characterization of two types of protein bodies in the rice endosperm. *Agric Biol Chem* 1980;44:1633–9.
82 Shewry PR, Miflin BJ. Seed storage proteins of economically important cereals. In: Pomeranz Y, ed. *Advances in Cereal Science and Technology.* VII. St Paul, Minnesota: American Association of Cereal Chemists, 1985:1–83.
83 Krishnan H, Okita TW. Structural relationships among the rice glutenin polypeptides. *Plant Physiol* 1986;81:748–53.
84 Kim WT, Okita TW. Nucleotide and primary sequence of a major rice prolamin. *FEBS Lett* 1988;231:308–10.
85 Kim WT, Okita TW. Structure, expression and heterogeneity of the rice seed prolamins. *Plant Physiol* 1988;88:649–55.
86 Matsumura T, Shibata D, Hibino T *et al.* cDNA cloning of an mRNA encoding a sulfur-rich 10k prolamin polypeptide in rice seeds. *Plant Mol Biol* 1984;12:123–30.
87 Esen A. A proposed nomenclature for the alcohol-soluble proteins (zeins) of maize (*Zea mays* L.). *J Cereal Sci* 1987;5:117–28.
88 Kirihara JA, Petri JB, Messing J. Isolation and sequence of a gene encoding a methionine-rich 10 kDa protein from maize. *Gene* 1988;71:359–70.
89 Pons M, Feliz M, Celma C, Giralt E. Conformational analysis of the repeated sequence of glutelin-2, a maize storage protein. *Magn Reson Chem* 1987;25:402–6.
90 Taylor JRN, Von Benecke R, Carlsson FHH. Distribution, purification and N-terminal amino acid sequence of sorghum-reduced soluble protein. *J Cereal Sci* 1989;9:169–77.
91 Ottoboni LMM, Leite A, Targon MLN, Crozier A, Arruda P. Characterization of the storage protein seed of *Coix lacryma-jobi* var. Adlay. *J Agric Food Chem* 1990;

38:631–5.

92 de Rose RT, Ma DP, Kwon IS, Hasnain SE, Klassy RC, Hall TC. Characterization of the kaffirin gene family from sorghum reveals extensive homology with zein from maize. *Plant Mol Biol* 1989;12:245–56.

93 Dicke WK. *Coeliac disease. Investigation of the harmful effects of certain types of cereals on patients with coeliac disease.* University of Utrecht: MD Thesis, 1950.

94 Dicke WK, Weijers HA, van de Kamer JH. Coeliac disease. II. The presence in wheat of a factor having a deleterious effect in cases of coeliac disease. *Acta Pediatr Scand* 1953;42:34–42.

95 van de Kamer JH, Weijers HA, Dicke WK. Coeliac disease. IV. An investigation into the injurious constituents of wheat in connection with their action on patients with coeliac disease. *Acta Pediatr Scand* 1953; 42:223–31.

96 Weijers HA, van de Kamer JH, Dicke WK. Celiac disease. In: Levine SZ, ed. *Advances in Pediatrics.* Chicago: Yearbook Publishers, 1957:277–318.

97 Hansted C. Effects of cereals in celiac disease. In: *8th International Congress of Pediatrics Exhibition.* 1956:137.

98 Simoons FJ. Celiac disease as a geographic problem. In: Walcher DN, Kretschmer N, eds. *Food, Nutrition and Evolution: Food as an Environmental Factor in the Genesis of Human Variability.* New York: Masson Publishing, 1981:179–99.

99 Baker PG, Read AE. Oats and barley toxicity in coeliac patients. *Postgrad Med J* 1976; 52:264–8.

100 Dissanayake AS, Truelove SC, Whitehead R. Lack of harmful effects of oats on small-intestinal mucosa in coeliac disease. *Br Med J* 1974;4:189–91.

101 Peterson DM, Brinegar AC. Oat storage proteins. In: Webster FH, ed. *Oats: Chemistry and Technology.* St Paul, Minnesota: American Association of Cereal Chemists, 1986:153–203.

102 Autran JC, Lew EJL, Nimmo CC, Kasarda DD. N-Terminal amino acid sequencing of prolamins from wheat and related species. *Nature* 1979;282:527–9.

103 Cole EW, Fullington JG, Kasarda DD. Grain protein variability among species of *Triticum* and *Aegilops*: quantitative SDS-PAGE studies. *Theor Appl Genet* 1981;60:17–30.

104 Lafiandra D, Benedetelli S, Margiotta B, Porceddu E. Chromosomal location of gliadin coding genes in *T. aestivum* ssp. *spelta* and evidence on the lack of components controlled by *Gli-2* loci in wheat aneuploids. *Theor Appl Genet* 1989;78:177–83.

105 Auricchio S, Greco L, Troncone R. Gluten-sensitive enteropathy in childhood. *Pediatr Clin N Am* 1988;35:157–87.

106 Shewry PR, Smith SJ, Lew EJL, Kasarda DD. Characterization of prolamins from meadow grasses: homology with those of wheat, barley and rye. *J Exp Bot* 1986;37:633–9.

107 Shewry PR, Parmar S, Pappin DJC. Characterization and genetic control of the prolamins of *Haynaldia villosa*: relationship to cultivated species of the Triticeae (rye, wheat and barley). *Biochem Genet* 1987; 25:309–25.

108 Dvorak J, Kasarda DD, Dietler MD *et al.* Chromosomal location of seed storage protein genes in the genome of *Elytrigia elongata. Can J Genet Cytol* 1986;28: 818–30.

109 Anderson CM, Frazer AC, French JM, Gerrard JW, Sammons HG, Smellie JM. Coeliac disease: gastro-intestinal studies and the effect of dietary wheat flour. *Lancet* 1952;i:836–42.

110 Sheldon W. Coeliac Disease. *Lancet* 1955; ii:1097–103.

111 Freedman AR, Galfre G, Gal E, Ellis HJ, Ciclitira PJ. Detection of wheat gliadin contamination of gluten-free foods by monoclonal antibody dot immunoblotting assay. *Clin Chim Acta* 1987;166:323–8.

112 Ciclitira PJ, Cerio R, Ellis HJ, Maxton D, Neluffer JM, Macartney JM. Evaluation of a gliadin-containing gluten-free product in coeliac patients. *Human Nutr: Clin Nutr* 1985;39C:303–8.

113 Holmes GKT, Prior P, Lane MR, Pope D, Allan RN. Malignancy in coeliac disease: effect of a gluten free diet. *Gut* 1989;30: 333–8.

114 van de Kamer JH, Weijers HA. Coeliac disease. V. Some experiments on the cause of harmful effect of wheat gliadin. *Acta Pediatr Scand* 1955;44:465–9.

115 Auricchio S, de Vizia B, Carta de Angelis L, Silano V. α-Amylase protein inhibitors from wheat in coeliac disease. *Lancet* 1974;i:98.

116 Frazer AC, Fletcher MB, Ross CAC, Shaw B, Sammons HG, Schneider R. Gluten-induced enteropathy: the effect of partially-digested gluten. *Lancet* 1959;ii:252–5.

117 Bronstein HD, Haeffner LJ, Kowlessar OD. Enzymic digestion of gliadin: the effect of the resultant peptides in adult celiac disease. *Clin Chim Acta* 1966;14:141–55.

118 Cornell HJ. Gliadin degradation and fractionation. In: Hekkens WThJM, Pena AS, eds. *Coeliac Disease*. Proceedings of the 2nd International Coeliac Symposium. Leiden: Stenfert Kroese, 1974:74–5.
119 Cornell HJ. Wheat proteins and coeliac disease. *Comments Agric Food Chem* 1988; 1:289–313.
120 Woodley JF. Pyrrolidonecarboxyl peptidase activity in normal intestinal biopsies and those from coeliac patients. *Clin Chim Acta* 1972;42:211–13.
121 Cornell HJ, Townley RRW. The toxicity of certain cereal proteins in celiac disease. *Gut* 1974;15:862–9.
122 Cornell HJ, Rolles CJ. Further evidence of a primary mucosal defect in coeliac disease. *Gut* 1978;19:253–9.
123 Cornell HJ, Maxwell RJ. Amino acid composition of gliadin fractions which may be toxic to individuals with coeliac disease. *Clin Chim Acta* 1982;123:311–19.
124 Townley RRW, Bhatal PS, Cornell HJ, Mitchell JD. Toxicity of wheat gliadin fractions in coeliac disease. *Lancet* 1973;i: 1363–4.
125 Cornell HJ, Auricchio S, de Ritis G *et al.* Intestinal mucosa of celiacs in remission is unable to abolish toxicity of gliadin peptides *in vitro* developing fetal rat intestine and cultured atrophic celiac mucosa. *Pediatr Res* 1988;24:233–7.
126 Cornell HJ. Amino acid composition of peptides remaining after '*in vitro*' digestion of a gliadin subfraction with duodenal mucosa from patients with coeliac disease. *Clin Chim Acta* 1988;176:279–90.
127 Bruce G, Woodley JF, Swan CHJ. Breakdown of peptides by intestinal brush borders from coeliac patients. *Gut* 1981;25:919–24.
128 Adibi SA, Kim YS. Peptide absorption and hydrolysis. In: Johnson LR, ed. *Physiology of the Gastrointestinal Tract*. Vol. 2. New York: Raven Press, 1981:1073–95.
129 van Roon JH, Haex AJCh, Seeder WA, de Jong J. Chemical and biochemical analysis of gluten toxicity. II. *Gastroenterologica* 1960;94:227–35.
130 Ewart JAD. Chemistry of wheat proteins. In: Booth CC, Dowling RH, eds. *Coeliac Disease*. Edinburgh: Churchill Livingstone, 1970:1–9.
131 Wrigley CW, Shepherd, KW. Electrofocusing of grain proteins from wheat genotypes. *Ann NY Acad Sci* 1973;209:154–62.
132 Hekkens WThJM, Haex AJCh, Willighagen PGJ. Some aspects of gliadin fractionation and testing by a histochemical method. In: Booth CC, Dowling RH eds. *Coeliac Disease*. Edinburgh: Churchill Livingstone, 1970:11–19.
133 Hekkens WThJM, Van der Aarsen CJ, Gilliams JP, Lems-Van Kan Ph, Bouma-Frolich G. α-Gliadin structure and degradation. In: Hekkens WThJM, Pena AS eds. *Coeliac Disease*. Proceedings of the 2nd International Coeliac Symposium. Leiden: Stenfert Kroese, 1974:39–45.
134 Hekkens WThJM. The toxicity of gliadin, a review. In: McNicholl B, McCarthy CF, Fottrell PE, eds. *Perspectives in Coeliac Disease*. Lancaster: MTP Press, 1978:3–14.
135 Kasarda DD. Structure and properties of α-gliadins. *Ann Technol Agric* (Fra) 1980;29: 151–73.
136 Kendall MJ, Cox PS, Schneider R, Hawkins CF. Gluten subfractions in coeliac disease. *Lancet* 1972;ii:1065–7.
137 Kumar PJ, Sinclair TS, Farthing MJG *et al.* Clinical testing of pure gliadins in coeliac disease. *Gastroenterology* 1984;86: 1147–52.
138 Falchuk ZM, Gebhard RL, Sessoms C, Strober W. An *in vitro* model of gluten-sensitive enteropathy. *J Clin Invest* 1974; 53:487–500.
139 Katz AJ, Falchuk ZM, Strober W, Schwachman H. Gluten-sensitive enteropathy: inhibition by cortisol of the effect of gluten protein *in vitro*. *N Eng J Med* 1976;295: 131–5.
140 Strober W. The genetic basis of gluten-sensitive enteropathy. In: King RA, Rotter JI, Motulsky A, eds. *The Genetic Basis of Common Diseases*. Oxford: Oxford University Press, in press.
141 Falchuk ZM, Nelson DL, Katz AJ *et al.* Gluten-sensitive enteropathy: influence of histocompatibility type on gluten sensitivity *in vitro*. *J Clin Invest* 1980;66:227–33.
142 Jos J, Charbonnier L, Mougenot JF, Mosse J, Rey J. Isolation and characterization of the toxic fraction of wheat gliadin in coeliac disease. In: McNicholl B, McCarthy CF, Fottrell PE eds. *Perspectives in Coeliac Disease*. Lancaster: MTP Press, 1978: 75–119.
143 Jos J, Charbonnier L, Mosse J, Olives JP, de Tand MF, Rey J. The toxic fraction of gliadin digests in coeliac disease. Isolation by chromatography on Biogel P-10. *Clin Chim Acta* 1982;119:263–74.
144 Howdle PD, Ciclitira PJ, Simpson FG, Losowsky MS. Are all gliadins toxic in

coeliac disease? An *in vitro* study of alpha, beta, gamma and omega gliadins. *Scand J Gastroenterol* 1984;19:41–7.

145 Ciclitira PJ, Evans DJ, Fagg NLK, Lennox ES, Dowling RH. Clinical testing of gliadin fractions in coeliac disease. *Clin Sci* 1984; 66:357–64.

146 Jos J, de Tand MF, Arnaud-Battandier JP, Popineau Y, Wajcman H. Separation of pure toxic peptides from a β-gliadin subfraction using high performance liquid chromatography. *Clin Chim Acta* 1983;134:189–98.

147 de Ritis G, Auricchio S, Jones HW, Lew EJL, Bernardin JE, Kasarda DD. *In vitro* (organ culture) studies of the toxicity of specific A-gliadin peptides in celiac disease. *Gastroenterology* 1988;94:41–9.

148 Kasarda DD, Adalsteins AE, Laird NF. γ-Gliadins with α-type structure coded on chromosome 6B of wheat (*Triticum aestivum*) cultivar Chinese Spring. In: Lasztity R, Bekes F, eds. *Gluten Proteins.* Proceedings of the 3rd International Workshop. Singapore: World Scientific Press, 1987:20–9.

149 Wieser H, Belitz HD, Ashkenazi A, Idar D. Isolation of coeliac active peptide fractions from gliadin. *Z Lebensm Unters Forsch* 1983;176:85–94.

150 Wieser H, Belitz HD, Ashkenazi A. Amino acid sequence of the coeliac active peptide B3242. *Z Lebensm Unters Forsch* 1984; 179:371–6.

151 Wieser H, Belitz HD, Idar D, Ashkenazi A. Coeliac activity of the gliadin peptides CT-1 and CT-2. *Z Lebensm Unters Forsch* 1986;182:115–17.

152 Okita TW, Cheesbrough V, Reeves CD. Evolution and heterogeneity of the α/β and δ-type gliadin DNA sequences. *J Biol Chem* 1985;260:8203–13.

153 Devery JN, Geczy CL, De Carle D, Skerritt JH, Krillis SA. Macrophage procoagulant activity as an assay of cellular hypersensitivity to gluten peptides in coeliac disease. *Clin Exp Immunol* 1990;82:333–7.

154 Skerritt JH, Devery JM, Hill AS. Gluten intolerance: chemistry, coeliac-toxicity and detection of prolamin in foods. *Cereal Foods World* 1990;35:638–44.

155 Kagnoff MF, Austin RK, Hubert JJ, Bernardin JE, Kasarda DD. Possible role for a human adenovirus in the pathogenesis of coeliac disease. *J Exp Med* 1984;1984:1544–57.

156 Rubenstein I, Geraghty DE. The genetic organization of zein. In: Pomeranz Y, ed. *Advances in Cereal Science and Technology.* III. St Paul, Minnesota: American Association of Cereal Chemists, 1986: 297–315.

157 Okita TW, Hwang YS, Hnilo J *et al.* Structure and expression of the rice glutelin multigene family. *J Biol Chem* 1989;264: 12573–81.

158 Pavone V, Rossi F, Pucci P *et al.* Studies on gliadin related peptides. *Int J Pept Protein Res* 1983;22:481–8.

159 Kasarda DD, Bernardin JE, Qualset CO. Relationship of gliadin protein components to chromosomes in hexaploid wheats. *Proc Natl Acad Sci USA* 1976;73:3646–50.

160 Kasarda DD, Qualset CO, Mecham DK, Goodenberger DM, Strober W. A test of toxicity of bread made from wheat lacking α-gliadins coded for by the 6A chromosome. In: McNicholl B, McCarthy CF, Fottrell PE, eds. *Perspectives in Coeliac Disease.* Lancaster: MTP Press, 1978:55–61.

161 Ciclitira PJ, Hunter JO, Lennox ES. Clinical testing of bread made from nullisomic 6A wheats in coeliac patients. *Lancet* 1980;ii: 234–6.

162 Strober W. An immunological theory of gluten-sensitive enteropathy. In: McNichol B, McCarthy CF, Fottrell PE, eds. *Perspectives in Coeliac Disease.* Lancaster: MTP Press, 1978:169–82.

163 Marsh MN. Studies of intestinal lymphoid tissue. XI. The immunopathology of cell-mediated reactions in gluten sensitivity and other enteropathies. *Scanning Microsc* 1988;2:1663–84.

164 Davidson AGF, Bridges MA. Coeliac disease: a critical review of aetiology and pathogenesis. *Clin Chim Acta* 1987;163: 1–40.

165 Bjarnason I, Marsh MN, Price A, Levi AJ, Peters TJ. Intestinal permeability in patients with coeliac disease and dermatitis herpetiformis. *Gut* 1985;26:1214–19.

166 Marsh MN, Bjarnson I, Shaw J, Ellis A, Baker R, Peters TJ. Studies of intestinal lymphoid tissue. XIV. HLA status, mucosal morphology, permeability and epithelial lymphocyte populations in first degree relatives of patients with coeliac disease. *Gut* 1990;31:32–6.

167 Weiser MM, Douglas AP. An alternative mechanism for gluten toxicity in coeliac disease. *Lancet* 1976;i:567–9.

168 Mitchell PJ, Tijian R. Transcriptional regulation in mammalian cells by sequence-specific DNA binding proteins. *Science* 1989;245:371–8.

169 Mermod N, O'Neill EA, Kelly TJ, Tjian R. The proline-rich transcriptional activator of CTF/NF-1 is distinct from the replication and DNA binding domain. *Cell* 1989;58: 741–53.

170 Courey AT, Tjian R. Analysis of Spl *in vivo* reveals multiple transcriptional domains, including a novel glutamine-rich activation motif. *Cell* 1988;55:887–98.

171 Hunt T. Cytoplasmic anchoring and the control of nuclear localization. *Cell* 1989; 59:949–51.

172 Campbell CS. The subfamilies and tribes of Gramineae (Poaceae) in the Southeastern United States. *J Arnold Arboretum* 1985; 66:123–99.

173 Bartels D, Altosar I, Harberd NP, Barker RD, Thompson RD. Molecular analysis of gamma-gliadin gene families at the complex *Gli*-1 locus of bread wheat (*T. aestivum* L.). *Theor Appl Genet* 1986;72:845–53.

174 Colot V, Thompson R, Flavell R. Molecular characterization of an active LMW glutenin gene and its relation to other wheat and barley prolamin genes. *Mol Gen Genet* 1989;216:81–90.

175 Forde BG, Heyworth A, Pywell J, Kreis M. Nucleotide sequence of a B1 hordein gene and the identification of possible upstream regulatory elements in endosperm protein storage genes from barley, wheat and maize. *Nucleic Acids Res* 1985;13:7327–39.

176 Forde BG, Kreis M, Williamson M *et al.* Short tandem repeats shared by B- and C-hordein cDNAs suggests a common evolutionary origin for two groups of cereal storage protein genes. *EMBO J* 1985;4:9–15.

177 Halford NG, Forde J, Anderson OD, Greene FC, Shewry PR. The nucleotide and deduced amino acid sequences of a HMW glutenin subunit from chromosome 1B of bread wheat (*Triticum aestivum* L.), and comparison with those of genes from chromosomes 1A and 1D. *Theor Appl Genet* 1987; 75:117–26.

178 Anderson OD, Litts JC, Gautier MF, Greene FC. Nucleic acid sequence and chromosomal assignment of a wheat storage protein gene. *Nucleic Acids Res* 1984;12:8129–44.

179 Shewry PR, Field JM, Kirkman MA, Faulks AJ, Miflin BJ. The extraction, solubility and characterization of two groups of barley storage proteins. *J Exp Bot* 1980;31: 393–407.

180 Kasarda DD, Nimmo CC, Bernardin JE. Structural aspects and genetic relationships of gliadins. In: Hekkens WThJM, Pena AS eds. *Coeliac Disease.* Proceedings of the 2nd International Coeliac Symposium. Leiden: Stenfert Kroese, 1974:25–34.

181 Shewry PR, Kreis M, Parmar S, Lew EJL, Kasarda DD. Identification of γ-type hordein in Barley. *FEBS Lett* 1985;190:61–4.

182 Field JM, Shewry PR, Miflin BJ, March JF. The purification and characterisation of homologous high molecular weight storage proteins from grain of wheat, rye and barley. *Theor Appl Genet* 1982;62:329–36.

183 Shewry PR, Field JM, Lew EJL, Kasarda DD. The purification and characterisation of two groups of storage proteins (secalins) from rye (secale cereale). *J Exp Bot* 1982; 33:261–8.

Chapter 12 / Whither coeliac disease?

MICHAEL N. MARSH

During the last 20 years a succession of international conferences has provided focus and fora for the presentation of new data, information and ideas for those whose interests lie with coeliac disease (CD). The vitality of those proceedings has resulted in five published symposia [1–5] which, although reflecting the ethos of each meeting, were never intended to provide smooth, balanced accounts of the subject in an easy, assimilable form. The aim of the current book, therefore, has been to produce a detailed overview of all current advances relevant to the broadest aspects of gluten sensitivity. So, in respect of these advances, whither CD?

Of its nature and definition

At its root is a primary host-mediated, genetically determined intestinal response to gluten proteins, comprising a series of well-defined, and dynamically interrelated patterns of mucosal change and injury [6–8]. That these represent T cell (lymphocyte)-mediated events is based on the striking parallelism between the spectrum of mucosal lesions elicited in experimental graft-versus-host (GVH) disease [8–10] and those shown to occur variously in patients with untreated CD and dermatitis herpetiformis (DH); in relatives of known coeliac patients, and in coeliacs in remission following graded oral challenges with gliadin digests. These similarities suggest a common immunopathological basis, not only in gluten sensitivity, but in other enteropathies including giardiasis, the tropical diarrhoea-malabsorption syndrome ('tropical enteropathy' and 'tropical sprue'), and food hypersensitivity reactions in youngsters.

In recognizing and redefining this spectrum of mucosal lesions as pre-infiltrative, infiltrative, infiltrative-hyperplastic, destructive, and irreversible hypoplastic-atrophic (see p. 138) we can, at last, begin to escape from the paralysing grip of the redundant terminologies of 'partial/subtotal villous atrophy' which have contributed little to our understanding of the basic immunopathology of this important group of enteropathies [6–11]. In addition, new vistas and precepts begin to emerge, such as (1) the recognition that gluten sensitivity may be associated with an end-stage and unresponsive form of intestinal failure, and (2) that the classic, textbook picture of 'CD', with its implicit galaxy of nutritional and absorptive defects, diarrhoea, weight loss and a flat mucosa, represents perhaps only 30–40% [12] of the entire spectrum of gluten-sensitized individuals. These two observations undermine traditional definitions of CD [13] which, in the light of newer advances, can now be seen to be unrepresentative of the individuals they were purported to encompass, and thus redundant.

Of its end-stage unresponsiveness

It should be remembered that the absence of a morphological response to gluten restriction by no means automatically implies that this small group of individuals, despite existing definitions, do not (or never did) have gluten sensitivity. Important clues scattered throughout the literature, as discussed here (see p. 144) and elsewhere [12] amply attest to the true underlying nature of this unresponsive phase of gluten-induced, end-stage intestinal failure. What should be avoided is the negative sense of resignation often felt by the attendant in these circumstances. Rather, when faced with this type of patient, he or she should grasp the nettle and ask useful questions as to why only certain coeliac patients develop this state of unresponsiveness and whether, for example, it could be due to sustained immunologically mediated 'suppressive' mechanisms as seen in chronic leishmaniasis and leprosy [14,15] or alternatively brought about and sustained by tumour growth, which invariably is the setting in which this complication arises and could be akin, perhaps, to the slowly progressive inanition that accompanies chronic GVH [10].

In attempting to adopt this kind of approach we might then be able to better define: (1) the mechanism(s) of unresponsiveness; (2) the factors responsible for the irreversible mucosal atrophy of the intestine; and (3) the causes of weight loss and progressive cachexia. Furthermore, it might also be possible to devise strategies that might: (1) reverse the unresponsiveness; (2) diminish the systemic effects of cytokines (e.g. tumour necrosis factor (TNF) or interferon (IFN)γ; or (3) immunize against malignant T cells providing oligoclonality, or restricted T cell receptor (TCR) usage, can be demonstrated.

Admittedly, some of these remarks may be slightly out of focus. Nevertheless, if we make some positive attempt to move forward (even though we may not have got it quite right!) at least we shall not remain fossilized by definitions and levels of thinking that characterize the 1960s and 1970s. For the 1990s, immunological techniques are probably sufficiently developed to permit us to answer some of these problems; in that way, we shall have advanced.

Of its latency

Much has been written in recent times of the alleged disappearance of childhood CD in northern Europe (but not, incidentally, in Sweden): this phenomenon may partly reflect altered feeding patterns, changes in environmental and other factors, and the current practice of restricting gluten-containing foods to infants over 2 years-of-age. However, biology is never that simplistic as is evident from studies of those families in which the handling pattern of the first-born coeliac child differed markedly from that of subsequent (coeliac) children in terms of breast feeding, weaning and concurrent introduction of solids [16]. Since genetic predisposition, and hence the number of individuals potentially liable to sensitization could not have changed in the short term, the permissive influence of environmental factors becomes readily apparent [17]; what we need to know is what has altered to effect such rapid and widespread falls in incidence.

Apart from these considerations, an increased perception and awareness of the concept of 'latent' gluten sensitivity is rapidly becoming necessary. Latency, originally denoting a mucosal deterioration in DH patients fed gluten [18], should now be applied to asymptomatic patients with any type of mucosal lesion (Type 0 through Type 4). The word 'latent' is an ideal term with which to designate this group of gluten-sensitized, but asymptomatic, individuals. (Oxford English Dictionary: latent, existing but not manifest.) If would only confuse the issue if attempts to further subdivide individuals within this group were proposed. Clearly, either a person is sensitized, or not. Given a state of sensitization, any type of mucosal lesion may develop in response to gluten ingestion and, irrespective of the degree and extent of mucosal involvement, the individual would be either symptomatic (i.e. have 'CD', whatever the lesion) or asymptomatic (i.e. be 'latent', whatever the lesion).

In general, it should be recalled that only ~30–40% gluten-sensitized individuals develop textbook features of classic CD malabsorption. The remainder comprise the submerged iceberg phenomenon which is numerically large (60–70%) perhaps representing 1 : 300 population [19]. Furthermore, it is important to remember that 50% of all CD relatives and an even greater proportion (80–90%) of DH patients with flat (Type 3) proximal jejunal lesions are asymptomatic [20].

How is it that so many of the latter with gluten sensitivity and a flat mucosa fail to present with malabsorption; or conversely, why do symptoms develop at all when the lesion is seemingly confined to the duodenum and upper jejunum only? For this would tend to conflict with experiences derived from other patients with massive enteric resections, or even extensive small bowel disease (Crohn's), who may often be asymptomatic, maintain their nutrition and fail to manifest the type of malabsorption and insufficiency that we have come to associate with textbook descriptions of CD. What does emerge is that development of clinical symptomatology, through unmasking of the latent condition and irrespective of the type of mucosal lesion present, is triggered by a variety of environmental factors, such as: (1) birth order, age of weaning and duration of breast feeding; (2) intercurrent infections (gastrointestinal or systemic); (3) stress-related events (operative, traumatic, metabolic, pregnancy); (4) concurrent nutritional deficiencies (dietary imbalance or low intake, especially of iron or folate); and (5) malignancy (obstruction, perforation, haemorrhage, progressive cachexia).

Corroboration of the importance of environment can be further gained from rediscovering, by reading the various contemporary reports, how gluten sensitivity has changed throughout this century. In its earlier decades, death, major chronic morbidity or invalidism from 'idiopathic steatorrhoea' was the typical scene. This was miraculously transformed by use of raw liver extract [21] in 1928, 2 years after its introduction had revolutionized treatment and survival in Addisonian pernicious anaemia [22]. At about the same time, yeast extract ('Marmite') was employed to provide another rich source of (what we now know as) exogenous folate. Other factors, apart from the gluten-free diet (1950 onwards), such as the statutory fortification of foods with vitamins and minerals have lessened the impact of malabsorption and poor diet and helped, to some extent, to guard against chronic debilitating and unreplenished deficiencies. In addition, and in a wider context the impressive effects of public health initiatives, governmental measures and newer therapeutic advances achieved throughout the century should not be underestimated such as the conquest of tuberculosis; control of atmospheric pollution; purification of water supplies; and the enforced legislation governing the processing and preparation of food products. The progressive improvement in the 'health and well-being' of society as a result of these medical and social changes has, indirectly, influenced the expression of gluten sensitivity.

Nowadays, to be given a diagnosis of CD is not to receive a death sentence. On the contrary, diagnosis is largely based on subtle hints, and in particular, on the clinician's need to develop a high degree of awareness (see p. 49). Indeed, cases have now been reported where an initial jejunal biopsy was normal, and only after several years was a flat mucosa subsequently demonstrated, sometimes in the continuing absence of major symptomatology, or nutritional insufficiency [23]. Thus, we have come to the point where diagnosis of gluten sensitivity is becoming increasingly difficult, and when the presence of a putatively 'normal' biopsy can no longer be taken as evidence by any physician that gluten sensitivity is not present, nor will erupt at some future date [12], especially in 'at-risk' subjects such as relatives of known CD individuals, patients with either ill-defined symptomatology or an atypical presentation, like growth defect, unexplained osteoporosis, osteomalacia or arthralgia (but not, apparently, rheumatoid arthritis), or with anomalous findings such as hyperglycaemia or unexplained elevated hepatic transaminase levels.

Nor should we any longer expect, nor continue to believe, that a diagnosis of CD simply means a flat mucosa and malabsorption (which the older definitions adhere to). Instead, we must be ever watchful, so that the more subtle histopathological mucosal changes are not overlooked, or regarded as 'non-specific', nor other trivial or unusual complaints glossed over and dismissed as 'psychological'.

Inevitably, there will always be some latent patients who will develop intercurrent infection, become nutritionally deprived, and even be subject to lymphoma (for which they are still much at risk because of chronic gluten exposure). Despite that, but aided by hindsight, it has become abundantly clear that gluten sensitivity, intrinsically, is an asymptomatic condition, a principle we can now propose as self-evident: Honi soit qui mal y pense.

This does raise further questions for the future, however. With our present knowledge, diagnosis can probably be achieved with a jejunal biopsy in a high proportion of cases, provided the subtle histological features of mucosal cell-mediated immunity (CMI) can both be recognized and acted upon, or a high percentage of γ/δ intraepithelial lymphocytes (IEL) can be demonstrated [24]. Some corroboration of diagnostic suspicion may also be secured by measurement of circulating, or locally secreted, antibody to α-gliadin with which diagnostic specificities and sensitivities of ~90% may be achieved, or to other connective tissue antibodies [25]. But this mode of approach is by no means foolproof, even given ease of access by the general physician or paediatrician to such a technical resource. Therefore, we must anticipate the use of probes based on major histocompatibility complex (MHC) class 2 specificities, T cell receptor genes, or cytokine profiles if, once categorized, they can be shown to exhibit an acceptable degree of exclusivity for gluten sensitivity, especially in population-based searches which include 'latent' subjects. Clearly, further advances along these lines can be anticipated. In saying that, however, it must be appreciated that at present, far too much effort is spent on the diagnosis, investigation and research into patients with classical coeliac malabsorption and a flat mucosa. This is no longer adequate; we are going to need highly discriminatory markers for latent gluten-sensitive disease that will identify individuals with early mucosal lesions, and this is where new prospective and collaborative initiatives should be directed and concentrated in the future.

Of T and B lymphocyte-mediated responses

The initiation of mucosal pathology seems to involve interactions between the absorbed disease-activating epitopes of gliadin and MHC class 2^+ antigen-presenting cells which, in turn, activate local $CD4^+$ cells [12]. That high titre interleukin 2R (soluble interleukin 2 receptors) are detectable in the circulation after gluten challenge [26] implies such an antigen-directed series of events, and which in turn inaugurate a widening cascade of inflammatory mediators (see p. 158). The future cloning of mucosal lymphocytes will hopefully permit study of these phenomena *in vitro* and permit elucidation of the cytokine profile of gluten-sensitized lymphocytes.

One further corollary derives from these considerations — that jejunal enterocytes are not the primary cause of CD, whether that is interpreted as due to: (1) their intrinsic failure to digest gluten protein; (2) expression of an abnormal glycoprotein receptor for gliadin; (3) a consequence of their upregulated MHC class 2 expression; or (4) a result of immune-mediated attack whether antibody-dependent, or cytolytic. The absence of ICAM-I within epithelium (despite its widespread disposition within the lamina propria [27]) provides firm evidence against any form of cytolytic activity towards surface enterocytes by lymphocytes.

Although anti-α-gliadin antibodies have been shown to play a valuable role in diagnosis [28] and also, apparently, in heralding an early phase in the temporal evolution of gluten sensitivity when mucosal architecture is still unchanged [29], there is little to suggest that either gluten sensitivity itself or the development of mucosal lesions have anything to do with the production of gliadin-specific antibodies. When examined *in vitro*, circulating antigliadin antibodies appear to react with whole gliadin, Frazer fraction 3, and low-molecular weight gluten, but exhibit little binding, if any, to smaller oligopeptides, such as peptide 1–53 (B1342 of Weiser [30]) or the 12-meric region spanning the adenovirus-12 E1B homology region [31,32]. Thus, while coeliac patients, presumably by virtue of their genetic background, respond abnormally to prolamins there is no qualitative difference in their spectrum of humoral responses compared with disease-control subjects [32]. This indicates that antibody is most unlikely to be a primary factor in aetiology or in terms of mucosal pathology, since high titre (luminal) anti-α-gliadin antibody can be produced [29] in the absence of any architectural, or cellular, damage. The high levels of IgG antibodies (see p. 253) and their ability to fix complement [33] could play some secondary role in mucosal inflammation, although this speculative idea still awaits some experimental proof. Recent work in this field [30,33,34] emphasizes a requirement for absolutely pure oligopeptide fragments, since minor degrees of cross-reactivity (often a big problem with chromatographic separation of peptides of very small molecular mass) will thwart the intended results of *in vitro* assays, and even *in vivo* challenges.

Of gliadin, and its immunopathological oligopeptides

There is a glimmer on the horizon to suggest a divarication between the non-specific antibody response to gliadin and the presumptive, specific role of small oligopeptides in evoking selective T cell-mediated responses (at least *in vitro*) [33,34]. Further evidence for the latter view is that pre-treatment of these oligopeptides with SDS reduces or abolishes their activity, i.e. T cells now fail to recognize the active, conformational epitope(s).

Considerable interest and effort has been invested in proteins and derivative oligopeptides in order to understand the molecular basis of immunogenicity, based on amino acid sequence, relevant secondary/tertiary conformational properties of epitopes, and identification of those residues which are critical for interaction with MHC alloantigens and thus T lymphocytes [11]. Peptides recognized by T cells are approximately 10–15 residues in size, and those gliadin excerpts shown to have T cell-activating potential contain either SPQQ, PQQP or QQQP tetrapeptide motifs (Table 12.1) [31–34]:

'active' H_2N-V_1R V P V P Q L Q P Q N P S Q Q Q P Q E Q V P L V Q Q Q Q F_{30}
'active' L_{31} G Q Q Q P F P P Q Q P Y P Q P Q P F P S Q Q P Y_{55}
'inactive' L_{56} Q L Q P F P Q P Q L P R_{68}

Note that QPFP[QP] is apparently an inactive sequence.

Based on primary amino acid sequence, algorithms have been used to predict T cell epitopes and employed with variable success [35,36]. Putative epitopes thereby predicted for the prolamins (Table 12.2) when compared against the two protein sequence databases (NBRF, Washington, DC, and Swiss-Prot, EMBO, Heidelberg, FRG) were all found to have marked homology with α/β, γ_2 and ω gliadins, and, to a lesser extent with hordeins (barley) and secalins (rye). There were homologies with other proteins in addition to adenovirus-12 (Ad12) E1B protein, including α-amylase and trypsin inhibitor, other adenoviruses, parovirus, napin-2 precursor-rape seed, glycinin maize gluten 2 protein, the 22 kDa α-zein precursor and high molecular weight (HMW) glutenin subunit precursor [33].

Studies of peptides A through G (Table 12.2) reveal most activity within the proline and glutamine rich N-terminus of α/β-gliadin, including oligomers containing the motif ^{13}PSQ^{16}Q and ^{50}PSQ^{53}Q. Activity was not seen with PQQP (peptide G) nor, surprisingly, with the Ad12 E1B sequence (211–217). Since inserts of the Ad12 viral

Table 12.1 Structural comparisons of grass storage proteins (prolamins) (N-terminal excerpts)

Prolamin	N-terminal sequence
Sulphur-rich prolamins	
γ-gliadin	N M Q V D P S S Q V Q W P Q Q Q P V P Q P H Q P F S Q Q P Q Q T F P Q P Q Q T F P H Q P Q Q Q F P Q P Q Q P Q Q Q F L Q
40 kDa secalin	N M Q V G P S G Q V E W P Q Q Q P L P Q
75 kDa secalin	N M Q V N P S G Q V Q W P Q Q Q P F P Q
γ-hordein	E M Q V N P S V Q V Q P P Q Q P P P Q S Q Q P F • • Q P Q • Q F P Q
β-hordein	Q Q Q P F P Q Q P I P Q Q P Q P Y P Q Q P Q P Y P Q Q P F P P Q Q P F P Q Q P V P Q Q P Q P Y P Q Q P F P P Q Q P F P Q
LMW gliadin	M K T F L V F A L I A V V A T S A I A Q M E T S C I S G L E R P W Q Q Q P L P P Q Q S F S Q Q P P F S Q Q Q Q Q P L P Q
α β γ1	V R F P V P Q L Q P Q N P S Q Q Q P Q E Q V P L V Q Q Q Q F L G Q Q Q P F P P Q Q P Y P Q P Q P F P S Q L P Y L Q L Q P
Sulphur-poor prolamins	
γ1 gliadin	R Q L N P S D Q E L Q S P Q Q L Y P Q Q P Y P Q Q P Y
γ2-gliadin	R E L N P S N K E L Q S P Q Q S F S H
γ-secalin	R Q L N P S E Q E L Q S P Q Q P V
C hordein	R Q L N P S S Q E L Q S P Q Q S Y L Q Q P Y P Y N P Y L P Q Q P F T V
High molecular weight	
20 HMW glutenin	E G E A S R Q L Q C E R E L Q E S S L E A C R Q V V D Q Q L A G R L P Q S T G L Q M R C C Q Q L R D V S A K C R P V A V
HMV secalin	E G E A S G Q L Q C E R E L Q Q S S L E A C R Q V V D Q Q L A G R L P W S T G L
D hordein	N I F L D S R S R Q L Q C E R E L Q • S • L E A C R R V V D Q Q L V G Q L P S S
Avenins (oats)	T T T V Q Y N P S E Q Y Q P Y P E Q Q E P F V Q Q Q P F V Q Q Q Q P F V Q Q Q Q M F L Q P L L Q Q Q L N P C K Q F L V
Zeins (maize)	F I I P Q C S L A P S A S I P Q F L P V T S M G F E H P A V Q A Y R L
Oryza (rice)	C R P L P S L M F L G Q S Y R Q Y Q L Q S P V L L Q Q Q V L S P Y N E F V R Q Q Y G I A A S P F L Q
Gamma grass (trypsicum)	F I I P Q C S Q L A P I A S L L Q P F Y L P V
Kafarin (sorghum)	F I I P Q C S L A P I A I A I Q F L P A L
Millet (pennisetum)	Y I S P V S A V A A T A S P L F W P Q A T S I A A T H P F V

The prolamins known to precipitate, or exacerbate, coeliac sprue disease (i.e. sulphur-rich or sulphur-poor prolamins of wheat, rye and barley; sulphur-rich and sulphur-poor prolamins, above) all contain recurring tetrapeptide motifs at their N-termini which are not seen in other phylogenetically distant, and disease-unrelated prolamins (high molecular weight glutenins, zeins (maize), and millet (pennisetum), above). Notice that avenins of oats (above) occupy a pivotal position, in that there are suggestions of motif homology to the more active prolamins in wheat etc. Finally, while low molecular weight (LMW) gliadin species carry similar motifs to gliadin, high molecular weight (HMW) species (glutenins, secalins and D hordein) do not, and are therefore unlikely to play any aetiological or pathogenetic role in gluten sensitivity.

genome have not been demonstrated in coeliac DNA, it is difficult to interpret two recent *in vitro* studies suggesting cellular activation by E1B protein and the homologous region of α-gliadin [37,38]. The inference is that PSQQ, *per se*, is insufficient to explain disease activity, but that in addition, the flanking P and Q residues abundant in domains I and II are also important and necessary but which are lacking in the homologous Ad12 proline-poor (domain V) region of α-gliadin.

To date, no crystallographic studies on the prolamins have been carried out, but analyses of synthetic peptides CT-1 (α-gliadin sequence 3–55 [28]); 3–19; 39–45 and 211–217 by circular dichroic spectroscopy [39] suggest the occurrence of β-reverse turn associated with PSQQ and (P)QQP. The relevance of such structures to recognition by MHC alloantigens and hence presentation to T cell receptor, nevertheless remains to be determined, although it is possible that some preliminary modelling, between presumptive epitopes and coeliac-associated MHC class 2 specificities, could soon be attempted.

Of genetic predisposition and background

The major predisposition for gluten sensitivity is expressed in 95% susceptible individuals as the 'DQ2' [40] serological haplotype. However, while concordance rates for identical twins are ~70%, those for HLA-identical siblings is 25–40% indicating a role for additional (non-MHC based) genes [41]. For insulin-dependent diabetes mellitus (IDDM) the corresponding figures are 50% and 20% respectively. Although DQ2 is highly represented in most coeliacs, and DQ3 in about 70% diabetics, similar haplotypes are seen in 25% 'normal' Caucasians; in other words, there are no MHC-specific, disease-associated genes [42].

Rather, it seems evident that a hierarchical system of multiple alleles operates competitively within any individual for 'peptide binding' (i.e. gliadin epitopes in gluten sensitivity) but so far unknown for other autoimmune diseases. Relative binding strengths ('affinities') for such disease-associated peptide epitopes determine the individual's susceptibility for that disease [43]. Conversely, a negatively associated haplotype would be deemed to outstrip any other potential disease-permissive haplotype and thus prevent onset of disease [41].

In this context much has been written about the so-called protective ^{57}D residue in the third hypervariable region (HVR) of the diabetogenic β1 domain of MHC [44]. Evidence against such an exclusive protective role is: (1) its presence in the genome of Oriental diabetics [45]; (2) that the $^{57}D^{+}$ DQβ gene failed to protect against diabetes when evaluated in family studies [46]; and (3) that a transmutated gene with a permissive ^{57}S (serine) in place of ^{57}D which was engineered on to the NOD $DQ\beta^{K}$ allele was not, alone, uniquely capable of conferring hyperglycaemia [47]. Thus, from these important studies [47,48], it is appar-

Table 12.2 Presumptive T cell epitopes of gliadin and related homologies [33]

Gliadins	Homologies			
Excerpts	Prolamines	Other proteins	References	Remarks
^{6}PQLQPQNPSQQQP^{20}E [A] α-gliadin (domain I), proline rich	α/β-gliadin 90%, γ-gliadin 65%, HMW glutenin 60%, C hordein 64%	Adenovirus h4 (Ed2) 67%, Varicella-zoster 55%, plasmodium (CSP-protein) 50%	Kitchingman [65] Davison [66] Lal [67]	Contains ^{13}PSQ^{16}Q of α-gliadin (amphipathic score; 5)
^{45}QPQPFPPSQQPYLQ^{58}L [B] α-gliadin (domain II), proline rich	α/β-gliadin 95%, γ-gliadin 60%, ω-gliadin 80%, B horzein 80%	Human retrovirus (GAG) 60%, fibronectin 60%, Human parovirus (coat protein) 50%	Ono [68] Pierschbacher [69] Shade [70]	Contains ^{51}PSQ^{54}Q of α-gliadin (amphipathic score; 11)
^{209}GSFRPSQQNPQAQ^{222}G [C], α-gliadin (domain V), proline poor	α/β-gliadin 95%	Adenovirus Ad12 (E1b) 80%	Kagnoff [31]	Contains ^{213}PSQ^{216}Q of α-gliadin
^{126}CHAVVLQQHNIAHGRS^{142}Q [D] α-gliadin (domain III), proline poor	α/β-gliadin 100%, 22 kDa zein 65%	Parovirus (coat protein) 55%	Rhode [71]	T cell epitope predicted by Rothbard* algorithm

^{169}CQAIHNVVHAIILH^{183}Q [E] α-gliadin (domain III), proline poor	α/β-gliadin 85%, γ-gliadin 85%, γ-secalin 90%, LMW glutenin 70%, 22 kDa zein 70%	Yeast (cell division protein) 50%	Camonis [72]	T cell epitope predicted by amphipathic helix algorithm† (amphipathic score; 30)
^{226}PQQLPQFEEIRNL^{239}A [F] α-gliadin (domain V), proline poor	α/β-gliadin 100%	Simia immunodeficiency virus (Gag-polyprotein) 60%	Fukasawa [73]	Predicted by amphipathic helix algorithm (amphipathic score; 24)
^{64}PFPQQPQQPYPQQ^{77}P [G] γ-gliadin (domain I), proline rich	α/β-gliadin 88%, γ-gliadin 80%, ω-gliadin 100%	Parovirus (coat protein) 50%, adenovirus h2 (hexon) 50%, 19 kDa zein protein 60%	Shade [70] Herisse [74] Marks [75]	Predicted by amphipathic helix algorithm (amphipathic score; 30)
^{172}CQQLAQIPQQLQC^{185}A [H] γ-gliadin (domain III), proline poor	α/β-gliadin 100%, γ-gliadin 100%, LMW gliadin 90%, β-hordein 75%, 22 kDa zein 60%	Adenovirus h4 (19 kDa protein) 60%, α-amylase (wheat) inhibitor 60%, maize (zein) 22 kDa 60%	Tokunga [76] Maeda [77] Marks [75]	Predicted by amphipathic helix algorithm (amphipathic score; 57)

* T cell epitope algorithm [36].
† Amphipathic helix [35].

Table 12.3 MHC class 2 β-chain (second exon) polymorphisms of third HVR

Current nomenclature	Previous specificities equivalents		S_1			S_2		S_3		H				
			95 (9)	97 (11)	99 (13)	114 (28)	116 (30)	123 (37)	124 (38)	142 (57)	146 (61)	152 (67)	155 (70)	156 (71)
Gluten sensitivity (subregion loci)														
• DRB1*0301	DR β 1	(w17)	E	S	S	D	Y	N	V		W	L	Q	[K]
• DRB3*0101	DR β 3	(52a)	E	R	S	D	Y	F	L		W	L	Q	[K]
• DQB1*0201	DQ β 1	(w2)	Y	F	G	S	S	I	V		W	I	R	[K]
DQB1*0301	DQ β 3.1	(w3)	Y	F	G	T	Y	Y	A		W	V	R	T
											(59)	(65)	(68)	(69)
DPB1*0201	DP β 2.1	(w2)	F	G	Q	E	Y	F	V		W	I	E	E
• DPB1*0101	DP β 1	(w1)	Y	G	Q	E	Y	Y	A		W	I	E	[K]
• DPB1*0301	DP β 3	(w3)	Y	L	Q	E	Y	F	V		W	I	E	[K]
• DPB1*0403	DP β 4.3	(w4)	F	G	Q	E	Y	F	V		W	I	E	[K]
• DPB1*0402	DP β 4.2	(w4)	F	G	Q	E	Y	F	A		W	I	E	[K]
Insulin-dependent diabetes mellitus														
DQB1*0301	DR4 DQ β	(w3.1)	Y	F	A	T	Y	Y	A	D	W	V	R	T
DQB1*0502	DR2 DQ β	(w1.2)	F	F	G	T	Y	Y	A	D	W	V	G	A
• DQB1*0302	DR4 DQ β	(w3.2)	Y	F	G	T	Y	Y	A	[A]	W	V	R	T
• DQB1*0501	DR1 DQ β	(w1.1)	Y	F	G	T	H	Y	V	[V]	W	V	R	A
• DQB1*0502	DR2 DQ β	(w1.AZH)	Y	F	G	T	H	Y	V	[S]	W	V	G	A

Rheumatoid arthritis																
Adult Type																
• DRB1*0401	DR4 Dw4	(w4)	E	V	H	F	D	Y	V	D		L	Q	K		
• DRB1*0404	DR4 Dw14	(w14)	E	V	H	F	D	Y	V	D		L	Q	R		
• DRB1*0405	DR4 Dw15	(w15)	E	V	H	F	D	Y	V	S		L	Q	R		
DRB1*0402	DR4 Dw10	(w10)	E	V	H	F	D	Y	V	n		I	D	E		
Juvenile Type											(59)	(65)	(68)	(69)	(70)	(71)
DPB1*0401	DP β 4.1	(w4)	F	G	Q	Y	Y	R	F		W	I	E	K	R	A
DPB1*0402	DP β 4.2	(w4)	F	G	Q	Y	Y	R	F		W	I	E	K	R	A
• DPB1*0201	DP β 2.1	(w2)	F	G	Q	Y	Y	R	F		W	I	E	E	R	A
Pemphigus Vulgaris																
• DQB1*0503	DRw6	DQβ1.3	V	F	G	T	H	Y	V	D	W	V	G	A		
DQB1*0501	DRw6	DQβ1.1	V	F	G	T	H	Y	V	V	W	V	G	A		

Polymorphisms of second exon illustrated for D subloci coding for gluten sensitivity, insulin-dependent diabetes mellitus, rheumatoid arthritis and pemphigus vulgaris. In gluten sensitivity, susceptibility is conferred, in part, by a K residue in place of E at position 156 (71 [DR,DQ]: or 69 [DP]). In diabetes A, V or S residues at position 142 (57 on β1 helix) confer some risk, compared with D. Similar alterations, such as K/R for E at position 156 (DR;71), or E for K (DP;69), or D for V at position 142 (DR;57) in pemphigus vulgaris, emphasize different conformations presented by each allelic variant into the peptide groove. Alleles predisposing to illness are denoted*. S_1, S_2, S_3 refer to positions within the first three turns of β-sheet, where minor polymorphisms occur on the β1 chain, while H refers to the important HVR on the β1 helix. Residue positions in parentheses indicate sequence of β1 chain; other positions refer to sequence in tandem with α1 chain. DP sequences are bracketed. Note apparent importance of residue at position 71 (156) involving switches between K or E residues, irrespective of disease background. (From [12], copyright American Gastroenterological Association.)

ent that while single codon substitutions in the β-chain can determine marked functional changes in its relationship to peptide binding and T cell receptor (TCR) interactions, the conclusion to be drawn is that other polymorphic sites (other than position 57) together with the polymorphism(s) and interactions of the associated α-chain jointly and ultimately determine the full functional properties of any one expressed human leucocyte antigen (HLA) heterodimer.

Structural studies of coeliac-associated MHC allelic specificities, mainly involving those of the third hypervariable region (HVR; residues 65–75) of β1 [49,50] reveal codon switches for residue K (lysine), vice E (glutamine), at position 71 DR, DQ and 69 (DP) (Table 12.3). Like IDDM, this single codon switch does not appear to be present in all individuals examined [49], indicating that the allelic structure of the whole β1 domain exerts an important influence. Since an identical switch occurs in dermatitis herpetiformis (DH), we are no further forward at this stage in understanding why, when considering its molecular basis, such patients invariably demonstrate far less mucosal damage, have a greater propensity to develop 'autoantibodies', and suffer from irritating gluten-driven skin blistering. Thus, while biochemical analysis of HLA gene products of D subloci have provided much useful information concerning β-chain polymorphisms relevant to many diseases, it has proved disappointing for failing (so far) to provide more illuminating insights into the molecular basis of disease susceptibility [51].

Other recent studies in the non-obese diabetic-prone (NOD) mouse indicate that at least three recessive autosomal genes [52,53] (of which one (Idd-1^s) is tightly linked to MHC (H-2) on murine chromosome 17, a second (Idd-2^s) on chromosome 9 and the third (Idd-3^s) at present unlocated) all contribute to disease susceptibility. Like their human counterparts, these mice (NOD) bear an H-2 I-A_β (i.e. 'MHC DQ-like') chain with an S residue at position 57 (A or V in humans) in the third HVR of β_1 and develop lymphocytic infiltrates of islets ('insulitis'), irrespective of clinical hyperglycaemia, between the 12th to 13th weeks of life after which they recede. By that time 70–80% females but only 10–20% males, will be diabetic; the rest survive unscathed despite the evanescent wave of pancreatic lymphoid infiltration.

Here the parallel with the evolution of the flat mucosal lesion is relevant – do those individuals (including asymptomatic family members [54] or DH patients [55] with only mucosal lymphoid infiltrates) invariably progress to a flat destructive lesion, or can those infiltrates regress (as in some NOD mice, or the second member of a diabetic twin [56]) and if so, after what period? The use of congenic animals has exemplified the difficulties in determining the genetic basis of the infiltrative insulitis, which is possibly caused by the non-H-2 linked (Idd-2^s) recessive gene [57], despite the permissive role of the MHC (H-2)-linked gene [53,57]. Nevertheless, until Idd-3^s locus is delineated, any proposal for an 'islet-lymphocyte-infiltrating' gene must remain tentative. From this, it can be seen that if there is an analogous non-MHC-linked gene for gluten-induced lymphocytic infiltration of intestinal epithelium, we are a long way from identifying it.

Finally, it should not be forgotten that gene penetrance is linked to other intrinsic interactions with sex steroids [58] and cytokines [59–61] in addition to extrinsic (environmental) agents which includes contact with infective microorganisms and food molecules [62,63]. Likewise, in gluten sensitivity, we are only at the threshold of exploring the molecular basis of prolamine antigenicity in terms of cross-reactive epitopes, and the structural basis of HLA-directed gluten susceptibilities. To these must also be added TCR that react with those MHC-peptide complexes. The indications are that '... the T cell response, even to fairly similar epitopes, is likely to be diverse [while] the relative contributions of HLA class 2 α- and β-chain polymorphisms to T cell recognition, and consequently to an *in vivo* immune response, are also likely to be extremely heterogeneous ...' [48].

CD, and the realm of gluten sensitivity, continue to intrigue the clinical and scientific mind alike. This is due to the fact that every advance in biomedical research has been successfully applied to one or other aspect of its many presenting facets — morphological, immunopathological, serological, biochemical and molecular [64]. For the future, monoclonal antibody production, DNA technology, cell cloning and other molecular approaches will continue to provide the basic tools for more productive research. The next decade will undoubtedly bring us nearer to a deeper understanding of the mechanisms underlying this fascinating condition.

References

1 Booth CC, Dowling RH. *Coeliac Disease.* Proceedings of the International Conference, Royal Postgraduate Medical School, London, 1969. London: Churchill Livingstone, 1970.

2 Hekkens WThJM, Peña AS. *Coeliac Disease.* Proceedings of the Second International Coeliac Symposium, Leeuwenhorst Congress Centre, Noordwijkerhont, The Netherlands, 1974. Leiden: Stenfert Kroese, 1975.

3 McNicholl B, McCarthy CF, Fottrell PF. *Perspectives in Coeliac Disease.* Proceedings of the Third International Symposium on Coeliac Disease, University College, Galway, Ireland, 1977. Lancaster: MTP Press, 1978.

4 Kumar PJ, Walker-Smith JA. *Coeliac Disease: One Hundred Years.* Proceedings of the Fourth International Symposium on Coeliac Disease, St Bartholomew's Hospital, London, UK, 1988. Leeds: University of Leeds Press, 1991.

5 Mearin ML, Mulder CJJ. *Coeliac Disease: 40 Years Gluten Free.* Proceedings of an International (5th) Symposium on Coeliac Disease, University Hospital, Leiden, The Netherlands. Dordrect: Kluwer Academic, 1991.

6 Marsh MN. Coeliac disease. In: Marsh MN, ed. *Immunopathology of the Small Intestine.* Chichester: Wiley, 1987:371–99.

7 Marsh MN. Studies of intestinal lymphoid tissue. XI. The immunopathology of cell-mediated reactions in gluten sensitivity and other enteropathies. *Scanning Microsc* 1988; 2:1663–84.

8 Marsh MN. Grains of truth: evolutionary

changes in small intestinal mucosa in response to environmental antigen challenge. *Gut* 1990;31:111–14.

9 Ferguson A. Models of immunologically-driven small intestinal damage. In: Marsh MN, ed. *Immunopathology of the Small Intestine*. Chichester: Wiley, 1987:225–52.

10 Mowat A McI, Felstein MV. Intestinal graft-versus-host reactions in experimental animals. In: Burakoff SJ, Ferrara H, eds. *Graft-Versus-Host Disease*. New York: Dekker, 1991:205–44.

11 MacDonald TT. T cell-mediated intestinal injury. In: Marsh MN, ed. *Coeliac Disease*. Oxford: Blackwell Scientific Publications, 1992:283–304.

12 Marsh MN. Gliadin, MHC and the small intestine. (A molecular and immunobiologic approach to the spectrum of gluten sensitivity ('celiac sprue'.)) *Gastroenterology* 1992;102: 330–54.

13 Cooke WT, Asquith P. Definitions. In: Cooke WT, Asquith P, eds. *Coeliac Disease*. Clinics in Gastroenterology. Philadelphia: Saunders, 1974;3:3–10.

14 Hirayama K, Matsushita S, Kikuchi I, Iuchi M, Ohta N, Sasazuki T. HLA-DQ is epistatic to HLA-DR in controlling the immune response to schistosomal antigen in humans. *Nature* 1987;327:426–30.

15 Matsushita S, Muto M, Suemura M, Saito Y, Sasazuki T. HLA-linked non-responsiveness to Cryptomeria japonica pollen antigen. I. Non-responsiveness is mediated by antigen-specific suppressor T cell. *J Immunol* 1987; 138:109–15.

16 Greco L, Auricchio S, Mayer M, Grimaldi, M. Case control study on nutritional risk factors in coeliac disease. *J Paediatr Gastroenterol Nutr* 1988;7:395–9.

17 Langman M. Can epidemiology help us prevent coeliac disease? *Gastroenterology* 1986;90:489–91.

18 Weinstein WM. Latent celiac sprue. *Gastroenterology* 1974;66:489–93.

19 Auricchio S, Greco L, Troncone R. What is the true prevalence of coeliac disease? *Gastroenterol Intern* 1990;3:140–2.

20 Marsh MN. Lymphocyte-mediated intestinal damage – human studies. In: Peters TJ, ed. *The Cell Biology of Inflammation in the Gastrointestinal Tract*. Hull: Corners Publications, 1989:203–29.

21 Bloomfield AL, Wyckoff HA. The treatment of sprue with liver extract. *Am J Med Sci* 1929;177:209–13.

22 Minot GR, Murphy WP. A diet rich in liver in the treatment of pernicious anaemia. *J Am Med Assoc* 1927;89:759–68.

23 Mäki M, Holm K, Koskimies S, Hällström O, Visakorpi JK. Normal small bowel biopsy followed by coeliac disease. *Arch Dis Child* 1990;65:1137–41.

24 Mäki M, Holm K, Collin P, Savilahti E. Increase in γ/δ T cell receptor bearing lymphocytes in normal small bowel mucosa in latent coeliac disease. *Gut* 1991;32:1412–4.

25 Mäki M, Hällström O, Marttinen A. Reaction of human non-collagenous polypeptides with coeliac disease autoantibodies. *Lancet* 1991; 338:724–5.

26 Penttila IA, Gibson CE, Forrest BD, Cummins AG, LaBrooy JT. Lymphocyte activation as measured by interleukin 2 receptor expression to gluten fraction III in coeliac disease. *Clin Exp Immunol* 1990;68:155–60.

27 Sturgess RP, Macartney JC, Mak MW, Hung GH, Ciclitira PJ. Differential upregulation of ICAM-1 in coeliac disease. *Clin Exp Immunol* 1990;82:489–92.

28 O'Farrelly C, Kelly J, Hekkens W *et al.* Alpha gliadin antibody levels: a serological screening test for coeliac disease. *Br Med J* 1983; 296:2007–10.

29 O'Mahony S, Ferguson A. Similarities in intestinal humoral immunity in dermatitis herpetiformis without enteropathy and in coeliac. *Lancet* 1990;335:1487–90.

30 Wieser H, Belitz H-D, Ashkenazi A. Coeliac activity of gliadin peptides CT-1 and CT-2. *Z Lebensm Unters Forsch* 1986;182:115–17.

31 Kagnoff MF, Paterson Y, Kumar P, Kasarda D, Austin RK. Evidence for the role of a human intestinal adenovirus in the pathogenesis of coeliac disease. *Gut* 1987;28: 995–1001.

32 Devery JM, LaBrooy JT, Krilis S, Davidson G, Skerritt JH. Antigliadin antibody specificity for gluten-derived peptides toxic to coeliac patients. *Clin Exp Immunol* 1989;76: 384–90.

33 Devery JM. *Identification of noxious gluten peptides in coeliac disease*. PhD Thesis, University of New South Wales, Australia, 1991.

34 de Ritis G, Auricchio S, Lew E, Bernardin J, Kasarda D. *In vitro* (organ culture) studies of the toxicity of specific A-gliadin peptides in celiac disease. *Gastroenterology* 1988;94: 41–9.

35 Maraglit H, Sponge JL, Cornette JL, Cease KB, Delisi C, Berzofsky JA. Prediction of

immunodominant helper T cell antigenic sites from the primary sequence. *J Immunol* 1987;138:2213–29.
36 Rothbard JB, Taylor WR. A sequence pattern common to T cell epitopes. *EMBO J* 1988;7: 93–100.
37 Karagiannis J, Jewell D, Priddle J. Cell-mediated immunity to a synthetic gliadin peptide resembling a sequence from Adenovirus 12. *Lancet* 1987;i:884–6.
38 Mantzaris G, Karagiannis J, Priddle J, Jewell D. Cellular hypersensitivity to a synthetic dodecapeptide derived from human adenovirus 12 which resembles a sequence of A-gliadin in patients with coeliac disease. *Gut* 1990;31:668–73.
39 Tatham AS, Marsh MN, Wieser H, Shewry PR. Conformational studies of peptides corresponding to coeliac-activating regions of wheat α-gliadin. *Biochem J* 1990;270: 313–18.
40 Sollid LM, Markussen G, Ek V, Gjerde HG, Vartdal F, Thorsby E. Evidence for a primary association of coeliac disease to a particular HLA-DQ α/β heterodimer. *J Exp Med* 1989; 169:345–50.
41 Monos DS, Spielman RS, Gogolin K *et al.* The HLA-DQw 3.2 allele of the DR4 haplotype is associated with insulin dependent diabetes; correlation between DQβ restriction fragments and DQβ chain variation. *Immunogenetics* 1987;26:299–303.
42 Erlich HA, Buguwan TL, Scharf S, Nepom GT, Tait B, Griffith RL. HLA-DQβ sequence polymorphism and genetic susceptibility to IDDM. *Diabetes* 1990;39:96–103.
43 Nepom GT. A unified hypothesis for the complex genetics of HLA associations with IDDM. *Diabetes* 1990;39:1153–6.
44 Todd JA, Bell JI, McDevitt HO. HLA-DQβ gene contributes to susceptibility and resistance to insulin-dependent diabetes mellitus. *Nature* 1987;329:599–604.
45 Awata T, Kuznya T, Matsuda A *et al.* High frequency of aspartic acid at position 57 of HLA-DQ β-chain in Japanese IDDM patients and non-diabetic subjects. *Diabetes* 1990;39: 266–9.
46 Nepom GT, Robinson DM. HLA-DQ and diabetes mellitus: a genetic and structural paradigm for models of disease susceptibility. In: Demaine AG, Banga J-P, McGregor AM, eds. *The Molecular Biology of Autoimmune Disease.* Berlin: Springer-Verlag, 1990: 251–62.
47 Miyazaki T, Masashi U, Masahiro U *et al.* Direct evidence for the contribution of the unique I-A^{nod} to the development of insulitis in non-obese diabetic mice. *Nature* 1990; 345:722–4.
48 Kwok W, Mickelson E, Masewicz S, Milner EC, Hansen J, Nepom GT. Polymorphic DQα and DQβ interactions dictate HLA class II determinants of allo-recognition. *J Exp Med* 1990;171:85–95.
49 Bugawan TL, Angelini G, Larvick J, Auricchio S, Ferrara GB, Erlich HA. A combination of a particular HLA-DP B allele and an HLA-DQ heterodimer confers susceptibility to coeliac disease. *Nature* 1989;339:470–3.
50 Kagnoff MF, Harwood JL, Buguwan LH, Erlich HA. Structural analysis of the HLA-DR, -DQ, -DP HLA-DR3 (DRw18) haplotype. *Proc Nat Acad Sci USA* 1989;86:6274–8.
51 Marsh MN. Biomolecular aspects of gluten-sensitivity: current trends. In: Cripps AW, ed. *Mucosal Immunology.* Newcastle: Newey and Beath, 1990:2–7.
52 Prochazkan M, Leiter EH, Serreze DV, Coleman DL. Three recessive loci required for insulin-dependent diabetes in nonobese diabetic mice. *Science* 1987;237:286–9.
53 Prochazkan M, Serreze DV, Worthen SM, Leiter EH. Genetic control of diabetogenesis in NOD/Lt mice: development and analysis of congenic stocks. *Diabetes* 1989;38: 1446–55.
54 Marsh MN, Bjarnason I, Shaw J, Ellis A, Baker R, Peters TJ. Studies of intestinal lymphoid tissue. XIV. HLA status, mucosal morphology, permeability and epithelial lymphocyte populations in first degree relatives of patients with coeliac disease. *Gut* 1990;31:32–6.
55 Marsh MN. Studies of intestinal lymphoid tissue. XV. Histopathologic features suggestive of cell-mediated reactivity in jejunal mucosae of patients with dermatitis herpetiformis. *Virchows Arch [A]* 1989;416:125–32.
56 Johnston C, Millward B, Hoskins P, Leslie R, Pyke D. Islet-cell antibodies as predictors of the later development of Type 1 (insulin-dependent) diabetes. *Diabetologia* 1989;32: 382–6.
57 Hattori M, Fukuda M, Ichikawa T, Baumgartl H-J, Katoh H, Makino S. A single recessive non-MHC diabetogenic gene determines the development of insulitis and the presence of an MHC-linked diabetogenic gene in NOD mice. *J Autoimmunity* 1990;3:1–10.
58 Makino S, Kunimoto K, Muraoka Y, Katagiri Y. Effect of castration on the appearance of

diabetes in NOD mouse. *Exp Anim* 1981;30: 137–40.
59 Serreze DV, Leiter EH. Defective activation of T suppressor cell function in nonobese diabetic mice: potential relation to cytokine deficiencies. *J Immunol* 1988;140:3801–7.
60 Jacob CO, Aiso S, Michie S, McDevitt HO, Acha-Orbea H. Prevention of diabetes in nonobese diabetic mice by tumour necrosis factor (TNF): Similarities between TNF-α and interleukin-1. *Proc Natl Acad Sci USA* 1990; 87:968–72.
61 Serreze DV, Hamaguchi K, Leiter EH. Immunostimulation circumvents diabetes in NOD/Lt mice. *J Autoimmunity* 1989;2: 759–76.
62 Sinha AA, Lopez T, McDevitt HO. Autoimmune diseases: the failure of self-tolerance. *Science* 1990;248:1380–8.
63 Yoon J-W, Ihm S-H, McArthur RG. Viruses as a triggering factor of autoimmune type 1 diabetes. In: Farid NR, Bona CA eds. *The Molecular Aspects of Autoimmunity*. New York: Academic Press, 1990:213–40.
64 Marsh MN, Loft DE. Celiac sprue: a centennial overview 1888–1988. *Dig Dis* 1988; 6:216–28.
65 Kitchingman GR. Sequence of the DNA-binding protein of a human subgroup E adenovirus (type 4): comparisons with subgroup A (type 12), subgroup B (type 7) and subgroup C (type 5). *Virology* 1985;146: 90–101.
66 Davison AJ, Scott JE. The complete DNA sequence of varicella-zoster virus. *J Gen Virol* 1986;67:1759–1816.
67 Lal AA, de la Cruz VF, Welsh JA *et al*. Structure of the gene encoding the circumsporozoite protein of Plasmodium yoelli. *J Biol Chem* 1987;262:2937–40.
68 Ono M, Yasunga T, Miayata T, Ushikubo H. Nucleotide sequence of human endogenous retrovirus genome related to the mouse mammary tumor virus genome. *J Virol* 1986;60:589–98.
69 Pierschbacher MD, Rooslahti E, Sundelin J. The cell attachment domain of fibronectin. Determination of the primary structure. *J Biol Chem* 1982;257:9593–7.
70 Shade RO, Blundell MC, Cotmore SF. Nucleotide sequence and genome organization of human parvovirus B19 isolated from the serum of a child during aplastic crisis. *J Virol* 1986;58:921–36.
71 Rhode SL, Paradiso PR. Parvovirus genoma: Nucleotide sequence of H-1 and mapping of its genes by hybrid-arrested translation. *J Virol* 1983;45:173–84.
72 Camonis JH, Kalekine M, Gondre B. Characterization, cloning and sequence analysis of the CDC25 gene which controls the cyclic AMP level of *Saccharomyces cerevisiae*. *EMBO J* 1986;5:375–80.
73 Fukasawa M, Miura T, Hasegawa A. Sequence of simian immunodeficiency virus from African green monkey, a new member of the HIV/SIV group. *Nature* 1988;333:457–61.
74 Herisse J, Courtois G, Galibert F. Nucleotide sequence of the EcoRI D fragment of adenovirus 2 genome. *Nucleic Acid Res* 1980;8: 2173–92.
75 Marks MD, Lindell JS, Larkins BA. Nucleotide sequence analysis of zein mRNAs from maize endosperm. *J Biol Chem* 1985;260: 16451–59.
76 Tokunga O, Yaegashi T, Lowe J. Sequence analysis in the E1 region of adenovirus type 4 DNA. *Virology* 1986;153:418–33.
77 Maeda K, Wakabayshi S, Matsubara H. Complete amino acid sequence of an alpha-amylase inhibitor in wheat kernal. *Biochim Biophys Acta* 1985;828:213–21.

Index